OPHTHALMOLOGY
for the
Primary Care Physician

OPHTHALMOLOGY
for the
Primary Care Physician

Edited by

DAVID A. PALAY, M.D.

Assistant Professor
Department of Ophthalmology
Emory University
Atlanta, Georgia

JAY H. KRACHMER, M.D.

Professor and Chairman
Department of Ophthalmology
University of Minnesota
Minneapolis, Minnesota

with 314 illustrations

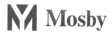 Mosby

St. Louis Baltimore Boston Carlsbad Chicago Minneapolis New York Philadelphia Portland
London Milan Sydney Tokyo Toronto

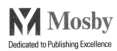

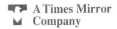

A Times Mirror
Company

Vice President and Publisher: Anne Patterson
Acquisition Editor: Laurel Craven
Senior Managing Editor: Kathy Falk
Project Manager: Linda McKinley
Designer: Renée Duenow
Manufacturing Manager: Linda Ierardi

Printed in the United States of America
Composition by Graphic World, Inc.
Lithography by ASAP, Inc.
Printing/binding by RR Donnelley & Sons, Inc.

Mosby–Year Book, Inc.
11830 Westline Industrial Drive
St. Louis, Missouri 63146

International Standard Book Number 0-8151-8898-6

97 98 99 00 01 / 9 8 7 6 5 4 3 2 1

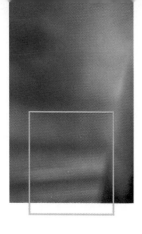

Consulting Editors

DOUGLAS D. BRUNETTE, M.D.
Senior Associate Physician
Department of Emergency Medicine
Hennepin County Medical Center;
Associate Professor
Program for Emergency Medicine
University of Minnesota School of Medicine
Minneapolis, Minnesota

JONATHAN J. MASOR, M.D.
Assistant Professor of Medicine
Department of Medicine
Emory University School of Medicine
Atlanta, Georgia

TIMOTHY J.J. RAMER, M.D.
Assistant Professor
Department of Family Practice and Community Health
University of Minnesota
Minneapolis, Minnesota

JOSEPH SNITZER, M.D.
Associate Professor of Pediatrics
Emory University School of Medicine
Atlanta, Georgia

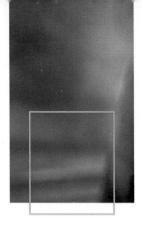

Contributors

ALLEN D. BECK, M.D.
Assistant Professor
Department of Ophthalmology
Emory University
Atlanta, Georgia

MICHAEL D. BENNETT, M.D.
Department of Ophthalmology
Emory Eye Center
Atlanta, Georgia

GEOFFREY BROOCKER, M.D., F.A.C.S
Associate Professor
Department of Ophthalmology
Emory University School of Medicine
Chief of Ophthalmology
Grady Memorial Hospital
Atlanta, Georgia

EMMETT F. CARPEL, M.D.
Clinical Professor
Department of Ophthalmology
University of Minnesota
Staff Physician
Hennepin County Medical Center
Health Partners
Minneapolis, Minnesota

MICHAEL C. DIESENHOUSE, M.D.
Clinical Lecturer
Department of Ophthalmology
University of Arizona
Tucson, Arizona

ARLENE V. DRACK, M.D.
Assistant Professor
Departments of Ophthalmology and Pediatrics
Emory University School of Medicine
Atlanta, Georgia

ANDREW R. HARRISON, M.D.
Department of Ophthalmology
University of Minnesota
Minneapolis, Minnesota

TERRY KIM, M.D.
Fellow in Cornea and External Disease
Department of Ophthalmology
Wills Eye Hospital
Philadelphia, Pennsylvania

JAY H. KRACHMER, M.D.
Professor and Chairman
Department of Ophthalmology
University of Minnesota
Minneapolis, Minnesota

Contributors

TIMOTHY J. MARTIN, M.D.

Assistant Professor
Department of Surgical Sciences/
    Ophthalmology
Wake Forest University Eye Center
Bowman Gray School of Medicine of
    Wake Forest University
Winston-Salem, North Carolina

TIMOTHY W. OLSEN, M.D.

Assistant Professor
Department of Ophthalmology
University of Wisconsin
Madison, Wisconsin

DAVID A. PALAY, M.D.

Assistant Professor
Department of Ophthalmology
Emory University
Atlanta, Georgia

WAYNE A. SOLLEY, M.D.

Chief Resident
Department of Ophthalmology
Emory Eye Center
Atlanta, Georgia

TED H. WOJNO, M.D.

Associate Professor
Department of Ophthalmology
Director
Oculoplastic & Orbital Surgery
Emory University School of Medicine
Atlanta, Georgia

This book is dedicated
to my wife, Debra, *my children,* Sarah and Matthew,
my sister, Deborah, *my parents,* Sandra and Bernard,
and my grandmother, Anne Kingloff,
and is in memory of Israel Palay, Ida Palay, *and* Jacob I. Kingloff.

DAVID A. PALAY

With great love and appreciation I dedicate this book
to my wife, Kathryn, *our children,* Edward, Kara, and Jill,
our parents, Paul and Rebecca Krachmer,
and Louis and Gertrude Maraist.

JAY H. KRACHMER

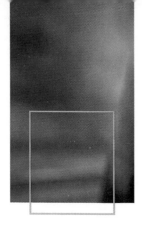

Preface

WITH the increasing role of managed care in the delivery of health care, primary care physicians are assuming a greater role in subspecialty care. In this book, we have attempted to provide the essential information that will allow the practicing physician to quickly diagnose ophthalmic disease and to treat if necessary or refer for further evaluation and treatment. More than just the primary care physician, this book is intended for anyone involved in direct patient care, including residents, medical students, optometrists, physician assistants, nurses, and nurse practitioners.

Ophthalmology is unique in that not only is it the study of visual disorders, but almost all the disorders of the eye can be directly visualized by the observer. We have complemented the text of this book with over 300 illustrations, almost all of these in color. A high percentage of figures underwent a variety of modifications such as labeling, magnified insets, and schematic illustrations to augment their educational value and emphasize desired features.

To achieve our goal of providing a practical guide to eye care, we have obviously omitted a wealth of information that is included in the training of ophthalmologists. Many diseases that are intrinsic to the eye were omitted from this text as the diagnosis and treatment were felt to be outside the realm of the primary care physician. The information in this book should not be substituted for a proper referral when necessary.

We tried to be as specific as possible when recommending treatment options. Drug dosages have been checked carefully; however, the reader is urged to check the *Physician's Desk Reference* or other source when prescribing medications that are unfamiliar.

We hope this book will serve as a valuable reference to all practitioners involved in delivering primary eye care. Please let us know what we missed so that we can consider it for a future edition.

DAVID A. PALAY, M.D.
JAY H. KRACHMER, M.D.

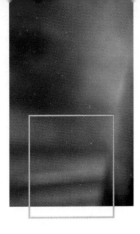

Acknowledgments

Wᴇ are extremely grateful to our many colleagues, associates, and friends who helped with the preparation of this book. We would like to credit and thank the following sources of material:

Maureen Bowers, COMT, Atlanta, Georgia (Fig. 9-24)

Antonio Capone Jr., M.D., Atlanta, Georgia (Figs. 9-28, 9-31, and 14-29)

James Gilman, CRA, Atlanta, Georgia (Figs. 1-14, 1-17, and 8-8)

Glaxo Wellcome (Fig. 1-1)

Harrington DO: *The Visual Fields: A Textbook and Atlas of Clinical Perimetry* (Fig. 11-1)

Edward J. Holland, M.D., Minneapolis, Minnesota (Fig. 4-20)

Scott Lambert, M.D., Atlanta, Georgia (Fig. 14-10)

Mark Mandel, M.D., Hayward, California (Figs. 7-7, 7-8, and 7-9)

Mark J. Mannis, M.D., Sacramento, California (Fig. 3-16)

Daniel F. Martin, M.D., Atlanta, Georgia (Figs. 8-10 and 14-2)

Robert A. Myles, CRA, Atlanta, Georgia (Fig. 9-27)

Maria Alexandra Pernetz, B.S., RDCS, Atlanta, Georgia (Fig. 9-17)

Dante Pieramici, M.D., Atlanta, Georgia (Fig. 8-5)

Spalton DJ, Hitchings RA, Hunter PA: *Atlas of Clinical Ophthalmology,* ed 2 (Figs. 1-5, 1-7, 1-13, 13-1, and 13-2)

Paul Sternberg Jr., M.D., Atlanta, Georgia (Fig. 9-29)

Ray Swords, CRA, Atlanta, Georgia (Figs. 9-1, 9-18, 9-25, and 9-26)

Keith P. Thompson, M.D., Atlanta, Georgia (Fig. 5-21)

Keith Walter, M.D., Winston-Salem, North Carolina (Fig. 4-10)

George O. Waring III, M.D., Atlanta, Georgia (Figs. 4-19, 8-2, and 8-9)

Watson PG, Ortiz JM: *Color Atlas of Scleritis* (Fig. 6-1)

We would also like to thank Linda McKinley and Kathy Falk at Mosby–Year Book, Inc. for their attention to detail and commitment to quality during the publishing of this book. We would especially like to express our gratitude to Deborah Vaughn, who coordinated many of the day-to-day activities related to this project and assisted with the typing of the manuscript.

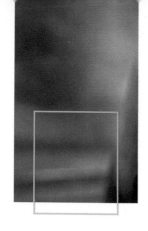

Contents

OPHTHALMOLOGY

for the

Primary Care Physician

General Eye Exam

Wayne A. Solley and Geoffrey Broocker

A structured approach is crucial in the evaluation of patients with ophthalmic complaints. This chapter introduces the primary care physician to a general approach to the eye exam in adult ophthalmic patients. Adherence to these basic steps minimizes the possibility of overlooking a serious ocular problem. (See Chapter 12 for details on the pediatric eye exam.)

ANATOMY

The cornea is located at the anteriormost aspect of the globe; along with the tear film, it is the major refracting surface of the eye (Fig. 1-1). Directly posterior to the cornea is the anterior chamber, a fluid-filled space in which blood, white blood cells, or fibrin may collect in injury, inflammatory disease, and infection. The iris is a pigmented structure comprising the sphincter and dilator muscles, connective tissue, and pigmented epithelium that lies just anterior to the crystalline lens and represents the posterior boundary of the anterior chamber. The lens is surrounded by a thin capsule. In cataract surgery (crystalline lens extraction), the capsule usually is left intact posteriorly and houses the intraocular lens implant. The lens is supported by small filaments termed *zonules* that attach to the periphery of the lens capsule and anchor at the ciliary processes of the ciliary body. Posterior to the lens is the vitreous body, a clear gel that is firmly attached to the inner eye at the area of the ora serrata (the anterior termination of the retina) and the optic nerve head (optic disc). The wall of the eye is composed of three layers: the sclera, choroid, and retina. The sclera is a firm collagenous layer that protects the intraocular structures, gives the globe its shape, and is the site of attachment of the extraocular muscles. The choroid is a highly vascular layer forming part of the uveal tract (iris, ciliary body, and choroid) that lies just inside the sclera. The ciliary body controls accommodation, is the site of aqueous production, and lies posterior and lateral to the iris. The retina is located anterior to the choroid and posterior to the vitreous body; it is composed of photoreceptors and neural tissues. The optic nerve is a congregation of approximately 1.2 million axons from the entire retina, and it exits the globe posteriorly and slightly nasally.

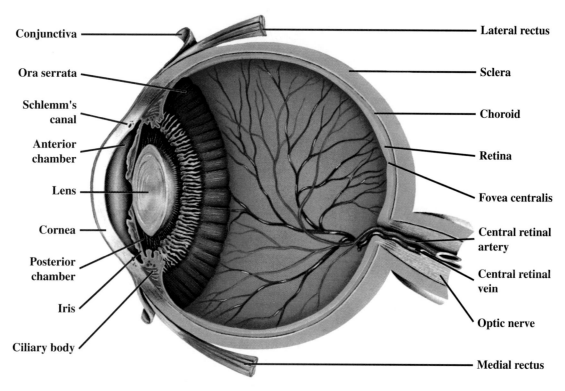

Conjunctiva — Lateral rectus

Ora serrata — Sclera

Schlemm's canal — Choroid

Anterior chamber — Retina

Lens — Fovea centralis

Cornea — Central retinal artery

Posterior chamber — Central retinal vein

Iris — Optic nerve

Ciliary body — Medial rectus

Fig. 1-1 The globe, looking down on the right eye, showing major anatomic structures.

THE OCULAR EXAM

Vision

Visual acuity is the "vital sign" in ophthalmology. Often the status of the patient's visual acuity is the first question the ophthalmologist asks the examining physician when consulted. Evaluation of this area should be the first step in the exam, preceding any diagnostic maneuvers (e.g., pupil evaluation, direct ophthalmoscopy, dilation, intraocular pressure evaluation). The examiner measures vision using a standardized visual acuity chart (Fig. 1-2) or near card (Fig. 1-3). If these tools are unavailable, the examiner can use newsprint, the patient's chart, or an ID badge or a nameplate. The examiner monitors the patient to ensure that no peeking through fingers or around an occluder occurs in an attempt to perform well on the vision "test." The physician evaluates each eye individually, not only with respect to visual acuity but also in every step of the eye exam. This is especially essential if trauma is involved; often the examining physician treats the obviously injured eye and overlooks injury in the "uninjured" eye.

When documenting visual acuity, the examiner should note whether optical correction (e.g., glasses) was used and which eye was tested. The abbreviation *OD* (oculus dexter) represents the right eye; *OS* (oculus sinister), the left eye; and *OU* (oculus uterque), both eyes. If a standard eye chart is used, the physician notes acuity by the line where most

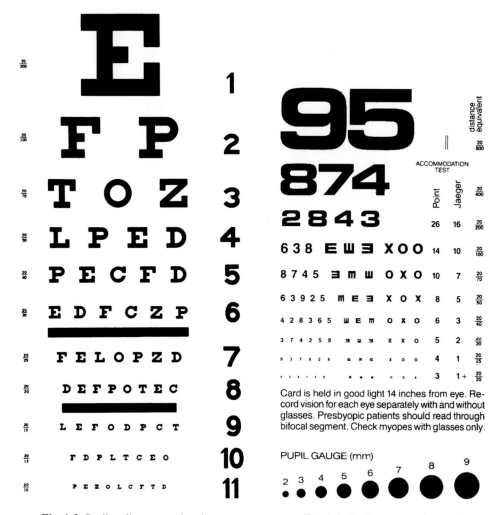

Fig. 1-2 Snellen distance acuity chart.

Fig. 1-3 Snellen near acuity card.

characters are read correctly. The corresponding vision (e.g., 20/20, 20/400) is documented for each eye. This notation is based on a standardized system in which a letter subtends 5 minutes of arc on the retina at a specified distance. For example, a "20/20 E" on a distance chart is designed to subtend 5 minutes of arc on the retina at a distance of 20 feet. A "20/40 E" is designed to subtend an arc of 5 minutes on the retina at 40 feet. A patient with 20/40 vision can discern at 20 feet what a patient with "normal," or 20/20, vision can discern at 40 feet. Near cards are designed for use at 14 to 16 inches, and these subtend the same distance as the distance acuity charts. Patients over 40 years old may require reading glasses or bifocals to overcome the normal loss of focusing ability caused by hardening of the crystalline lens (presbyopia). For patients with less than 20/400 vision, the examiner can use the notations "count fingers" (CF), "hand motions" (HM), "light perception" (LP), and "no light perception" (NLP) vision.

Emmetropia, Myopia, Hyperopia, Astigmatism, and Pinhole Effect

Emmetropia is the refractive state of an eye in which parallel rays of light entering the eye are focused on the retina, creating an image that is perceived as crisp and in focus. Myopia, hyperopia, and astigmatism are abnormalities of this desired condition (Fig. 1-4). In myopia, or nearsightedness, the refractive power of the eye exceeds the refraction necessary for the axial length of the eye. This results in an image that is focused in front of the retina. Most commonly, this occurs from axial myopia, a condition in which the eye is abnormally long, but other causes are an abnormally steep cornea, lens abnormalities (cataract), and a combination of these factors. Correction is obtained by placement of a "minus" or concave lens in front of the eye, thus adding divergence to the incoming light rays and moving the focused image onto the retina.

Hyperopia, or farsightedness, is a refractive condition of the eye in which the axial length is too short, the cornea is too flat, or the lens has too little refractive power to focus the image on the retina. The image is therefore focused posterior to the retina. This con-

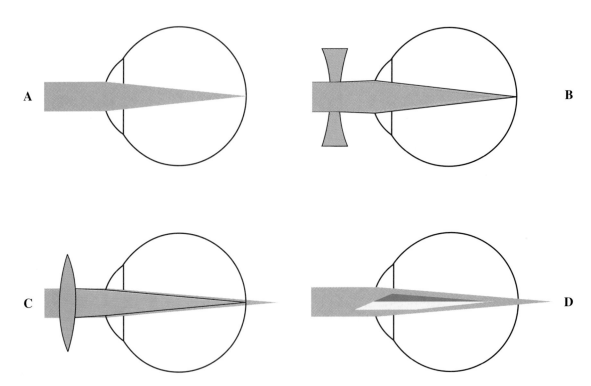

Fig. 1-4 A, Emmetropia. Parallel light rays entering the eye are focused on the retina, providing a sharp image. **B,** Myopia. Parallel light rays entering the eye are converged anterior to the retina, which is perceived as a blurred image *(orange).* This is corrected by addition of a minus lens, which creates divergence in the rays and causes the image to focus on the retina *(blue).* **C,** Hyperopia. Parallel light rays are focused posterior to the retina *(orange).* This is corrected by addition of a converging or plus lens to the eye, placing the image on the retina *(blue).* **D,** Astigmatism. Parallel light rays are focused at two different planes because of unequal corneal or lenticular curvature in separate (usually perpendicular) meridians. This is corrected by addition of a cylindrical lens in the proper meridian.

dition is corrected by addition of a "plus" or convex lens to the optical system, which provides additional convergence to the light rays entering the eye, thus moving the image forward onto the retina.

In astigmatism the refractive power of the eye in one plane (or meridian) is different from the refractive power in a different meridian. This results in essentially two focal planes from these two meridians, causing a blurred, distorted image. This is corrected by placement of a cylindrical lens in front of the eye.

If the visual acuity is poor because of a refractive error, the examiner reevaluates the patient's vision using a pinhole aperture. (One may be fashioned from a 3 × 5 inch card with several tiny holes placed in it with a sharp pencil.) Pinhole testing generally corrects any uncorrected refractive errors. If correction is not seen, the examiner must ascertain whether a pathologic cause of decreased visual acuity such as unclear ocular media (e.g., a cataract), optic nerve disease, or retinal disease is present.

Pupils

The pupil exam is one of the most important determinants of the integrity of the anterior visual pathway. Too often the acronym PERRLA (*p*upils *e*qual, *r*ound, *r*eactive to *l*ight and *a*ccommodation) is noted and substituted for an accurate assessment of pupil function. The first step to examining the pupils is to measure pupil size in dim light with the patient fixating on a distant object. The examiner directs a penlight at each pupil, and notes the rapidity and amount of pupil constriction in each eye. Anisocoria, or a difference in pupil size, may be normal (physiologic or essential anisocoria) but may also be a sign of ocular or neurologic disease (see Chapter 2). As a general rule, the pupil that reacts poorly to direct light is abnormal.

The relative afferent pupillary defect (RAPD, or Marcus Gunn pupil) has both ocular and neurologic significance. The swinging flashlight test is an essential component of the pupillary evaluation (Fig. 1-5). In a dimly lit room the patient fixates on a distant object. The

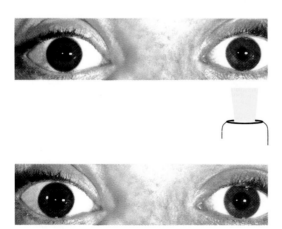

Fig. 1-5 A right afferent pupillary defect is present in this patient. Stimulation of the left eye *(top)* produces bilateral pupillary constriction. Transfer of the light to the right eye *(bottom)* produces a relative dilation of the pupil in both eyes.

examiner swings a penlight back and forth over the bridge of the nose and between both pupils. When the light focuses on one eye, the pupil constricts (direct response), as does the contralateral pupil because of the crossing fibers in the midbrain (consensual response). When the light reaches the contralateral eye, this eye now manifests the direct response and the first eye constricts consensually. If a condition exists in one eye that markedly limits the amount of light the midbrain perceives, both direct and consensual responses are decreased because the relative "input" to the system (the light) is perceived to have decreased. In this case, shining the light in the "good" eye elicits a brisk, healthy pupillary response in both eyes. When swinging the light back and forth between the two eyes and observing the direct response of each eye, the examiner will find that the diseased eye reacts much less briskly or even dilates when the light shines in it. This reaction must not be mistaken for hippus (a rhythmic wavering pupil), which is a normal finding. In addition, in cases of severe bilateral disease, both eyes may react equally. In this case, no "relative" afferent pupil defect exists.

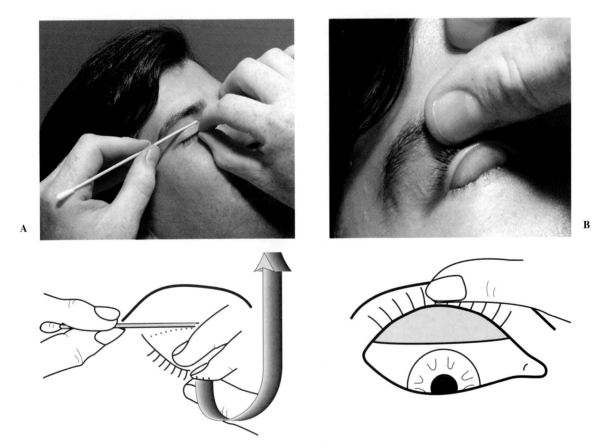

A

B

Fig. 1-6 A, For eversion, the examiner places a wooden applicator stick at the superior edge of the superior tarsal plate, firmly grasps the lashes of the upper eyelid, and gently moves the applicator stick inferiorly while pulling up on the lashes slightly. **B,** The examiner removes the stick while holding the eyelid in place (often with the cotton-tipped end). Administration of a topical anesthesia (proparacaine) may make this a slightly more comfortable procedure but is not essential.

External Exam

A general inspection of the periorbital region, eyelids, globe position, and lid margin is the next step in the ocular exam. The examiner who omits this inspection and instead proceeds to the slit lamp or fundus exam may miss key findings. For example, protrusion of the eye (known as *proptosis* or *exophthalmos*) alerts the examiner to possible orbital disease (e.g., Graves' disease, orbital tumor or pseudotumor, orbital cellulitis, retrobulbar hemorrhage), and a sunken eye (known as *enophthalmos*) is often seen in fractures of the orbital floor. Both are noted during the general inspection.

The examiner inspects the conjunctiva superiorly and inferiorly and everts the upper lids for a better view of the superior cul-de-sac and examination of the superior eyelid conjunctiva. Both areas may hide a retained foreign body. To perform lid eversion, the examiner grasps the upper eyelashes, pulls the upper lid away from the globe, and uses a small, narrow object (such as an applicator stick) to press the region of the superior tarsal plate inferiorly (Fig. 1-6). The examiner also inspects the lids and especially the lid margins for any signs of disease such as erythema, crusting, lash loss, chalazia, and irregularity and notes the presence of a droopy eyelid (ptosis).

Motility, Position, and Extraocular Muscles

The six ocular muscles (superior, inferior, medial, and lateral recti and superior and inferior obliques) are responsible for movements of the globe (Fig. 1-7). Cranial nerve VI innervates the lateral rectus, which is responsible for abduction (turning out) of the eye. Cranial nerve IV innervates the superior oblique, which abducts, depresses, and intorts (rotates in) the eye. Cranial nerve III innervates the medial rectus, inferior rectus, superior rectus, and inferior oblique muscles. The medial rectus adducts the eye (turning in), the inferior rectus depresses the eye, the superior rectus elevates the eye, and the inferior

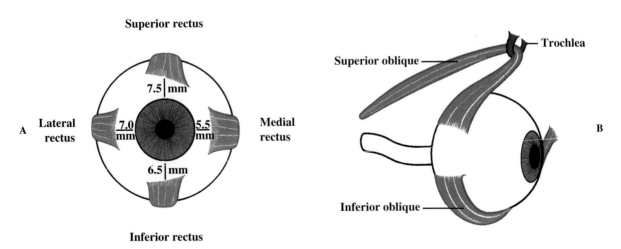

Fig. 1-7 A, The four recti muscles and their insertions into the right globe. **B,** The insertion of the oblique muscles into the right globe. The oblique muscles exert their action from the anteromedial part of the orbit. The superior oblique arises from the posterior orbit, and its tendon passes through the trochlea, the small, cartilaginous pulley on the frontal bone. The inferior oblique arises from the anterior medial orbit.

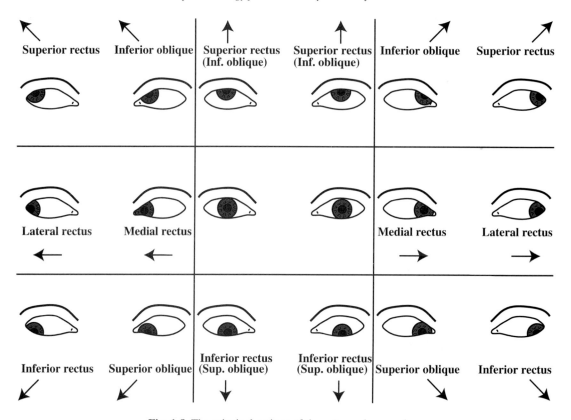

Fig. 1-8 The principal actions of the extraocular muscles.

oblique abducts, elevates, and extorts (rotates out) the eye. Cranial nerve III also innervates the levator muscle, which is responsible for lid elevation. (The cardinal movements of the eye are shown in Fig. 1-8.)

The examiner must carefully note the position of the eyes and their excursions relative to each other in patients with complaints of diplopia, those with strabismus (misalignment of the eyes), and those with suspected neurologic or orbital disease. The extraocular movements involve complex coordination of frontomesencephalic and cerebellomesencephalic interactions via the third, fourth, and sixth cranial nerves. Any disturbance in intracranial processing, midbrain or cranial nerve function, or intraorbital muscle pathology may result in an ocular position imbalance. Abnormalities may be seen in the primary gaze (straight ahead) or congruity of gaze in the six cardinal positions (left, right, up and right, up and left, down and right, and down and left). The examiner can identify esodeviations (cross-eyes) and exodeviations (walleyes) by seeing a light reflex temporal to the central cornea (Fig. 1-9) or nasal to the central cornea (Fig. 1-10), respectively. A cover/uncover test can help document esodeviations, exodeviations, and hyperdeviations. In this test the patient remains fixated on a distant object while the examiner covers and uncovers each eye. The deviated eye straightens when the normal eye is covered (opposite the direction of the original deviation). An esotropic (cross-eyed) eye moves temporally to pick up fixation when

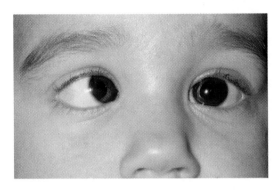

Fig. 1-9 Esodeviation, or cross-eyes, is most easily seen by observing the corneal light reflex differences in the two eyes. In an esotropic eye (turned in toward the nose), the corneal light reflex is temporally displaced.

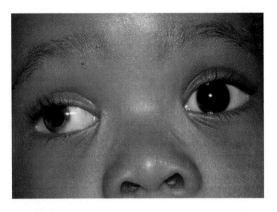

Fig. 1-10 Exodeviation, or walleyes, is also seen by observing the corneal light reflexes. The nasal displacement of the light reflexes is diagnostic of an exodeviation.

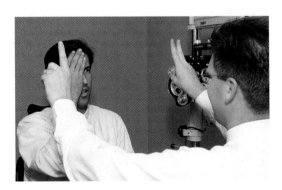

Fig. 1-11 Confrontation visual fields. If the patient cannot see an object that is visualized in the examiner's field, a visual field defect is probably present.

the straight, fixating eye is covered. An exotropic (walleyed) eye moves nasally when the straight, fixating contralateral eye is covered. The examiner can also identify vertical deviations using this method, with the higher eye labeled as hypertropic. Determining the origin of the motility disturbance is a challenge because the condition may be inherited, acquired, neural, muscular, or a combination of these factors.

Visual Fields

The examiner tests the integrated functioning of the separate parts of the visual system during the visual field evaluation. Defects in visual field testing can indicate injury at any point along the visual pathway from retinal damage to occipital lobe injury. Confrontation visual field testing provides gross evaluation of the integrity of the visual field. In this test the patient covers one eye and the examiner faces the patient, positioned approximately 3 feet in front of the uncovered eye. The examiner then moves the fingers or uses a small, red object to test the peripheral and central fields of each eye (Fig. 1-11). This method

Ophthalmology for the Primary Care Physician

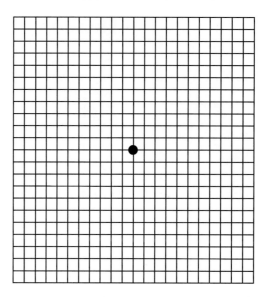

Fig. 1-12 The Amsler grid.

detects gross hemianopic defects (blindness in one half of the visual field) and isolated defects. The examiner can use an Amsler grid to test the central 10 degrees of the visual field of each eye (Fig. 1-12). When the patient fixates on the black central dot of the white checkerboard, the grid is projected onto the central retina (macula). The patient maps wavy lines (metamorphopsia), blind spots (scotomata), and other irregularities in the checker-board; these findings can guide the examiner toward a certain region to look for disease. Amsler grid testing can sometimes identify hemianopic defects.

Color Vision

Although formal color vision testing is not performed in the nonophthalmic setting, gross comparison of the two eyes can provide useful localizing information. Taken together, the macula and optic nerve are essentially a color processing system: defects in basic color sensitivity can localize disease to these anatomic locations. The most appropriate test in the primary care setting is the central red saturation/desaturation test. Using a penlight shining through the cap of a bottle of a cycloplegic/mydriatic (dilating) agent, the exam-iner asks the patient to quantify the "degree" of redness seen by each eye. If the response indicates less than full saturation in one eye as compared with the other, optic nerve or macular disease may be present.

Slit Lamp Exam

The anterior segment of the eye is best examined with the slit lamp biomicroscope (Fig. 1-13). This part of the exam is essential in any condition requiring an accurate and highly magnified view of the anterior and posterior segments of the eye. The patient places the chin on the chin rest and the forehead against the forehead rest. The examiner adjusts the height for comfort and for the appropriate range of excursion of the lamp, which is best accomplished by aligning the patient's eyes with the black line on the vertical pole next to

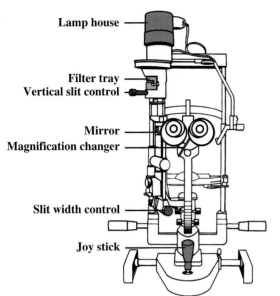

Lamp house

Filter tray
Vertical slit control

Mirror
Magnification changer

Slit width control

Joy stick

Fig. 1-13 A slit lamp and its optics. Light arising from a filament lamp in the lamp house passes through a condenser to a variable slit mechanism that allows the length and width of the slit to be altered. Below this is a tray for various filters to be inserted in the light path. The beam is directed into the eye by a mirror and focused so that the focal plane is the same as that for the viewing microscope. The angle between the illuminating beam and the viewing microscope can be varied at will. The microscope incorporates a two-stage magnification changer that alters the objective lenses without moving the focal plane. Height and focusing are altered by means of a joy stick.

the patient's face. The examiner sets the oculars (eyepieces) at zero and adjusts their width to equal the examiner's interpupillary distance, such as with binoculars. With a hand on the base of the lamp, the examiner moves the chassis forward and backward and achieves fine focus with small forward and backward movements of the joy stick. The light source is approximately 45 degrees to the patient/examiner axis, and the examiner adjusts the width of the beam from full (circular) to a very thin slit. Up/down control is on the joy stick or a separate wheel depending on the model of the slit lamp. The magnification is adjustable as well, usually beginning at low power and progressing to higher power if needed. With this setup a thin beam can show the separate layers of the cornea and intraocular contents. The examiner must use a systematic approach to slit lamp examination, usually beginning with the eyelids and moving posteriorly to examine the conjunctiva, cornea, anterior chamber, iris, lens, and anterior vitreous cavity.

Eyelids. The examiner inspects lid margins for lacerations, eversion (ectropion), inversion (entropion), abnormal lash growth toward the cornea (trichiasis), chalazia, meibomian gland dysfunction, and lash loss.

Conjunctiva. The examiner evaluates the conjunctiva for discharge, follicles, fluid accumulation (chemosis), and hyperemia. Conjunctival lacerations must be carefully examined to note whether the underlying sclera is also injured. The slit lamp greatly facilitates foreign body removal, usually accomplished with topical anesthesia and a moistened cotton swab (see Chapter 15). For patients with foreign body sensation or corneal abrasions, eversion of the upper lid at the slit lamp, although more difficult to achieve than on the external exam, provides a magnified view of the superior lid (palpebral) conjunctiva and cul-de-sac. Often a tiny foreign body can be found embedded in the conjunctiva in this location.

Cornea. The examiner inspects the epithelium for abrasions, edema, ulcers, and foreign bodies. A single drop of fluorescein stains areas of denuded epithelium. Once rotated into position, the cobalt blue filter highlights the stained areas. Tiny dots of green across the corneal surface signify punctate epithelial keratopathy (PEK), an indicator of diffuse epithelial disease (e.g., dry eyes, toxic epitheliopathy). Large areas of intense green staining indicate abrasions. The examiner evaluates the stroma for scars, edema (thickening), and foreign bodies. Keratic precipitates (collections of white blood cells and macrophages) on the endothelium, which is the internal layer of the cornea, are a hallmark of iritis and are easily seen with the slit lamp. The examiner may also find pigment and adhesions of iris to the cornea (anterior synechiae) in eyes subjected to prior trauma or surgery.

Anterior chamber. The anterior chamber is an aqueous-filled chamber bounded by the iris posteriorly and the corneal endothelium anteriorly. The slit beam can identify inflammatory cells floating in the aqueous in iritis and flare (light scatter caused by inflammatory proteins in the aqueous). Red or white cells may be present in the anterior chamber. Red blood cells usually result from trauma, and the layering of these cells in the anterior chamber is a hyphema. The layering of white cells in iritis or infection is a hypopyon.

Iris and lens. In the iris and lens exam the examiner notes pupil abnormalities, which may include traumatic tears in the iris sphincter and adhesions of the iris to the anterior lens capsule (posterior synechiae). The iris may plug corneal lacerations or be torn at its insertion (iridodialysis). Very few blood vessels are normally seen on the iris, and none are usually visible at the pupillary margin. Any fine blood vessels seen at the pupillary margin (rubeosis iridis) should prompt referral for ophthalmologic evaluation for possible neovascular glaucoma. Opacities of the lens (i.e., cataract) may result from aging or a number of secondary causes. Injury to the capsule of the lens in penetrating trauma causes the lens to hydrate rapidly and become densely white (cataractous).

Vitreous. While the eye is dilated, the examiner focuses the slit beam posterior to the lens into the anterior vitreous. In inflammatory conditions involving the posterior segment of the eye, the examiner will note a cellular reaction in the vitreous, much like the cells seen in the anterior chamber in iritis. Vitreous hemorrhage may also result in the presence of numerous red blood cells.

Intraocular Pressure

Measurement of intraocular pressure (IOP) in assessment of the eye is analogous to measurement of blood pressure in assessment of the cardiovascular system. Normal values are 8 to 21 mm Hg but may range anywhere from 0 (in cases of ruptured globe, hypotony after glaucoma surgery, and severe intraocular inflammation) to 70 or 80 mm Hg (in cases of angle-closure glaucoma). IOP may be measured by several different methods.

Applanation tonometry. The applanation tonometer is accurate and easy to use; it can be found on most slit lamps. The Perkins tonometer is a handheld applanation model for patients unable to move into the proper position at the slit lamp (e.g., those in wheelchairs or stretchers, small children). To perform applanation tonometry, the examiner instills a drop of anesthetic (proparacaine) and a drop of fluorescein dye in the eye and sets the applanation tension at mid-range, approximately 15 to 20 mm Hg. The examiner gently holds the eyelids open, taking care to not put any pressure on the globe while holding the lids. Even negligible pressure of the examiner's fingers resting on the globe can cause a significant increase in IOP. The examiner rotates the cobalt blue filter into place and turns up the light intensity. The light is directed at the tonometer tip, which is also rotated into position, and the examiner moves the tonometer directly in front of the patient's cornea.

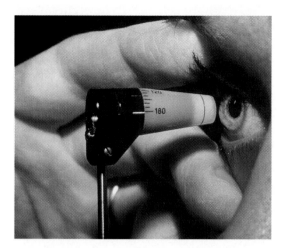

Fig. 1-14 Applanation tonometry. The tonometer head has an area such that the surface tension force of the tear film and the elastic tension within the cornea are equal and cancel each other. The prismatic doubling head of the applanator splits the tear meniscus into two identifiable mires for measurement of the IOP when gently touched to a patient's cornea.

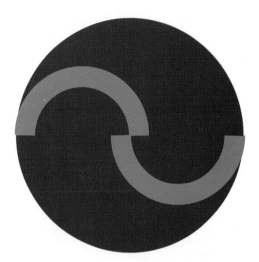

Fig. 1-15 Tonometric mires. The fluorescein rings just overlap, producing the endpoint at which IOP is measured.

The examiner instructs the patient to open both eyes wide and slowly moves the tonometer forward until it gently touches the cornea (Fig. 1-14). Because of the prismatic effect of the tonometer tip, two green half circles are seen when the tonometer tip is fully applanated (Fig. 1-15). These are known as *tonometric mires* and shift in relation to each other as the tonometer scale is rotated. The goal is to align the mires so that the inside edge of one just touches the inside edge of the other. At this point the examiner reads the IOP from the scale. The scale is marked in centimeters of mercury; for conversion to millimeters of mercury (standard notation), the scale reading is multiplied by 10.

Tonometer pens. A tonometer pen (Tono-Pen) is an electronic device that is very easy to use and relatively accurate (Fig. 1-16). The accuracy diminishes as the pressure moves farther outside the normal range. Drawbacks include expense and fragility of the pens, but they are extremely effective for obtaining the IOP in emergency situations.

Pneumotonometers. Although effective and easy to use, pneumotonometers are not portable. They are also expensive to maintain and must be calibrated often. Like the tonometry pens, pneumotonometers are effective in dealing with patients who have abnormal corneal surfaces and irregular tear films, rendering applanation impossible.

Schiøtz (indentation) tonometry. The Schiøtz tonometer is cumbersome, can spread infection, and may create its own trauma. Because the preceding methods are much easier and safer, it is seldom used (Fig. 1-17).

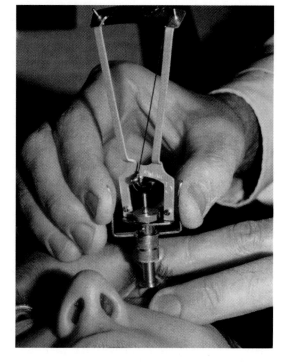

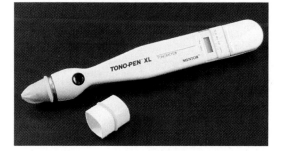

Fig. 1-16 A handheld tonometry pen (Tono-Pen). **Fig. 1-17** Schiøtz tonometry.

Manual assessment. Manual assessment provides only a crude measure and is extremely inaccurate when performed by nonophthalmologists. The examiner palpates the globe through closed lids using a gentle ballotting motion and compares the eyes. The examiner's eye may be used as a control. Although only a gross assessment of IOP, manual assessment can be extremely useful in cases such as the evaluation of a red eye that is thought to represent angle-closure glaucoma. The involved eye is markedly firm to palpation when compared with the fellow eye. This method should be avoided in recently operated eyes or in cases of a suspected ruptured globe.

Fundoscopic Evaluation

A direct ophthalmoscope is invaluable for the primary care physician. The light source is bright enough to evaluate the pupils, a cobalt blue filter often is built into the instrument for use with fluorescein staining, and an excellent evaluation of the fundus is achieved. If an abnormality in the posterior pole is suspected, the eyes may be dilated.

The physician should use a weak mydriatic agent after vision assessment and pupillary exam. Tropicamide 0.5% or 1% and phenylephrine 2.5% are good choices; both reverse effects in 4 to 6 hours. Atropine drops should not be used because they produce dilation for as long as 1 to 2 weeks. Pupil dilation causing an attack of angle-closure glaucoma is extremely uncommon.

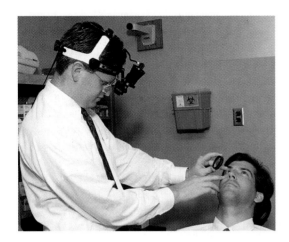

Fig. 1-18 Indirect ophthalmoscopy. The examiner views the retina through a handheld lens that is coaxial with the headset loupes and light source. This provides an exceptional view of the entire retina.

Documenting the time of dilation and the agents used for dilation in the chart is an important step. Even in undilated eyes, examination with the direct ophthalmoscope can give useful information pertaining to the clarity of the ocular media and refractive error. A diminished red reflex or irregularities in the red reflex may result from cloudy media (e.g., corneal or lens opacities, vitreous blood) and unusual refractive errors. The -2 to -3 diopter lens on the ophthalmoscope (the red 2 or 3) usually generates a comfortable view of the fundus. If the examiner has difficulty seeing the fundus, different lenses may be rotated into position until a clear image appears. The direct ophthalmoscope evaluates the optic nerve head, retinal vessels, and macula. For examination of the periphery, an ophthalmologist must use an indirect ophthalmoscope (Fig. 1-18).

The examiner's right eye is used to assess the patient's right eye, and the examiner's left eye assesses the patient's left eye. The optic nerve head is most easily seen by having the patient look straight ahead and approaching with the ophthalmoscope from a slightly temporal angle. The examiner is looking for abnormalities in shape and color. The margins should be sharp and vessels crisp as they cross the edge of the disc. If this is not seen, the disc may be edematous. The examiner notes any hemorrhages or infarctions of the nerve fiber layer (cotton-wool spots) near the nerve head. Pallor of the nerves (resulting from optic atrophy) may indicate an old optic neuropathy and should be evaluated by an ophthalmologist. Increased intracranial pressure (papilledema) is one cause of disc edema. Marked or asymmetric cupping of the nerve is a possible sign of glaucoma.

The best view of the macula occurs when the patient looks directly at the examining light. (The macula is examined last because of the patient's light sensitivity.) A small reflex of light seen hovering directly over the fovea (the foveal light reflex) is one indicator of normal foveal anatomy. Hemorrhage, exudates, microaneurysms, and areas of edema are findings in microvascular disease. The examiner should note whether these signs are localized to one area of the retina (as in a vascular occlusion), diffusely scattered throughout one retina (as in ocular ischemia or radiation retinopathy), or a generalized finding in both eyes (as in systemic diseases such as diabetes and hypertension). The depth of hemorrhage is difficult to determine; however, deep hemorrhages tend to be small and irregular (dot and blot), whereas superficial hemorrhages follow the nerve fiber layer and are flame shaped. Retinal edema gives the retina a grayish appearance and also is present in areas of vascular occlusion. In central retinal artery occlusions and conditions in which the nerve fiber layer is thickened, a red spot (cherry-red spot) is usually present in the central macular region. This phenomenon occurs as the normal choroidal blood flow is viewed through the fovea centralis, the only area of the retina lacking ganglion cells and a nerve fiber layer. Cherry-red spots also occur in metabolic storage diseases (e.g., Tay-Sachs disease) as a result of the retina accumulating the products of abnormal enzyme pathways.

Evaluation of the retinal circulation is difficult with the direct ophthalmoscope, but dilation of the pupil facilitates observation of the vessels. Venous occlusions have associated retinal hemorrhages, exudates, and retinal thickening from edema. Arteriovenous nicking is present in hypertensive retinopathy. In atherosclerotic disease (especially carotid disease), cholesterol emboli may lodge in the retinal arterioles at their bifurcations and are therefore noticeable on ophthalmoscopic examination. These small refractile bodies in the lumen of the vessels are known as *Hollenhorst plaques.*

ADDITIONAL DIAGNOSTIC TESTS

Gonioscopy

In the anterior chamber angle of the eye, aqueous drains from the anterior chamber. This area is not accessible for viewing with routine slit lamp examination because of the optical properties of the cornea. A slit lamp–magnified view through a contact gonioscopic lens (along with a topical anesthetic such as proparacaine) provides access. Goldmann and Zeiss lenses are equipped with periscopic mirrors through which the angle is examined with reflected light (Fig. 1-19). Gonioscopy is useful in differentiating various forms of glaucoma (e.g., open angle, narrow angle, closed angle, neovascular, angle recession) and for viewing pathologic conditions in the angle (e.g., peripheral iris anomalies, tumors, foreign bodies, trauma to the angle).

Tear Function Test

Schirmer's tear test with and without anesthesia evaluates tear adequacy and often aids in the diagnosis of dry eye syndrome. Schirmer's test without anesthesia measures basal tear secretion and reflex tear secretion. Schirmer's test with anesthesia measures basal tear secretion only by eliminating the irritation that causes reflex tearing. To perform the test, the examiner first dries the inferior cul-de-sac with a cotton swab and places one end of Whatman 41 filter paper strips (5 × 30 mm) over the lateral third of the lower lid (Fig. 1-20). The patient may continue blinking normally or keep the eyes closed. After 5 minutes the examiner removes the strips and measures the length of strip wetted by tears. Without anesthesia, wetting of less than 15 mm of a Schirmer's strip indicates dry eyes. With anesthesia the interpretation is as follows: 0 to 5 mm of wetting, severe dry eyes; 5 to 10 mm of wetting, moderately dry eyes; 10 to 15 mm of wetting, mildly dry eyes; and greater than 15 mm of wetting, normal tear function.

Primary Dye Test

The primary dye test evaluates tear drainage function (e.g., patency of puncta, canaliculi, lacrimal sac, nasolacrimal duct). The examiner instills fluorescein dye into the lower cul-

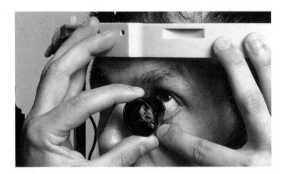

Fig. 1-19 Gonioscopy. A Goldmann gonioscope lens being placed on the patient's eye. The indirect gonioscope lens is a solid contact lens within which a small mirror is mounted, allowing the anterior chamber angle structures to be easily viewed. The full circumference of the angle may be viewed by 360-degree rotation of the lens.

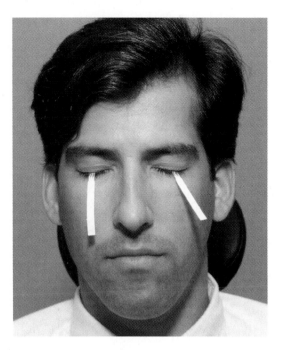

Fig. 1-20 Schirmer's tear test. Patients may keep eyes open or closed.

de-sac and places a small, cotton-tipped applicator approximately 3.5 to 4 cm into the nose under the inferior meatus. After 2 minutes the examiner removes the cotton swab. If the swab is stained with fluorescein, the system is patent. If no dye is present, either the cotton tip was in the wrong position or the system is blocked at some point.

A shortcut to this test is the "dye disappearance test," which grossly evaluates the patency of the nasolacrimal system. The examiner instills a single drop of fluorescein in each eye. If one eye retains fluorescein dye after 3 to 5 minutes while the other eye clears, asymmetry of nasolacrimal drainage is indicated.

Exophthalmometry

A Hertel exophthalmometer measures the amount of anterior protrusion of the globes (Fig. 1-21). The examiner faces the patient, palpates the patient's lateral orbital rims, places the concave sites on the side of the Hertel instrument over each rim, and records the base (or distance between these two points) from the instrument. This measurement is the baseline for accurately assessing the degree of protrusion in future examinations. For example, in Graves' disease and orbital tumors this measurement changes depending on the progression of the disorder. The examiner observes the mirror on the side of the patient's right eye while the patient fixates the right eye on the examiner's left eye or left ear. The front of the cornea lines up with the scale and the distance is in millimeters. The process is repeated for the left eye looking at the examiner's right eye or ear. Normal ranges are 12 to 20 mm, and no asymmetry greater than 2 mm should be seen.

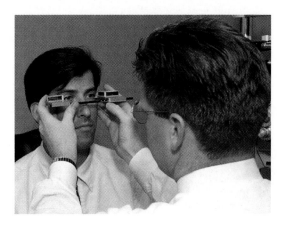

Fig. 1-21 Hertel exophthalmometry.

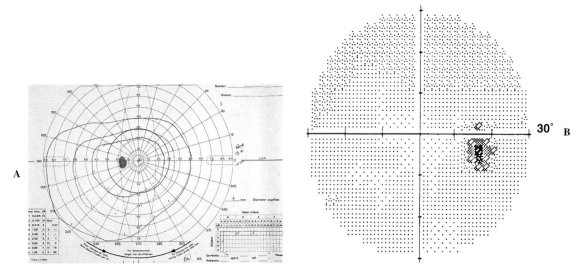

Fig. 1-22 Formal perimetry testing (visual fields). **A,** Normal Goldmann visual field. **B,** Normal Humphrey visual field.

Perimetry

The next step in evaluating abnormal confrontation visual field findings, perimetry provides an accurate assessment of the extent of a patient's visual field. Kinetic testing (Goldmann perimetry) involves the examiner moving a light of varying intensity from areas outside the visual field toward fixation, with the patient responding when the light is seen. Automated or static perimetry is computerized and involves variable intensity lights that are flashed at different locations in the visual field. The patient again acknowledges each time the light is seen. A printout of this assessment of the visual field is obtained for each time the test is performed, which enables the clinician to follow the disease state (Fig. 1-22).

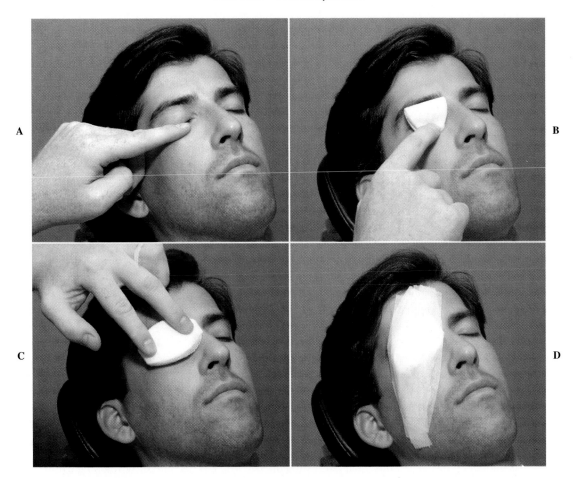

Fig. 1-23 Applying a pressure patch. **A,** The patient closes both eyes; the examiner must ensure good closure of the eyelids. **B,** The examiner applies an eye pad to the closed eyelids, either lengthwise or folded in half *(shown)*. **C,** The examiner places a second patch lengthwise over the first patch. **D,** Finally, the examiner secures the patches with tape placed from the center of the forehead to the angle of the jaw across the patched eye. Usually, an antibiotic ointment is applied before patching, and the patient's progress should be followed daily.

Eye Patching

When properly applied, patching helps promote epithelial wound healing (Fig. 1-23). Usually an antibiotic ointment such as erythromycin or polymyxin B/bacitracin (e.g., Polysporin) is instilled before patching. The lids must be closed, and the patch must be snug enough to keep the lids from opening underneath the patch, thus causing an iatrogenic corneal abrasion. Indiscriminate patching may be harmful, especially in cases of possible infection, because a warm, protected environment under a patched lid can facilitate bacterial growth. Some researchers advocate patching in patients with extremely large abrasions only.

EYEDROPS

When dilated pupils are seen in patients in the emergency room setting, pharmacologic agents are often the cause. Transdermal patches (e.g., scopolamine) and aerosolized medications (e.g., albuterol) are possible offending agents, and the patient may not realize their effects. Instillation or ingestion of ophthalmic medications belonging to other family members can also result in dilated pupils. "Red-top" ocular medications are mydriatic and cycloplegic agents (i.e., dilate and block accommodation).

Gentamicin ophthalmic drops and ointments are quite toxic to the corneal epithelium. Neomycin ophthalmic drops and ointments can cause an allergic reaction in up to 10% of patients treated. Better choices for routine broad-spectrum antibiotic coverage are fluoroquinolones (e.g., Chibroxin, Ciloxan, Ocuflox), polymyxin B/trimethoprim (Polytrim), and sulfacetamide drops or erythromycin and polymyxin B/bacitracin (e.g., Polysporin) ointments. These agents are much less damaging to the cornea and therefore more appropriate for routine coverage when epithelial regrowth is desired (e.g., in cases of corneal abrasion).

Examiners should *never* prescribe or hand a bottle of topical anesthetic drops to the patient and must always keep track of the bottle after instilling it into the patient's uncomfortable eye. Patients often want to keep the bottle of the "good drops" and will steal it without the examiner's knowledge. Topical anesthetic abuse can lead to more serious injury of the eye (because of the anesthesia) and also retards wound healing as a toxic effect.

FREQUENCY OF EXAMINATION

How often should patients have their eyes examined? The primary care physician must take an active role in reminding patients to obtain periodic exams; this is often the only way to identify potentially serious eye disease (e.g., glaucoma, macular degeneration, diabetic retinopathy). Individuals with ocular complaints should be examined and treated as outlined previously. Those without symptoms but with risk factors for developing eye problems (e.g., patients taking certain medications, especially corticosteroids, Plaquenil, and Mellaril; those with diabetes mellitus; those with a family history of glaucoma, cataracts, strabismus, retinal detachments, or any familial eye condition; patients over 65 years of age) should be examined regularly depending on their age.

Newborns. All newborns should have a general screening exam while in the nursery. High-risk characteristics for ocular disease in newborns include maternal rubella, venereal or AIDS-related infections, and a family history of retinoblastoma, metabolic or genetic disease, or congenital eye disorders. Screening for retinopathy of prematurity is needed for newborns weighing 1500 g or less, those with a gestational age of 33 weeks or less, and those receiving oxygen therapy for more than 48 hours.

Preschool children. Every child should receive a screening ocular examination by 3½ years of age. Amblyopia is the most common ocular problem among preschool children; this is the failure of the visual system to develop in one or both eyes because the brain receives a blurred or distorted image. This is often caused by a large asymmetry in refractive errors between the two eyes, cataract formation in one eye, or strabismus (misalignment of the eyes). Diminished visual acuity in a young child warrants an ophthalmic search for these disorders.

School-aged children. Children who have no evidence of ocular disease or special risk factors for disease should be seen at a frequency determined by the ophthalmologist. In general, every 2 to 3 years is the preferred interval.

Adults. The frequency of significant eye disease in the adult population under 35 years of age is low. A routine glaucoma evaluation at age 35 is advisable for normal patients. Periodic reevaluations should be performed approximately every 2 to 5 years for normal adults. Patients at special risk for eye disease should have examinations in intervals determined by an ophthalmologist. Patients with diabetes are generally seen at diagnosis and annually thereafter. Patients at risk for glaucoma are seen annually. Adults aged 65 years and older should be examined every 2 years.

Once the patient gains access to the ophthalmologist, regular follow-up examinations are arranged. The primary care provider can play a crucial role in helping reduce the incidence of serious eye disease by reminding patients of the need for periodic evaluations and promptly referring any patient at risk for developing ocular problems.

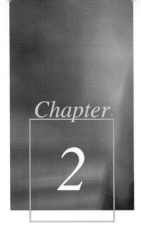

Chapter 2

Ophthalmic Differential Diagnosis

David A. Palay

THIS chapter presents an overview of the common symptoms and signs associated with ocular disorders. A more in-depth discussion can be found in other chapters of this book. The text here attempts to present clinical "pearls" that will quickly guide the reader to the appropriate diagnosis.

SYMPTOMS

Visual Loss

Visual loss is a common symptom of ophthalmic conditions. However, the patient's subjective description of visual loss often correlates poorly with the examiner's objective measurements. Some patients with profound visual loss contact the physician long after the onset of symptoms, and their subjective complaints may be relatively minor. In contrast, patients with relatively minor objective visual loss may be seen immediately after the onset of symptoms and overstate complaints. For this reason, obtaining an accurate visual acuity measurement in each eye is essential. The physician should perform confrontational visual field tests because substantial field loss can be present with normal visual acuity. Patients with hemianopic defects (blindness in one half of the visual field) often relate the disease to the eye on the side of the defect rather than the true abnormality of the right or left hemifield. Finally, the physician should evaluate color vision because its loss is specific for central retinal or optic nerve dysfunction.

More recent visual loss requires more urgent evaluation, so the physician should determine the duration of the visual loss. Bilateral visual field loss that respects the vertical meridian is almost always associated with cerebral lesions including or posterior to the optic chiasm. Uniocular visual field loss results from direct involvement of the eye or optic nerve anterior to the optic chiasm. Patients sometimes mistake uniocular disease for binocular disease. For example, if a patient has unrecognized poor vision in one eye caused by a chronic disease and the contralateral eye is unaffected, a loss of vision in the good eye is sometimes interpreted as acute visual loss in both eyes.

Acute, painless loss of vision. In cases of acute, painless loss of vision, no injection of the conjunctiva occurs. The following provides information on these types of disorders:

ADDITIONAL HISTORY	KEY EXAM FEATURES
Vitreous hemorrhage Patients report the sensation of spider webs clouding their vision or have recent-onset floaters. Associated systemic diseases include diabetes, sickle cell anemia, and blood dyscrasias.	If the vitreous hemorrhage is extensive, decreased red reflex and poor visualization of the retina are found. Mild vitreous hemorrhages may be difficult to see with the direct ophthalmoscope.
Retinal detachment Retinal detachment commonly occurs in highly nearsighted individuals or may occur after eye surgery or trauma. The onset may be preceded by acute symptoms of flashes or floaters. Patients report a loss of visual field or a curtain covering part of their vision.	Detachment may be difficult to recognize with the direct ophthalmoscope. Indirect ophthalmoscopic evaluation is indicated.
Retinal artery occlusion Occlusion is caused by emboli and may be associated with carotid artery disease and valvular heart disease. It may be associated with previous episodes of a cloud interfering with the vision that eventually clears (amaurosis fugax). The visual loss is abrupt and almost complete.	With central retinal artery occlusion, vision is often limited to hand motions or light perception. Emboli may be visualized in the retinal arterioles. With central retinal artery occlusion, diffuse retinal whitening occurs and a cherry-red spot is present in the macula.
Retinal vein occlusion Occlusion is most commonly associated with hypertension and rarely with blood dyscrasias.	Occlusion results from a thrombosis of the retinal veins. Ophthalmoscopic findings include numerous retinal hemorrhages and occasional cotton-wool spots. The veins are tortuous and dilated.

ADDITIONAL HISTORY	KEY EXAM FEATURES

Exudative macular degeneration

Macular degeneration usually occurs in older individuals (over the age of 60 years) and may progressively worsen over several days. It is associated with an abnormal distortion of straight lines (metamorphopsia).

Retinal hemorrhage is noted in the macular region.

Ischemic optic neuropathy

Visual loss is usually sudden. The disorder is often associated with giant cell arteritis, and patients may have symptoms of jaw claudication, scalp tenderness, neck pain, and weight loss (age usually 60 years or older). It may also be associated with hypertension and diabetes (age usually 40 years or older).

An afferent pupillary defect is present. The optic nerve head is swollen on ophthalmoscopic examination.

Optic neuritis

Visual loss usually occurs over several days. Pain with eye movement may be present. The disorder is usually associated with multiple sclerosis (in patients 15 to 45 years of age).

An afferent pupillary defect is present. Two thirds of patients have a normal optic disc; one third have optic disc edema.

Cerebral infarct

A history of previous vascular disease or strokes may be reported.

A bilateral loss of visual field usually occurs. If the infarct involves the occipital lobe, visual acuity may be reduced. Ocular examination findings are normal.

Functional visual loss

A history of recent stress or earlier psychologic problems is usually reported.

Examination findings are normal.

Acute, painful loss of vision. The following group of disorders cause acute visual loss and are associated with severe pain. In addition, marked injection of the conjunctiva often occurs as a result of ocular inflammation:

ADDITIONAL HISTORY | KEY EXAM FEATURES

Corneal ulcer

A history of recent trauma or contact lens wear is usually reported. Sleeping in contact lenses greatly increases the risk of developing an infectious corneal ulcer.

The penlight exam may show a corneal abrasion, but an early corneal infiltrate can be difficult to identify. As the infection progresses, a white infiltrate is seen in the cornea. With extensive infections, a layering of white cells may be seen in the anterior chamber (hypopyon).

Uveitis

The origin of uveitis is often idiopathic. Common systemic associations include sarcoidosis, syphilis, tuberculosis, and HLA-B27–associated disorders (e.g., Reiter's syndrome, ankylosing spondylitis, inflammatory bowel disease, psoriasis). A history of sensitivity to light is also noted.

The pupil may be small, sluggish, or nonreactive to light. A circular injection of the eye surrounding the cornea (circumlimbal flush) is seen. The red reflex may be diminished, particularly with corneal edema and vitreous inflammation. Uveitis is usually unilateral but may affect both eyes.

Acute angle-closure glaucoma

Acute angle-closure glaucoma usually occurs in older individuals and more commonly in those who are farsighted. It may be precipitated by an advancing cataract. A full-blown attack may be preceded by a history of blurred vision, halos around lights, and pain precipitated by dark conditions (e.g., after being in a movie theater). Markedly elevated intraocular pressure can cause a headache and nausea and vomiting. Systemic symptoms may be out of proportion to visual symptoms, so patients can be misdiagnosed.

In its acute form, it is always unilateral. The eye is red, and the pupil is middilated and nonreactive. Vision is usually diminished initially because of corneal edema, but it may be subsequently diminished by optic nerve damage from prolonged elevated intraocular pressure. Intraocular pressure is usually elevated to levels above 50 mm Hg.

Endophthalmitis

Most cases of endophthalmitis are associated with recent eye surgery. Rarely, patients may develop endophthalmitis (e.g., fungal endophthalmitis) from another source of infection in the body.

In addition to markedly decreased vision and injection of the eye, a mucopurulent discharge may be present. A layering of white cells in the anterior chamber (hypopyon) is common. The red reflex is diminished because of vitreous inflammation. In fungal endophthalmitis, the anterior segment exam may be entirely normal.

Chronic, progressive loss of vision. The following disorders cause chronic, progressive loss of vision:

ADDITIONAL HISTORY	KEY EXAM FEATURES
Refractive error The patient may already wear contacts or glasses.	The visual acuity is near normal when the patient looks through a pinhole.
Cataract Cataract is one of the most common causes of chronic, progressive visual loss and may be associated with a family history of cataracts, diabetes, or chronic corticosteroid use. Patients may complain of multiple images when looking with only one eye. As the cataract progresses, objects become blurred and distinguishing objects up close and at a distance is difficult.	The visual acuity may be slightly improved with the pinhole. Pupil responses are normal. The normal red reflex is diminished, and visualizing the fundus with a direct ophthalmoscope can be difficult.
Open-angle glaucoma Open-angle glaucoma is more common in patients with a family history of glaucoma, nearsighted patients, patients with diabetes, and African-American patients. Visual acuity may remain normal until very late in the disease process, so patients with severe glaucoma may be relatively asymptomatic.	Elevated intraocular pressure greater than or equal to 22 mm Hg and increased optic nerve cupping of 0.6 or greater are significant.
Atrophic macular degeneration Atrophic macular degeneration is usually seen in patients older than age 60 years. It may be associated with a family history of macular degeneration.	With early disease, multiple hyaline nodules (drusen) are seen in the fundus. With advancing disease, retinal atrophy occurs, leaving a large scar or an atrophic area in the central macula.
Brain tumor Headache, nausea upon awakening, and variable neurologic symptoms and signs can be seen.	The pattern of visual field loss varies with the location of the tumor. Tumors posterior to the optic nerve chiasm do not produce optic nerve atrophy or afferent pupillary defects. Tumors involving the chiasm or intrinsic to the optic nerve produce afferent pupillary defects and optic nerve atrophy.

Distorted Vision (Metamorphopsia)

Metamorphopsia is the perception that straight lines are distorted or bowed. This usually results from macular dysfunction and can be tested with an Amsler grid (see Fig. 1-12). Conditions that elevate the retina (fluid under the retina) such as exudative macular degeneration cause the lines on an Amsler grid to bow in, which is termed *micropsia*. In contrast, conditions that pull the retina together such as an epiretinal membrane cause bowing out of the lines, which is termed *macropsia*.

Transient Visual Loss

A common patient complaint is vision that tends to fluctuate when the eyes blink. This commonly results from a poor tear film on the ocular surface, with dry eyes as the causative factor. Blinking reestablishes the tear film momentarily and can lead to a sudden improvement in vision that deteriorates as the tear film dissipates. Excessive mucus production from dry eyes may also cloud the vision. Fluctuation in vision may be associated with new-onset diabetes. Elevations in blood glucose level cause swelling of the lens and progressive nearsightedness. As patients pass age 40, they have more difficulty accommodating and focusing on near objects. Alterations in distance may also be difficult, such as when patients suddenly change focus from close objects to far objects and vice versa. This condition is termed *presbyopia*. An embolus to the retinal circulation temporarily interfering with ocular blood flow may cause the sensation that a curtain or cloud has come over the vision. This is termed *amaurosis fugax*. If the embolus does not clear, a central or branch retinal artery occlusion occurs. An impending thrombosis of the central retinal or a branch retinal vein can cause transient visual loss. Carotid artery or vertebrobasilar insufficiency can also cause transient visual symptoms that may be associated with movements in the neck. Papilledema caused by increased intracranial pressure may result in transient bilateral visual loss lasting a few seconds. Many systemic medications can cause transient visual symptoms, particularly those with hypotension as a possible side effect.

Night Blindness

The examiner must distinguish a patient's decreased ability to function in the dark from true night blindness. Young patients with uncorrected myopia often complain of decreased ability to function, particularly when driving at night. Commonly, they are unable to see street signs until they are close to them. This can usually be corrected with glasses. Similarly, patients with cataracts may complain of having difficulty driving at night because of excessive glare and visual distortion. True night blindness can occur with retinitis pigmentosa, vitamin A deficiency, and systemic medications such as phenothiazines. Patients with true night blindness have difficulty seeing any stars in the sky on a clear night and may be unable to ambulate without assistance in a dark environment such as a movie theater.

Flashes

The sudden onset of flashes in the peripheral visual field suggests traction of the vitreous on the peripheral retina. This phenomenon may occur during the evolution of a posterior vitreous detachment or as the vitreous pulls on a tear in the retina. Retinal tears and detachments are more common in highly nearsighted individuals and patients who have undergone intraocular surgery. The flashes may be more pronounced in the dark and especially apparent with rapid eye movement. In addition, retinal flashes may be associated with the sudden onset of floaters, which can indicate debris or blood in the vitreous cavity. Because a tear in the retina can lead to a retinal detachment, urgent consultation with an ophthalmologist is required.

A second type of flashing light can occur with a migraine. These flashes have a distinct quality and are often described as scintillations or zigzagging lights that march across the visual field. They may last a few minutes or as long as 30 minutes and can be associated with transient visual field loss. Headache may not follow the visual symptoms, and the patient may have a prior history of migraines without any visual symptoms. Often a family history of migraines or a history of carsickness as a child is reported. Hormonal changes such as occurs with pregnancy, menopause, use of birth control pills, and the menstrual cycle may trigger an attack, as can stress and alcohol use.

Floaters

Many patients report seeing floaters, particularly when they look at a bright, white background or into the blue sky. These floaters are caused by small aggregates in the vitreous cavity, which result from a normal aging process of the vitreous (syneresis). The acute onset of vitreous floaters may be associated with uveitis affecting the vitreous cavity or the sudden onset of bleeding in the vitreous cavity. Disorders associated with vitreous hemorrhage include diabetes and sickle cell anemia. The acute onset of floaters, particularly if associated with flashing lights, may be a sign of a posterior vitreous detachment or a retinal tear with an impending retinal detachment. Therefore urgent ophthalmic referral for indirect ophthalmoscopy is essential. Detection of a retinal tear with direct ophthalmoscopy is almost impossible; most tears occur in the peripheral retina.

Photophobia

Photophobia, particularly if associated with eye pain, redness, and decreased vision, is a symptom of uveitis. The same symptoms may occur 3 or 4 days after an acute ocular injury as a result of traumatic iritis. Photophobia and increased sensitivity to loud noises can be associated with an acute migraine. Meningeal irritation may also cause photophobia.

Halos around Lights

Cataracts commonly cause patients to see halos around lights, particularly when they are driving at night. Episodic decreased vision, redness, and halos around lights may be symptoms of impending angle-closure glaucoma. Conditions that cause corneal edema can also result in halos.

Double Vision (Diplopia)

The examiner must distinguish monocular from binocular diplopia. Binocular diplopia results from a misalignment of the eyes: when one eye fixates on a target, the other eye sees the image slightly displaced from the image in the fixating eye. For this reason, binocular diplopia disappears when *either* eye is covered. If the images are side by side, the disorder is termed *horizontal diplopia*. If the images are up and down, it is termed *vertical diplopia.*

In monocular diplopia the image is split within the eye and focuses poorly on the retina, resulting in a double image or ghosting of the image. Because monocular diplopia is intrinsic to the eye, it persists when the uninvolved eye is covered.

Monocular diplopia. Common causes of monocular diplopia include (1) uncorrected refractive error, (2) dry eye with irregular corneal surface, (3) corneal scar, and (4) cataract.

Binocular diplopia. The following disorders cause binocular diplopia:

ADDITIONAL HISTORY	KEY EXAM FEATURES
Third nerve palsy	
Third nerve palsy may be associated with aneurysm, microvascular infarct (particularly with diabetes or hypertension), tumor, trauma, and uncal herniation. Some patients may experience pain.	A droopy eyelid is seen on the involved side. The pupil may be fixed and dilated. If the pupil is involved, the cause of the disorder is probably an aneurysm (of the posterior communicating artery). If the pupil is not involved, microvascular ischemia is usually the cause. Because the third nerve controls superior, inferior, and medial movements, the eye is usually pointed down and out.
Fourth nerve palsy	
The fourth nerve controls vertical eye movement, so fourth nerve palsy causes vertical diplopia. Some patients report difficulty reading but may have no symptoms. This palsy may occur with trauma, microvascular infarct (particularly with diabetes or hypertension), tumor, and aneurysm.	The involved eye is higher than the uninvolved eye. The deviation may be so slight that detecting the difference on gross examination is difficult. Patients may have a head tilt that eliminates the double vision.
Sixth nerve palsy	
The sixth nerve controls lateral eye movements. Patients therefore complain of horizontal diplopia. Sixth nerve palsy may be associated with trauma, microvascular infarct (from diabetes or hypertension), increased intracranial pressure, temporal arteritis, cavernous sinus tumor, and aneurysm.	An inability to move the eye outward with the involved eye pointing in (esotropia) is significant.
Decompensated strabismus	
The patient may report a history of strabismus or previous eye muscle surgery.	Horizontal (esotropia/exotropia) or vertical deviation may be present depending on the muscles involved.

Myasthenia gravis

Patients may have the typical symptoms of myasthenia gravis, including fatigue, weakness, and difficulty swallowing, chewing, and breathing; these symptoms may fluctuate during the day. The double vision also tends to fluctuate during the day and worsens with fatigue.

Droopy eyelids that become worse toward the end of the day or when the individual is fatigued are significant. With sustained upgaze, the droopy eyelids may worsen. Systemic edrophonium chloride (Tensilon) often improves the eyelid droop and/or double vision. Weakness of the facial muscles and limb muscles may occur, but no pupil abnormalities are present.

Thyroid eye disease

Eye disease is usually associated with hyperthyroidism; however, patients may have a normal functioning thyroid gland. The eye disease may be present even when the systemic disease is under good control.

Unilateral or bilateral proptosis may be present, and the conjunctiva can be injected or filled with fluid (chemosis). Eye movement may be limited, particularly up and out. When the patient looks down slowly, the upper eyelids may lag behind the eye movement such that the superior sclera is visible (lid lag). The proptosis may lead to an inability to fully close the lids, causing dry eye signs and symptoms.

Orbital pseudotumor

Patients report severe pain and redness, usually in one eye.

The conjunctiva is usually injected, and swelling of the conjunctiva (chemosis) may occur. The eyelids are often red and swollen. Proptosis and restriction of movement in one eye occur, and a palpable orbital mass may be present. The vision in the involved eye may be decreased.

Blow-out fracture

Blow-out fracture is associated with a history of blunt trauma to the orbit.

Restricted eye movement, particularly in upgaze and/or lateral gaze, is significant. Subcutaneous air (crepitus) and numbness in the distribution of the infraorbital nerve, which involves the cheek and upper lip, are possible.

Itching and Burning

Itching and burning are nonspecific complaints that can be associated with many diseases of the lids and conjunctiva. Any acute conjunctivitis can be associated with itching and burning. Chronic itching and burning is most commonly associated with allergic conjunctivitis, blepharitis, and dry eyes.

Foreign Body Sensation

Foreign body sensation, or the feeling that a grain of sand is in the eye, is a common ocular complaint. The most common cause is dry eyes. In severe cases, superficial punctate staining of the corneal epithelium is possible. Lashes rubbing on the eye from an entropion or misdirected lashes (trichiasis) can cause a foreign body sensation. Most corneal abrasions cause severe pain, but minor abrasions may be associated with a foreign body sensation. An arc welder burn causes a punctate corneal keratopathy, and foreign body sensation may be a prominent symptom. Conjunctival and corneal foreign bodies also produce this symptom.

Severe Eye Pain

As stated, corneal ulcer, uveitis, acute angle-closure glaucoma, and endophthalmitis are disorders that cause severe eye pain and are associated with acute loss of vision. Injection of the conjunctiva and sclera with severe ocular pain but with an otherwise normal eye exam usually results from scleritis. Episcleritis has a similar clinical presentation but is associated with only a mild degree of pain. Any defect in the corneal epithelium caused by contact lens wear, trauma, or recurrent erosion syndrome is associated with a severe burning pain in the eye. The instillation of topical anesthesia eliminates the pain and can be a useful diagnostic test for the physician to establish whether the pain is caused by one of these entities. Orbital pseudotumor is an inflammatory disease of the orbit associated with severe orbital pain. Important signs include proptosis, restriction of ocular motility, injection and edema of the conjunctiva and lids, optic nerve swelling, and in some cases, visual loss.

Excessive Tearing

An overflow of tears from the eye onto the cheek is termed *epiphora*. Impairment of tear drainage can occur with lid malposition. Ectropion is an outward turning of the lid that results in an inability of the tears to enter the puncta. Obstructions of the nasolacrimal drainage system distal to this area can also result in excessive tearing in both adults and children. External ocular irritation can cause reflex tearing and an overflow of tears from the eye. Two common examples include turning in of the lids (entropion) and abnormal lashes rubbing on the cornea (trichiasis), stimulating tear production. Dry eyes produce less tear volume, which results in drying of the cornea and conjunctiva. This can cause pain and inflammation, stimulating lacrimal gland production of tears, and can result in paradoxical tearing despite a dry eye. In the neonate, excessive tearing can be the earliest sign of congenital glaucoma, necessitating urgent ophthalmologic examination.

Eyelid Twitching

Any irritation of the conjunctiva or cornea can cause eyelid twitching. Occasional twitching of the lids is usually associated with stress. Caffeine or other stimulants can cause a similar reaction. Severe spasm of the lids with a functional impairment is termed *benign essential blepharospasm*. Rarely, multiple sclerosis is associated with lid spasm.

SIGNS

Conjunctivitis

Any type of ocular inflammation can be associated with a secondary conjunctivitis. Corneal ulcers, angle-closure glaucoma, endophthalmitis, and uveitis are associated with conjunctival inflammation. Conjunctivitis, as opposed to scleritis and episcleritis, usually involves the entire conjunctiva (not just a section), is usually associated with a discharge, and is usually not associated with pain. (Table 2-1 outlines common ophthalmic disorders that manifest primarily as a conjunctivitis.)

Table 2-1

Ophthalmic disorders associated with conjunctivitis

ACUTE OR CHRONIC	UNILATERAL OR BILATERAL	KEY SYMPTOMS	DEGREE OF INJECTION	DISCHARGE TYPE	OTHER FEATURES
Viral conjunctivitis					
Acute	Bilateral, possibly asymmetric	Itching, burning, soreness	4+	Watery	Preauricular lymphadenopathy
Bacterial conjunctivitis					
Acute	Unilateral or bilateral	Burning, general irritation	3+	Heavy, muco-purulent	Lids possibly adherent
Herpes simplex conjunctivitis					
Acute	Unilateral	Photophobia, mild irritation	1-2+	None	Dendrite on the cornea or vesicles on the lid possible
Adult chlamydial conjunctivitis					
Subacute/ chronic	Usually unilateral	Burning, general irritation	2+	Scant, muco-purulent	Usual occurrence in young, sexually active adults
Allergic conjunctivitis					
Chronic	Bilateral	Itching	2+	Stringy, mucoid	Usual occurrence in atopic individuals, possible seasonal symptoms
Blepharitis					
Chronic	Bilateral	Itching, burning, foreign body sensation	1-2+	Usually none	Inflammation and crusting of lid margins
Dry eye					
Chronic	Bilateral	Foreign body sensation	1+	Mucoid in severe cases	Punctate fluorescein staining of the cornea
Cavernous sinus AV fistula					
Chronic	Unilateral	Double vision, audible bruits	1-4+	None	Elevated intraocular pressure, proptosis, possible vision loss

AV, Arteriovenous.

Table 2-2

Disorders causing ptosis

History	Degree of ptosis	Motility	Pupil
Third nerve palsy Double vision, possible severe pain	Moderate to severe	Decreased elevation, depression, and medial movement	Dilated and unreactive or normal
Horner's syndrome Asymptomatic	Mild	Normal	Small
Myasthenia gravis Fatigue, difficulty swallowing or breathing, double vision	Variable, possible worsening on sustained upgaze	Any abnormality or no abnormality	Normal
Senile ptosis Possible history of recent eye surgery	Variable	Normal	Normal

Eyelid Swelling and Erythema

Patients with blepharitis often complain of fullness or swelling in the eyelids, although the lids may not appear thick on clinical evaluation. Examination of the lid margin often shows inflammation and crusting along the lashes. A chalazion is an acute inflammation of the meibomian glands and can cause diffuse erythema and inflammation of one eyelid. The examiner can often palpate a nodule in the center of the area of inflammation. Patients with preseptal and orbital cellulitis are often seen with erythema and swelling of the eyelids. In contrast to an acute chalazion, both lids are involved and the inflammation extends to the skin beyond the lids. In addition, patients usually have a fever and an elevated white blood cell count. Contact dermatitis with secondary lid swelling may develop after prolonged use of a topical medication. Clinically, erythema and an eczematous reaction of the skin are present. Symptoms include itching and irritation.

Ptosis (Droopy Eyelid)

Table 2-2 details disorders that result in ptosis.

Small Pupil

When one pupil is smaller than the other, the disparity between pupils is greater in darkness than in well-lit conditions. It can occur in Horner's syndrome and is associated with ptosis on the same side. Tertiary syphilis is associated with Argyll Robertson pupils. These bilaterally small pupils react poorly to light. When the patient fixates on a near target, the pupils constrict normally (light-near dissociation). The use of miotic drops (e.g., pilocarpine), traumatic iritis, uveitis, and recent eye surgery may be associated with a small pupil.

Large Pupil

With an abnormally large pupil, the disparity between pupil size is greater in light than in darkness. Inadvertent deposition of any α-adrenergic or anticholinergic agent into the

Table 2-3
Disorders resulting in proptosis

ACUTE OR CHRONIC	UNILATERAL OR BILATERAL	CONJUNCTIVAL INJECTION (REDNESS)	PAIN	FEVER	OTHER FEATURES
Thyroid eye disease					
Subacute	Bilateral but possibly asymmetric	0-4+, variable depending on extent of disease	None	No	Possible association with systemic thyroid abnormalities
Orbital pseudotumor					
Acute	Usually unilateral	3-4+	Severe pain, particularly with eye movement	No	Possible decreased vision and diplopia
Optic nerve tumor					
Chronic	Unilateral	0	None	No	Slow-onset visual field loss
Cavernous sinus AV fistula					
Acute onset, chronic course	Unilateral	1-4+, variable depending on flow rate	Variable	No	Elevated intraocular pressure, double vision, possible visual loss, audible bruit or pulsating exophthalmos
Cellulitis					
Acute	Unilateral	4+	Moderate to severe	Yes	Most common association with sinusitis, elevated white blood cell count

AV, *Arteriovenous.*

eye can cause a large pupil. The unilateral use of dilating drops is a common cause of an abnormally large pupil. Scopolamine patches for the control of seasickness can cause a fixed, dilated pupil if the patient rubs the eye after touching the patch. With eye trauma, the iris sphincter muscle can be damaged and an abnormally large pupil can result. Tears in the iris sphincter can sometimes be appreciated with a slit lamp exam. Third nerve palsy may cause a dilated pupil and is associated with ptosis, decreased elevation, decreased depression, and decreased medial movement of the eye. Adie's pupil is an idiopathic abnormality of the pupil that results in unilateral dilation. The pupil is hypersensitive to weak cholinergic drops such as pilocarpine 0.125%. Traumatic iritis, uveitis, angle-closure glaucoma, and recent eye surgery may be associated with a large pupil.

Proptosis
Proptosis is an abnormal protrusion of the eye (Table 2-3).

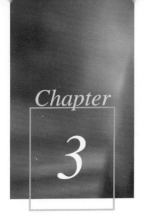

Chapter

3

Eyelid Abnormalities

Ted H. Wojno

ANATOMY

In adults the upper lid usually rests at a point between the upper limbus (corneoscleral junction) and upper pupillary border. The lower lid margin usually rests along the inferior limbus. A small amount of scleral show (visibility of the sclera between the lid and limbus) is not abnormal in the lower lid but is in the upper lid. In most individuals the upper lid has a distinct crease where fibers from the levator muscle insert; this is covered by a small fold of skin. A lower lid crease is sometimes present and less well defined than that in the upper lid. The upper and lower lids join at the medial and lateral canthi (Fig. 3-1).

The tarsal plates are composed of dense, collagenous tissue that forms the skeleton of the lids. Vertically oriented meibomian oil glands within the tarsi have orifices visible just posterior to the lashes (Fig. 3-2). The tarsal plates are attached to the orbital rims by the medial and lateral canthal tendons.

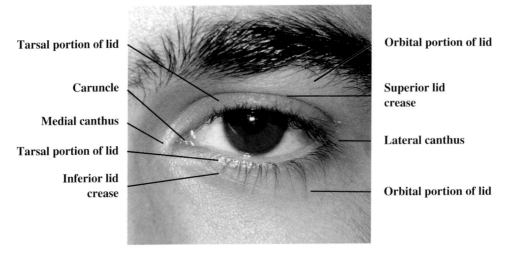

Fig. 3-1 The eyelids.

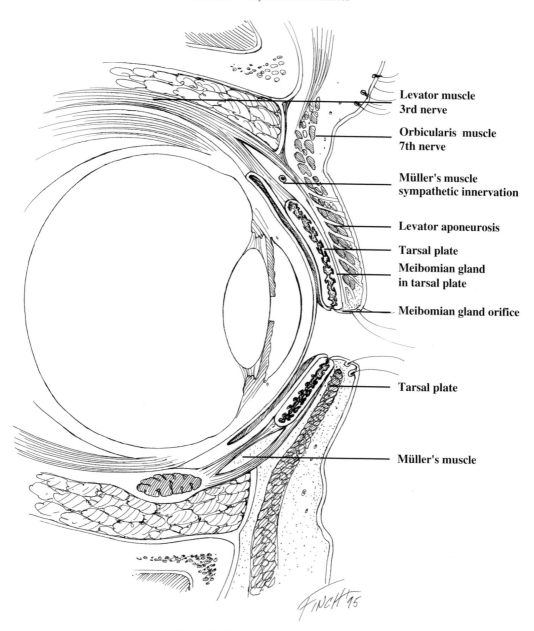

**Levator muscle
3rd nerve**

**Orbicularis muscle
7th nerve**

**Müller's muscle
sympathetic innervation**

Levator aponeurosis

Tarsal plate

**Meibomian gland
in tarsal plate**

Meibomian gland orifice

Tarsal plate

Müller's muscle

Fig. 3-2 Side view of eyelid anatomy.

Elevation of the upper lid is primarily the work of the levator muscle (innervated by the third cranial nerve) and is assisted by Müller's muscle (through sympathetic innervation). Third nerve palsy results in a moderately droopy lid (at least 3 mm lower than usual), known as *ptosis,* whereas sympathetic palsy results in a mildly droopy lid (1 to 2 mm lower than usual).

The orbicularis muscle, innervated by the seventh cranial nerve, is responsible for involuntary blinking and forceful lid closure. The lids are separated from the orbit by the orbital septum, a fibrous membrane that functions to prevent the spread of superficial infections into the orbit. Thinning of the septum with age allows the orbital fat to prolapse anteriorly, causing characteristic bulges, or "bags," in the lids.

ECTROPION

Symptoms

- Irritation, burning, and foreign body sensation occur.
- Tearing results from punctal malposition.

Signs

- An out-turned lower lid margin occurs, often with a visible space between the globe and lid (Fig. 3-3).

Etiology

- Involutional—The disorder is caused by lower lid laxity, which occurs with aging.
- Cicatricial—The disorder is caused by a scar on the lower lid skin.
- Paralytic—The disorder is caused by a seventh nerve palsy.
- Mechanical—The disorder is caused by a mass on the lower lid or cheek.
- The disorder rarely has a congenital origin.

Treatment

- Surgery is performed to correct any causative abnormality.

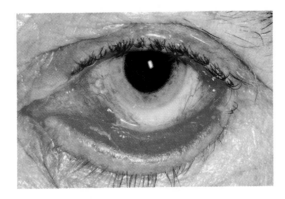

Fig. 3-3 Involutional ectropion.

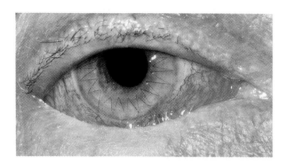

Fig. 3-4 Involutional entropion. Note that this patient has undergone corneal transplantation.

ENTROPION

Symptoms

- Irritation, burning, and foreign body sensation occur.
- Tearing results from lashes abrading the globe.

Signs

- An in-turned lower lid margin is present (Fig. 3-4).

Etiology

- Involutional—The disorder is caused by lower lid laxity, which occurs with aging.
- Cicatricial—The disorder is caused by a scar on the conjunctival surface such as from a chemical burn.
- The disorder rarely has a congenital origin.

Treatment

- Surgery is performed to correct any causative abnormality.

TRICHIASIS

Symptoms

- Irritation, burning, and foreign body sensation occur.
- Tearing results from lashes abrading the globe.

Signs

- Lashes on a normally positioned lid margin are posteriorly misdirected (Fig. 3-5).

Etiology

- Spontaneous—The disorder usually affects an isolated lash or two and often occurs at the site of a previous stye.
- An inflammatory process of the conjunctiva results from injuries such as a chemical burn or a disease such as ocular cicatricial pemphigoid.

Associated Diseases

- The disorder may coexist with cicatricial entropion.

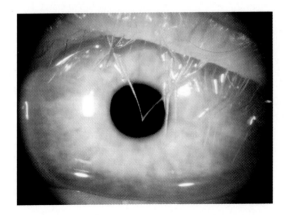

Fig. 3-5 Trichiasis.

Treatment

■ Isolated lashes are removed with forceps.

■ Extensive lash abnormalities are corrected with surgery.

LAGOPHTHALMOS

Symptoms

■ Irritation, burning, and foreign body sensation occur.

■ Tearing is caused by failure of the "lacrimal pump."

Signs

■ The patient cannot completely close the eye (Fig. 3-6).

Etiology

■ Possible causes include the following:
  • Severe lower lid laxity
  • Seventh nerve palsy
  • Proptosis
  • Overcorrected ptosis repair or blepharoplasty
  • Scarring changes in upper or lower lid

Treatment

■ The following applies to seventh nerve palsy:
  • Mild—Artificial tears or tear ointments are used. The eye is taped shut at night.
  • Moderate to severe—Lid margins are sutured together (tarsorrhaphy).
  • Permanent—A gold weight is surgically inserted into the upper lid.
■ For other causes the primary problem is treated.

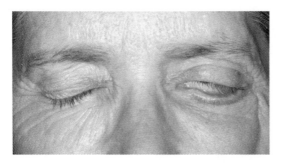

Fig. 3-6 Lagophthalmos of the left eye due to seventh nerve palsy.

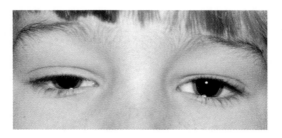

Fig. 3-7 Ptosis of the right upper lid.

PTOSIS

Symptoms

- Obstruction of the superior visual field occurs.
- Reading is difficult, with acquired ptosis usually worse in downgaze.
- The patient is concerned about the cosmetic appearance of the lid.
- If the ptosis is congenital or acquired in early childhood, amblyopia often is present.

Signs

- The upper lid margin is in an abnormally low position (Fig. 3-7).

Etiology

- Congenital—The disorder usually results from a malformed levator muscle.
- Acquired—A thinning or detachment of the levator aponeurosis is present.
- Horner's syndrome—The disorder involves 1 to 2 mm of ptosis with a small pupil on the same side (see Chapter 11).
- Third nerve palsy—With ophthalmoplegia, more than 3 mm of ptosis is present (see Chapter 11).
- Myasthenia gravis—Ptosis varies and may worsen with sustained upgaze (see Chapter 11).

Treatment

- For congenital or acquired lesions, surgery is performed to tighten the levator aponeurosis or resect the levator muscle.
- For other causes the primary problem is treated.

FLOPPY EYELID SYNDROME

Symptoms

- Irritation, burning, foreign body sensation, and discharge occur.

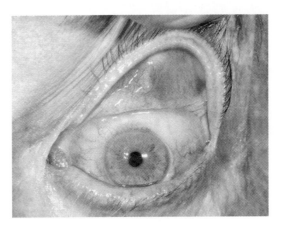

Fig. 3-8 Floppy eyelid syndrome demonstrating ease with which upper lid is everted.

Signs

- The disorder is usually unilateral or asymmetric.
- Chronic conjunctivitis that is nonresponsive to topical antibiotics is present.
- A giant papillary reaction (papillae >1 mm in size) of the tarsal conjunctiva occurs, giving the surface a red cobblestone or velvety appearance.
- A characteristic finding is the ability to evert the patient's upper lid by simply pulling upward from the lateral brow area (Fig. 3-8).

Etiology

- There is an abnormal laxity of the lateral canthal tendon and tarsal plate.
- The upper lid everts during sleep and rubs against the pillow, leading to severe irritation of the conjunctiva and mucus secretion.

Treatment

- A Fox shield (plastic or metal shield usually worn after cataract surgery) is taped over the eye at night to prevent the lid rubbing on the pillow.
- Surgery is necessary to tighten the upper and lower lids horizontally; the procedure may need to be repeated after several years.

SEBORRHEIC KERATOSIS

Symptoms

- Patients are usually symptom free.
- Occasional itchiness occurs.

Signs

- The lesion is usually well demarcated with variable pigmentation, a "stuck-on" appearance, and a cerebriform surface (Fig. 3-9).
- A lobulated papillary or pedunculated frond is sometimes present at the lid margin.

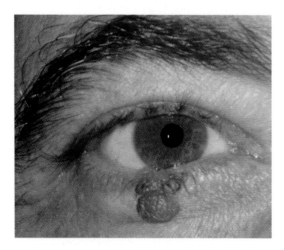

Fig. 3-9 Seborrheic keratosis.

Differential Diagnosis

■ Differential diagnoses include the following:
- • Nevus
- • Basal cell carcinoma
- • Melanoma

Treatment

■ Seborrheic keratoses are benign lesions, usually requiring no treatment.
■ A superficial shave biopsy or an excision can be performed if lesions are cosmetically undesirable.

ACTINIC KERATOSIS

Symptoms

■ Patients are usually symptom free.
■ Occasional itchiness occurs.

Signs

■ The disorder varies from a flat, scaly lesion to a papilloma to a cutaneous horn (Fig. 3-10).

Etiology

■ The disorder results from overexposure to actinic radiation.

Differential Diagnosis

■ Differential diagnoses include the following:
- • Squamous cell carcinoma
- • Verruca
- • Seborrheic keratosis

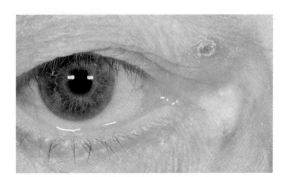

Fig. 3-10 Actinic keratosis.

Associated Factors and Diseases
- The disorder is more common in fair-skinned individuals.
- The disorder may develop into squamous cell carcinoma.

Treatment
- The three treatment options are as follows:
  - Surgical excision is performed.
  - Patients undergo cryotherapy.
  - Topical 5-fluorouracil (e.g., Efudex) is prescribed.

XANTHELASMA
Symptoms
- Patients are usually symptom free.
- The disorder is a cosmetic deformity.

Signs
- A bilateral, plaquelike, yellow lesion usually is present (Fig. 3-11).
- The lesion is found in the medial upper and lower lids.

Etiology
- The origin is usually idiopathic.

Associated Factors and Diseases
- The disorder affects middle-aged to elderly individuals and predominantly women.
- The disorder is occasionally associated with hyperlipidemia or diabetes.

Treatment
- Surgical excision of the involved skin is performed.
- A skin graft is often necessary for a large lesion.

EPITHELIAL INCLUSION CYST
Symptoms
- Patients are usually symptom free.

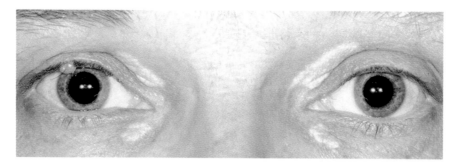

Fig. 3-11 Xanthelasma of all four lids. The patient also has an intradermal nevus of the right upper lid margin.

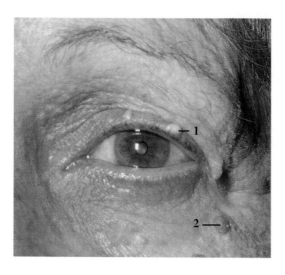

Fig. 3-12 Epithelial inclusion cyst *(1)* of the left upper lid. The patient also has a seborrheic keratosis *(2)* of the lower lid and lateral canthus.

Signs

- The cyst is slow growing, white, round, and firm (Fig. 3-12).
- The diameter of the cyst is usually smaller than 1 cm.

Etiology

- The cyst results from traumatic implantation of epidermis into the dermis.

Differential Diagnosis

- Differential diagnoses include the following:
  - Milium (small retention cyst of a hair follicle)
  - Syringoma (adenoma of an eccrine sweat gland)
  - Hydrocystoma (cyst of an eccrine sweat gland)
  - Trichoepithelioma (squamous cell cyst of a hair follicle)
  - Basal cell carcinoma

Associated Diseases

■ The disorder is rarely associated with Gardner's syndrome.

Treatment

■ Excision or marsupialization of the cyst is performed.

BASAL CELL CARCINOMA

Symptoms

■ Patients are usually symptom free.

Signs

■ Nodular—Most commonly, a solid, pearly lesion is covered with telangiectatic vessels and a central ulceration (Fig. 3-13).
■ Infiltrative—Rarely, a superficial, erythematous patch is present.
■ The most common locations are the lower lid and medial canthus.

Etiology

■ The disorder results from overexposure to actinic radiation.

Differential Diagnosis

■ Differential diagnoses include the following:
  • Milium (small retention cyst of a hair follicle)
  • Syringoma (adenoma of an eccrine sweat gland)
  • Hydrocystoma (cyst of an eccrine sweat gland)
  • Trichoepithelioma (squamous cell cyst of a hair follicle)

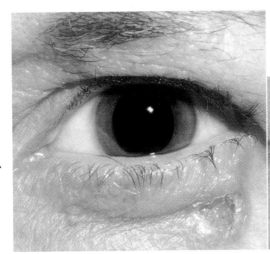
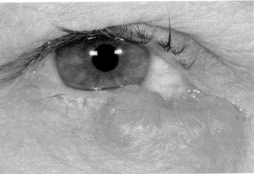

A   B

Fig. 3-13 A, A relatively flat basal cell carcinoma. **B,** A typical nodular basal cell carcinoma.

Associated Factors and Diseases

- It is the most common primary eyelid malignancy, occurring in 80% to 90% of cases.
- The disorder is more common in basal cell nevus syndrome and xeroderma pigmentosum.
- The carcinoma rarely metastasizes but is locally destructive.

Treatment

- The preferred technique is Mohs' removal followed by reconstruction; this results in a high cure rate (98%) and spares as much normal tissue as possible. Surgical excision with frozen section control is an acceptable alternative with a high cure rate (95%).
- Radiation therapy (80% to 90% cure rate) is usually reserved for patients unable or unwilling to have surgery.

Follow-Up

- The site is examined for recurrence.
- Sun-exposed body parts are inspected for additional lesions.

SQUAMOUS CELL CARCINOMA

Symptoms

- Patients are usually symptom free.

Signs

- An infiltrative, erythematous patch often with ulceration is a common sign of squamous cell carcinoma (Fig. 3-14).
- A nodular, erythematous lesion often with ulceration is an uncommon finding.

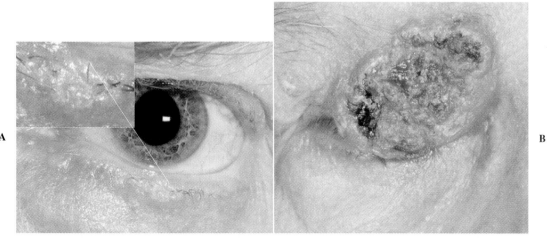

Fig. 3-14 A, A typical small squamous cell carcinoma. **B,** A large nodular squamous cell carcinoma.

Etiology

■ The disorder results from overexposure to actinic radiation.

Differential Diagnosis

■ Differential diagnoses include the following:
  • Basal cell carcinoma
  • Actinic keratosis
  • Verruca

Associated Factors and Diseases

■ It is the second most common primary eyelid malignancy (5% to 10% of cases).

■ It is more common in fair-skinned individuals.

■ It is more common in patients with xeroderma pigmentosum, those who have undergone radiation therapy, and immunosuppressed patients (such as those with human immunodeficiency virus [HIV] infection).

■ The carcinoma may metastasize.

Treatment

■ Surgery as for basal cell carcinoma is performed.

■ Radiation is usually ineffective.

Follow-Up

■ Follow-up involves the same procedures as for basal cell carcinoma.

BLEPHARITIS

Symptoms

■ Irritation, burning, and foreign body sensation occur.

■ Excessive tearing (epiphora), photophobia, and intermittent blurred vision are present.

Signs

■ Erythema of the lid margin occurs.

■ Dandrufflike deposits on the lashes (scurf) are found.

■ Fibrinous scales surround individual lashes (collarettes).

■ Lash loss occurs.

■ Recurrent, mild conjunctivitis is present.

■ Thick, cloudy secretions from the meibomian orifices result with digital pressure on the lid.

Etiology

■ Three distinct types of blepharitis may occur:
  • Seborrhea (Fig. 3-15, *A*) is often associated with dandruff of the brows and scalp.
  • Staphylococcal infection (Fig. 3-15, *B*) is often associated with styes (hordeola).
  • Meibomian gland dysfunction (posterior lid margin disease and meibomianitis) (Fig. 3-15, *C*) is often associated with chalazia.

■ A combination of any of the three types can cause the disorder.

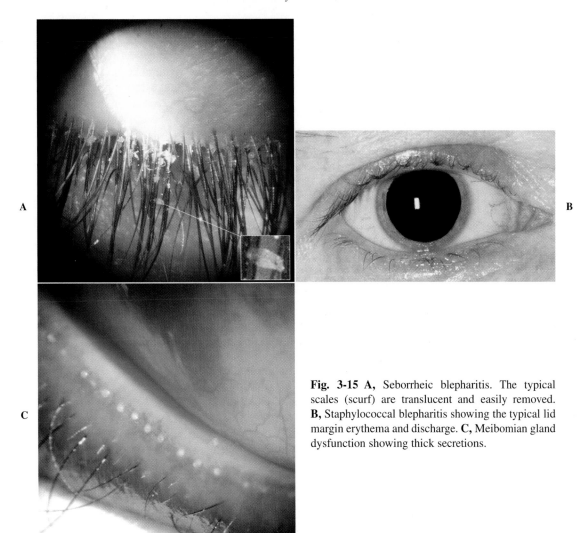

Fig. 3-15 A, Seborrheic blepharitis. The typical scales (scurf) are translucent and easily removed. **B,** Staphylococcal blepharitis showing the typical lid margin erythema and discharge. **C,** Meibomian gland dysfunction showing thick secretions.

Differential Diagnosis

■ Differential diagnoses include the following:
  • Infiltrative lid neoplasm (e.g., squamous cell carcinoma, sebaceous cell carcinoma)
  • Discoid lupus erythematosus

Treatment

■ The lid margins are scrubbed daily with a cotton-tipped applicator dipped in dilute baby shampoo to remove scurf, collarettes, and bacteria. Massage of the lid margins may help express the abnormal meibomian secretions.

■ Antibiotic treatment consists of the following:
  • A topical antibiotic ointment such as erythromycin or polymyxin B/bacitracin (e.g., Polysporin) is applied to the lid margins at night if lid scrubs are ineffective.
  • A 6-week course of doxycycline (50 to 200 mg/day) is added to improve meibomian gland function. Doxycycline is contraindicated in children, pregnant women, and breastfeeding mothers.

Follow-Up
■ The disorder frequently recurs and is sometimes recalcitrant to treatment.

STYE (HORDEOLUM)
Symptoms
■ The subacute onset of a painful nodule or pustule of the eyelid occurs.

Signs
■ A painful, erythematous, often pointed nodule is present on the skin surface (external stye) (Fig. 3-16) or conjunctival surface (internal stye).

Etiology
■ Usually the disorder is caused by a staphylococcal infection of a sebaceous gland of the lid.

Differential Diagnosis
■ Differential diagnoses include the following:
  • Chalazion
  • Inclusion cyst
  • Lid tumor

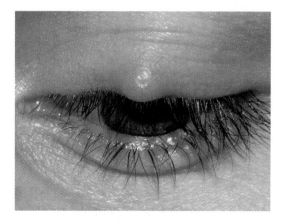

Fig. 3-16 External stye.

Treatment

- Warm compresses and topical antibiotic drops such as fluoroquinolones (e.g., Chibroxin, Ciloxan, Ocuflox) or polymyxin B/trimethoprim (Polytrim) are applied 3 to 4 times a day.
- Incision and drainage is performed if compresses and antibiotics fail or the patient wants rapid relief of symptoms.

Follow-Up

- The focus of follow-up is to ensure that preseptal cellulitis does not occur.

CHALAZION

Symptoms

- Patients are usually symptom free or have a minimally tender nodule of the lid.

Signs

- A firm, well-demarcated nodule just below the lid margin occurs (Fig. 3-17, *A*).
- Usually a grayish discoloration is visible on the conjunctival surface (Fig. 3-17, *B*).

Etiology

- A chronic, lipogranulomatous inflammation of a meibomian gland is present.
- The disorder is more common with meibomian gland dysfunction.

Differential Diagnosis

- Differential diagnoses include the following:
  - Hordeolum
  - Inclusion cyst
  - Lid tumor

A 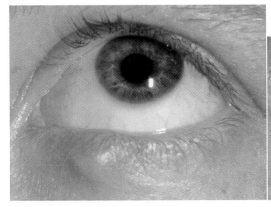 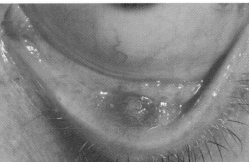 B

Fig. 3-17 A, A typical chalazion appearing as a pea-sized nodule. **B,** The conjunctival appearance of the same chalazion.

Treatment

- Early treatment (first 5 days) consists of application of frequent, warm compresses to open the inflamed gland.
- Intermediate treatment (first 2 to 3 weeks) consists of injection of triamcinolone. Steroid injections can result in depigmentation and are contraindicated in darkly pigmented individuals.
- Late treatment (after 1 month) entails marsupialization of the encysted meibomian gland using a conjunctival approach.

MOLLUSCUM CONTAGIOSUM

Symptoms

- Irritated skin, conjunctivitis, and keratitis secondary to viral shedding into the tear film occur.

Signs

- Round, umbilicated, pearly-white lesions of the skin are present (Fig. 3-18).
- Lesions are usually multiple.

Etiology

- The disorder is caused by a poxvirus.

Differential Diagnosis

- Differential diagnoses include the following:
  - Verruca
  - Herpes zoster
  - Herpes simplex

Associated Factors and Diseases

- It is more common in children, sexually active adults, and patients with HIV.

Treatment

- The lesion is destroyed using excision, curettage, electrocautery, or cryotherapy.

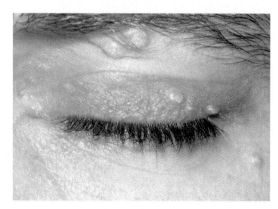

Fig. 3-18 Multiple molluscum contagiosa.

HERPES SIMPLEX DERMATITIS

Symptoms

■ Mild to moderately painful blepharitis occurs.

Signs

■ Vesicular eruption on the skin of the lids or lid margin is present (Fig. 3-19).
■ The eruption progresses to an ulcerative lesion with escharification.

Etiology

■ The disorder is commonly caused by infection with herpes simplex virus I.
■ Infection with herpes simplex II is uncommon.

Differential Diagnosis

■ Differential diagnoses include the following:
   • Molluscum
   • Verruca
   • Herpes zoster

Workup

■ A viral culture is performed if necessary.

Treatment

■ In mild cases, good hygiene is encouraged to prevent secondary bacterial infection.

A

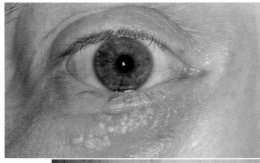

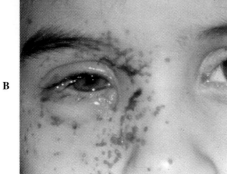

B

Fig. 3-19 A, Herpes simplex dermatitis of the eyelids. **B,** Herpes simplex dermatitis of the face and eyelids.

■ In moderate to severe cases the following apply:
  • Topical polymyxin B/bacitricin (e.g., Polysporin) ointment to prevent secondary bacterial infection
  • Trifluridine (Viroptic) drops to prevent secondary herpetic keratitis
  • Oral acyclovir

Follow-Up

■ The patient is referred to an ophthalmologist, who monitors for subtle signs of herpetic keratitis.

CONTACT DERMATITIS

Symptoms

■ Generalized pruritic or painful eyelid occurs.

Signs

■ In acute cases, erythema and edema of the eyelid occur (Fig. 3-20).
■ In chronic cases, acute findings as well as scaling and lichenification are present.
■ Generally, the inflammation has a well-demarcated border.

Etiology

■ Pollen, dust, chemicals, and cosmetics are causative agents.

Differential Diagnosis

■ Differential diagnoses include the following:
  • Atopic dermatitis
  • Seborrheic dermatitis
  • Psoriasis
  • Preseptal cellulitis

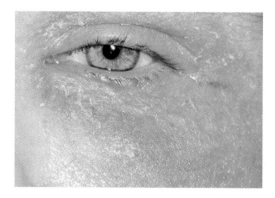

Fig. 3-20 Contact dermatitis from tape used to secure an eye patch.

Workup

- A thorough history of the exposure is obtained.
- The possibility of infection is excluded.
- Patch testing may be necessary.

Treatment

- Patients are advised to avoid contact with the suspected cause.
- A topical corticosteroid such as fluorometholone 0.1% ophthalmic ointment is applied to the lids. Prolonged use of such agents can be associated with glaucoma and cataracts.

ESSENTIAL BLEPHAROSPASM

Symptoms

- Irritation, burning, and foreign body sensation occur.
- An inability to keep the eyes open, frequent blinking, and photophobia are present.

Signs

- Obvious, frequent blinking and an inability to open the eyes are evident (Fig. 3-21).

Etiology

- The disorder probably results from an abnormality of the basal ganglia or midbrain.

Differential Diagnosis

- Any secondary cause of blepharospasm such as iritis, corneal foreign body, or keratitis is identified.

Associated Factors and Diseases

- The disorder is often associated with other dystonic movements of the face and neck (Meige's syndrome).

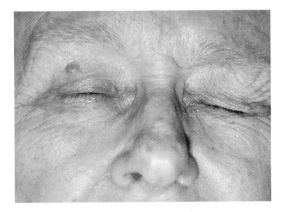

Fig. 3-21 A patient with essential blepharospasm.

- The disorder is sometimes associated with peripheral dystonias of the legs, arms, and back and Parkinson's disease.
- A family history of the disorder is occasionally reported.

Treatment

- Botox (botulinum toxin) injections into the eyelids and other affected facial muscles are administered. Botox produces a positive response in approximately 90% of patients.
- Oral medication with clonazepam (Klonopin) if Botox is ineffective or not maximally effective.
- Surgery (orbicularis myectomy or differential section of the seventh nerve) is performed if administration of Botox and oral medication fail.

Follow-Up

- Botox injections usually need to be repeated every 2 to 3 months.

Conjunctival Abnormalities

David A. Palay

ANATOMY

The conjunctiva is a thin, transparent mucous membrane that lines the inner surface of the lids and outer surface of the eye. The portion of the conjunctiva on the eye is the bulbar conjunctiva, and the portion of the conjunctiva on the lid is the palpebral conjunctiva. The point of transition between these two zones is the fornix. An inferior and a superior fornix are normally present (Fig. 4-1). Glands in the conjunctiva produce the components of the tear film; a healthy conjunctiva is therefore essential for maintaining a healthy corneal surface. The conjunctiva also serves as a barrier against infection. Medially, the two important conjunctival structures are the plica semilunaris and caruncle (Fig. 4-2).

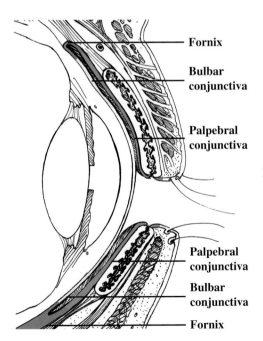

Fornix

Bulbar
conjunctiva

Palpebral
conjunctiva

Fig. 4-1   The region of the conjunctiva.

Palpebral
conjunctiva

Bulbar
conjunctiva

Fornix

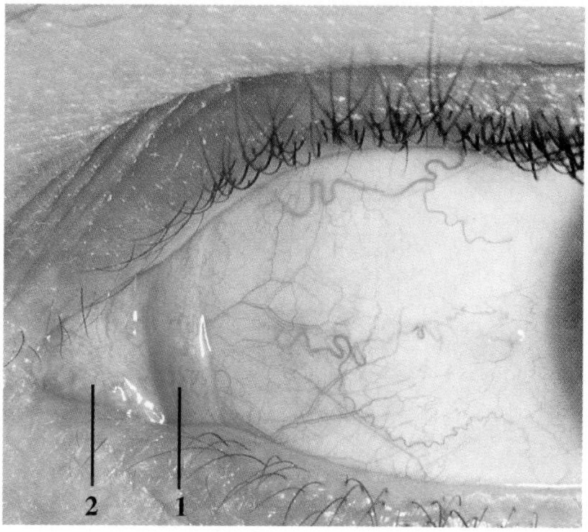

Fig. 4-2 Conjunctiva, normal anatomy. The medial fold in the conjunctiva is the plica semilunaris *(1)*. The caruncle *(2)* is an elevated mass that has features of both skin and conjunctiva.

VIRAL CONJUNCTIVITIS

Symptoms

- The onset of the disorder is acute.
- Redness, watering, soreness, and general discomfort occur.
- The second eye is usually involved 3 to 7 days after the first, and the symptoms are less severe in most cases.

Signs

- Diffuse injection of the conjunctiva with a watery discharge is present (Fig. 4-3).
- In severe cases, erythema and edema are often found in the lids (Fig. 4-4).
- A follicular response in the conjunctiva is evident in most cases (Fig. 4-5).
- Preauricular adenopathy is common; patients may report tenderness in this region. Bacterial conjunctivitis is almost never associated with preauricular adenopathy, which can be a differentiating feature.
- Subepithelial infiltrates can develop in the cornea 2 to 3 weeks after the acute infection (Fig. 4-6). They result from the body's immune response to viral antigens and can cause decreased vision and photosensitivity.

Etiology

- Adenovirus infection (epidemic keratoconjunctivitis) is usually the cause.

Treatment

- The disease is self-limiting.
- Patients' symptoms are treated, usually with cold compresses, artificial tears, and a vasoconstrictor/antihistamine (e.g., Naphcon-A, Vasocon-A) 4 times a day if the itching is severe.
- Patients are counseled about the highly contagious nature of this viral infection. Infected persons involved in patient care should be excused from work until the acute signs and symptoms have resolved (usually in 5 to 14 days).

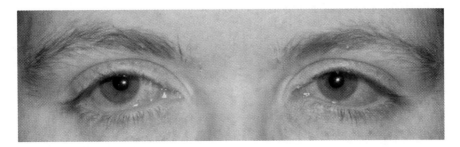

Fig. 4-3 Diffuse injection of the conjunctiva with a watery discharge is evident in this case of viral conjunctivitis.

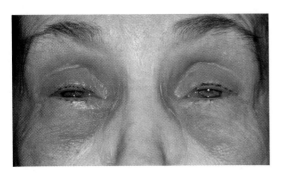

Fig. 4-4 In this severe case of viral conjunctivitis, erythema and swelling of the lids and periocular skin are noted in addition to the diffuse injection of the conjunctiva.

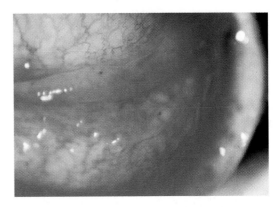

Fig. 4-5 Small, elevated, cystic-appearing lesions termed *follicles* commonly occur on the palpebral conjunctiva in viral conjunctivitis.

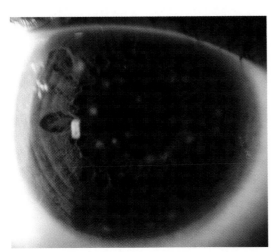

Fig. 4-6 Subepithelial infiltrates can occur in the cornea 2 to 3 weeks after the acute viral infection.

Ophthalmology for the Primary Care Physician

BACTERIAL CONJUNCTIVITIS

Symptoms

- Redness, irritation, and adhesion of the lids (especially in the morning) occur.

Signs

- A mucopurulent exudate is found in the fornix and on the lid margin (Figs. 4-7 and 4-8).
- In cases of diffuse conjunctivitis, erythema and edema of the lids is sometimes observed.
- *N. gonorrhoeae* and *N. meningitidis* cause a "hyperacute" conjunctivitis characterized by an exuberant mucopurulent discharge (Fig. 4-9). Because the organism can rapidly invade the cornea, causing tissue destruction and ocular perforation, infection with *Neisseria* species results in a potentially serious form of conjunctivitis (Fig. 4-10).

Etiology

- Any bacteria can cause conjunctivitis; *Staphylococcus aureus, Haemophilus* species, *Streptococcus pneumoniae,* and *Moraxella* species are the most common agents. *N. gonorrhoeae* and *N. meningitidis* are rarely the cause.

Workup

- Gram's stain and conjunctival culture are performed in any cases suggestive of conjunctivitis caused by *Neisseria* species.
- Most cases do not require extensive workup because broad-spectrum antibiotics eradicate the infection.

Treatment

- A broad-spectrum antibiotic such as a fluoroquinolone (e.g., Chibroxin, Ciloxan, Ocuflox), polymyxin B/trimethoprim (Polytrim), or sulfacetamide drops is administered 4 to 6 times a day.

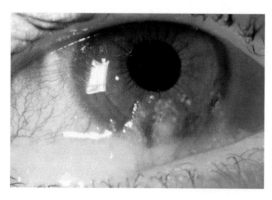

Fig. 4-7 Diffuse injection of the conjunctiva with a thick, purulent discharge is evident in this case of bacterial conjunctivitis.

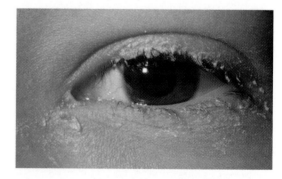

Fig. 4-8 In this case of bacterial conjunctivitis the purulent material has dried and created a thick crust of material on the lid and lid margin.

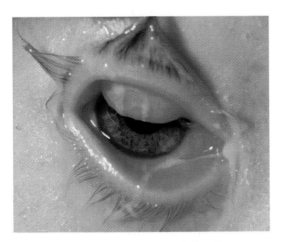

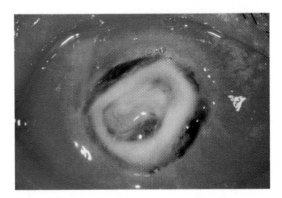

Fig. 4-9 Bacterial conjunctivitis resulting from infection with *Neisseria gonorrhoeae* showing a thick, mucopurulent discharge on the conjunctiva and lids.

Fig. 4-10 In this case of bacterial conjunctivitis resulting from infection with *Neisseria gonorrhoeae,* the patient has a central corneal perforation and retina plugs the perforation site.

- Drops are preferred over ointments because the latter can cause blurring of the patient's vision.
- For conjunctivitis caused by *Neisseria* species, the following apply:
  - Urgent referral to an ophthalmologist is necessary.
  - The eyes are irrigated with saline solution and the lids are cleansed 4 to 6 times a day.
  - Topical antibiotics (e.g., bacitracin, erythromycin ointment) are applied 4 to 6 times a day.
  - A single-dose (1 g) of ceftriaxone (Rocephin) is injected intramuscularly in adults. In patients with severe penicillin allergy, medication with an oral fluoroquinolone (e.g., ciprofloxacin) for 3 to 5 days may be effective.
  - A twice-a-day oral dose of doxycycline (100 mg) is administered for 2 to 3 weeks to treat a concomitant chlamydial infection that may be present. Tetracycline and doxycycline are contraindicated in children, pregnant women, and breastfeeding mothers.
  - Sexual partners are counseled and treated.

ADULT CHLAMYDIAL CONJUNCTIVITIS

Symptoms

- The onset of the disorder is acute or subacute.
- Redness, foreign body sensation, tearing, and photosensitivity occur.

Signs

- The conjunctivitis is more often unilateral than bilateral.

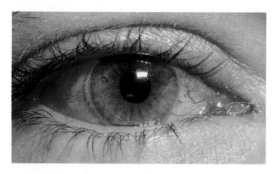

Fig. 4-11 Diffuse injection of the conjunctiva is evident in this case of adult chlamydial conjunctivitis.

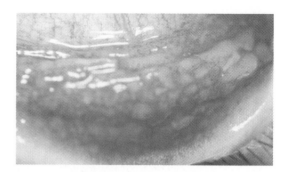

Fig. 4-12 The inferior palpebral conjunctiva has multiple cystic-appearing lesions (follicles) in adult chlamydial conjunctivitis.

Fig. 4-13 An epithelial cell from a conjunctival scraping obtained from a patient with adult chlamydial conjunctivitis shows basophilic inclusion bodies *(1)*, the cell cytoplasm *(2)*, and the cell nucleus *(3)*.

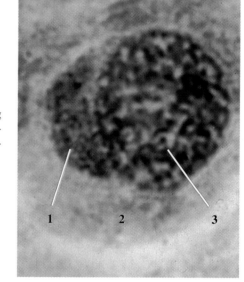

Etiology

- Ocular inoculation usually results from chlamydial infection of the genitalia.
- Diffuse injection of the conjunctiva with a scant mucopurulent discharge is present (Fig. 4-11).
- A follicular response in the conjunctiva is usually present (Fig. 4-12).
- Preauricular adenopathy is possible.

Workup

- Giemsa stain of a conjunctival scraping may show basophilic inclusion bodies (Fig. 4-13).
- Direct fluorescent antibody staining of conjunctival scrapings can be useful; however, a high incidence of false-negative results has been reported.

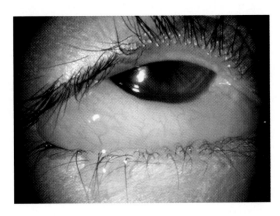

Fig. 4-14 Acute allergic conjunctivitis caused by an airborne allergen. A diffuse conjunctivitis with swelling of the conjunctiva (chemosis) is present.

Treatment

- Medication entails oral tetracycline (250 mg) 4 times a day for 3 weeks or oral doxycycline (100 mg) 2 times a day for 3 weeks. Tetracycline and doxycycline are contraindicated in children, pregnant women, and breastfeeding mothers. If tetracyclines are contraindicated or not tolerated, oral erythromycin (250 mg) 4 times a day for 3 weeks is an effective alternative.
- Topical treatment consists of application of erythromycin ointment 2 to 4 times a day for 3 weeks.
- Sexual partners also are treated.

ALLERGIC CONJUNCTIVITIS

Symptoms

- The prevalent symptom is intense itching.

Signs

- The conjunctivitis is almost always bilateral.
- Mild conjunctival injection is present.
- A stringy mucoid discharge is evident.

Associated Factors and Diseases

- The disorder is usually seasonal, often occurring in individuals with a history of atopic disease.
- Some airborne allergies (e.g., animal dander, dust, plant pollens, ragweed, mold spores) can incite a type-I hypersensitivity reaction with acute swelling of the conjunctiva (chemosis) (Fig. 4-14).

Treatment

- Systemic allergy evaluation is performed with consideration of desensitization treatment and removal of allergens from the patient's environment.
- Systemic antihistamines are administered.

- Several topical preparations may be useful:
  - Topical vasoconstrictor/antihistamine combinations (e.g., Naphcon-A, Vasocon-A) can be used 4 times a day for several days, but their chronic use can be associated with a worsening of the conjunctivitis from rebound vasodilation after discontinuation of the vasoconstrictor.
  - Topical antihistamines (e.g., Livostin) are applied 4 times a day as the symptoms warrant.
  - Mast cell stabilizers (e.g., Crolom, Alomide) are applied 4 times a day. These agents require 10 to 14 days of use to reach their maximal effectiveness.
  - Topical nonsteroidal agents (e.g., Acular) are applied 4 times a day as symptoms warrant.
- If these treatments fail, patients should be referred to an ophthalmologist for further treatment and consideration of topical corticosteroid treatment.

CONJUNCTIVITIS ASSOCIATED WITH BLEPHARITIS

Symptoms

- Burning, itching, and foreign body sensation occur.
- Unlike dry eyes, in which symptoms are worse as the day progresses, symptoms in this disorder are usually worse in the morning. However, blepharitis is often associated with dry eyes; therefore this distinction may not be useful in patients with severe dry eyes associated with blepharitis.

Signs

- Diffuse injection and inflammation of the lid margin involving the meibomian glands is present (Fig. 4-15).
- Moderate conjunctival injection is found.
- In rare cases, vascularization of the cornea occurs (Fig. 4-16).
- The disorder is usually bilateral but may be asymmetric.

Etiology

- Three distinct types of blepharitis may occur and cause conjunctivitis:
  - Seborrhea is often associated with dandruff of the brows and scalp.
  - Staphylococcal infection is often associated with styes (hordeola).

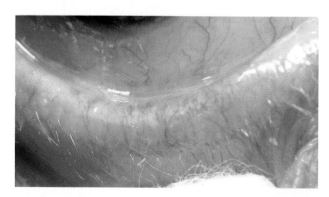

Fig. 4-15 In blepharitis the lid margin is thickened, and vascularization of the lid margin occurs.

• Meibomian gland dysfunction (posterior lid margin disease and meibomianitis) is often associated with chalazia.
• Any combination of these causes is possible.

Associated Factors and Diseases

■ Blepharitis is one of the most common causes of chronic conjunctivitis.
■ Meibomian gland dysfunction is a disorder of the sebaceous glands frequently associated with rosacea, which is a sebaceous gland dysfunction of the skin (Fig. 4-17).

Treatment

■ The underlying blepharitis is treated (see Chapter 3).

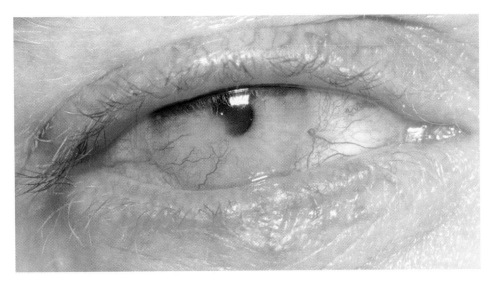

Fig. 4-16 In severe blepharitis with rosacea the lid margins and conjunctiva are inflamed and corneal vascularization and scarring are present.

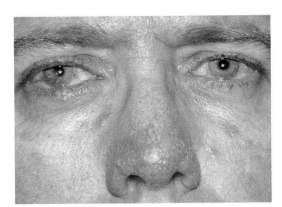

Fig. 4-17 Occurring with greater frequency in females, rosacea often involves erythema, telangiectasia, and acne as common dermatologic findings.

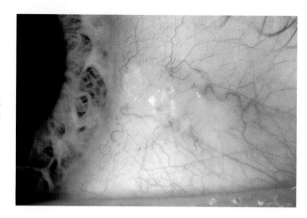

Fig. 4-18 Pinguecula are elevated, fleshy conjunctival masses located in the interpalpebral region, most commonly on the nasal side. They are yellow or light brown.

PINGUECULA
Symptoms
- Patients are symptom free.

Signs
- An elevated, fleshy conjunctival mass is located on the sclera adjacent to the cornea (Fig. 4-18).
- The pinguecula is yellow or light brown.
- Rarely, the pinguecula can become acutely inflamed.

Etiology
- The disorder is usually associated with chronic actinic exposure, repeated trauma, and dry and windy conditions.

Treatment
- No treatment is usually necessary; in rare cases in which the pinguecula is chronically irritated or cosmetically undesirable, resection is performed.

NEVI
Symptoms
- Patients are symptom free.

Signs
- Benign pigmented lesions of the conjunctiva are found (Fig. 4-19).
- The nevi usually occur on the conjunctiva covering the globe.
- The lesions are freely mobile over the sclera.
- In rare cases, nevi progress to a malignant melanoma (Fig. 4-20).

Workup
- A biopsy of nevi that show documented growth or change in appearance is done.

Treatment
- Resection of suspicious lesions is performed.

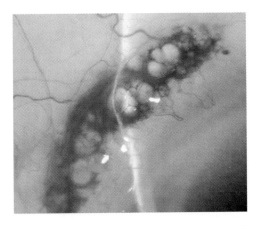

Fig. 4-19 Nevi are benign pigmented lesions of the conjunctiva. Occasionally they develop clear cystic spaces.

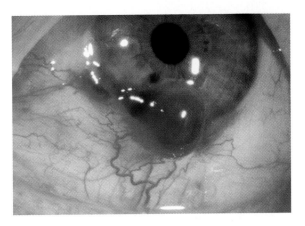

Fig. 4-20 In this case of malignant melanoma of the conjunctiva, the tumor is elevated, pigmented, and highly vascular.

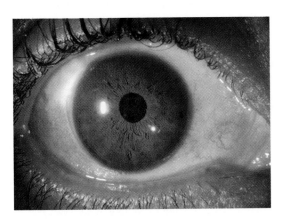

Fig. 4-21 In racial melanosis a flat, deeply pigmented lesion of the conjunctiva is commonly found near the limbus.

RACIAL MELANOSIS

Symptoms
■ Patients are symptom free.

Signs
■ This lesion of the conjunctiva is flat and deeply pigmented (Fig. 4-21).
■ The lesion is usually found on the conjunctiva overlying the globe.
■ The disorder occurs primarily in darkly pigmented patients and has no malignant potential.

Treatment
■ If the lesion is cosmetically undesirable, resection is performed.

Chapter 5

Corneal Abnormalities

David A. Palay

ANATOMY

The cornea is the primary refractive element of the eye, and any disturbance in corneal clarity results in visual impairment. The cornea has five layers: the epithelium, Bowman's layer, the stroma, Descemet's membrane, and the endothelium (Fig. 5-1). The epithelium is four to six layers thick and composed of nonkeratinized, stratified squamous epithelium. Bowman's layer is a thin, acellular area composed of collagen fibers. The stroma constitutes 90% of the corneal thickness and is composed primarily of keratocytes, collagen, and proteoglycans. Descemet's membrane is a thin, collagenous layer produced by the endothelium. The endothelium is one cell layer thick and is responsible for removing fluid from the cornea, thereby preventing corneal edema. The cornea is approximately 12 mm in diameter and has a central thickness of 0.5 mm. The peripheral cornea is 0.65 mm thick (Fig. 5-2).

DRY EYE

Symptoms

- Foreign body sensation, irritation, dryness, and mild redness occur.
- Patients may report symptoms out of proportion to the signs present.
- Symptoms worsen as the day progresses and may be exacerbated by smoke, cold, low humidity, wind, prolonged use of the eye without blinking, and contact lens wear.

Signs

- The disorder is usually bilateral, although it may be slightly asymmetric.
- Mild conjunctival injection occurs primarily medially and laterally.
- Excessive mucus production is evident (Fig. 5-3).
- Punctate staining of the cornea is found with fluorescein dye (Fig. 5-4).

Associated Factors and Diseases

- Most cases of dry eye are idiopathic and occur in older individuals. In younger individuals, contact lens wear may precipitate dry eye signs and symptoms.
- Any eyelid abnormality resulting in poor lid closure such as seventh nerve palsy and ectropion can lead to exposure and drying of the cornea (Fig. 5-5).
- Graft-versus-host disease can cause severe dry eyes.

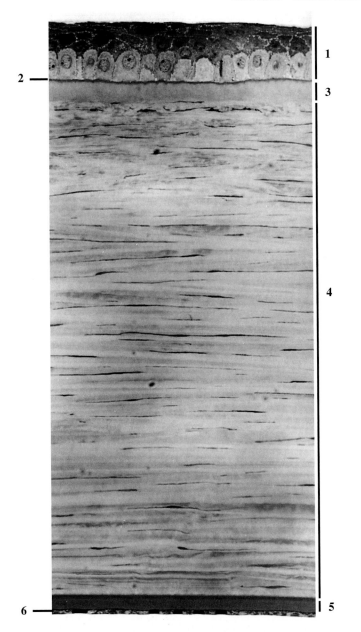

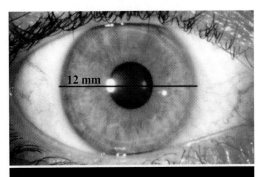

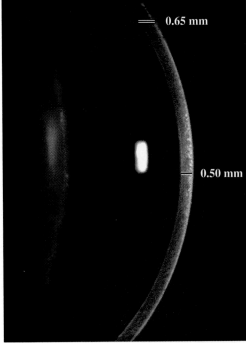

Fig. 5-1 The normal cornea. The epithelium *(1)*, epithelial basement membrane *(2)*, Bowman's membrane *(3)*, stroma *(4)*, Descemet's membrane *(5)*, and endothelium *(6)*.

Fig. 5-2 *Top,* The normal cornea is 12 mm in diameter. *Bottom,* The central thickness is 0.5 mm, and the peripheral thickness is 0.65 mm.

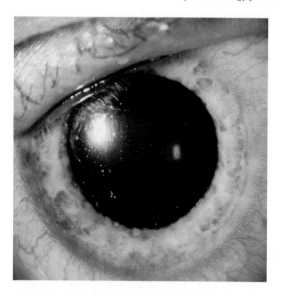

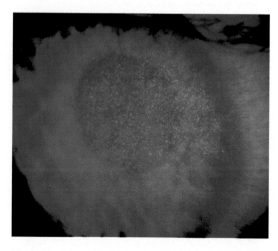

Fig. 5-3   In this case of dry eye the corneal surface is dry and mucus on the surface is observed.

Fig. 5-4   Punctate staining of the cornea with fluorescein dye in dry eye. The areas of abnormal epithelium stain green.

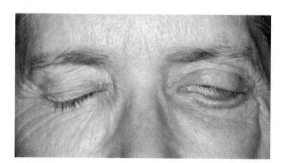

Fig. 5-5   In seventh nerve palsy the inability to close the lids and the out turning of the lower lid (ectropion) can cause dry eye.

- Collagen vascular diseases such as rheumatoid arthritis and systemic lupus erythematosus are often associated with dry eyes. The combination of dry eyes and dry mouth is termed *primary Sjögren's syndrome.* The combination of dry eyes, dry mouth, and collagen vascular disease, most commonly rheumatoid arthritis, is termed *secondary Sjögren's syndrome.*
- The disorder is often associated with blepharitis.
- Sarcoidosis can cause infiltration of the lacrimal gland and is associated with dry eyes.
- Many systemic medications are associated with dry eyes. Drugs with anticholinergic properties are often implicated.

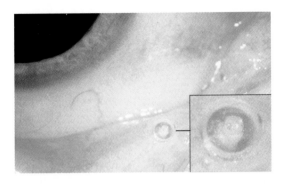

Fig. 5-6   A silicone punctal plug *(inset)* has been placed in the right inferior punctum. The plug increases the volume of the tear film by decreasing tear outflow.

Workup—Schirmer's Test

- Schirmer's test can be performed with or without the instillation of anesthesia. (The procedure is described in Chapter 1.)
  - With anesthesia this test provides an indication of the basal tear secretion, that is, the amount of tears being produced without any noxious stimuli to the eye, which is probably a more accurate measure of tear production.
  - Without anesthesia this test measures the ability of the lacrimal gland to produce tears in response to a noxious stimulus; a false-negative result can occur, particularly in patients in whom the diagnosis is not clear.

Treatment

- For mild cases, preserved artificial tears (e.g., Hypotears, Tears Naturale II) are used as symptoms warrant. Excessive use of artificial tears (e.g., every 1 to 2 hours) can result in toxic effects from the preservatives.
- For more severe cases a nonpreserved artificial tear preparation (e.g., Bion Tears, Refresh, Hypotears preservative free) are administered. These can be used as frequently as necessary and do not cause toxic effects to the eye from preservatives.
- Artificial tear ointments (e.g., Refresh PM, Hypotears ointment, Lacri-Lube) are used at bedtime and during the day if necessary. Ointments provide a longer lasting effect than drops; however, they will blur a patient's vision.
- Insertion of punctal plugs decreases the outflow of tears through the nasolacrimal system (Fig. 5-6).

HERPES SIMPLEX KERATITIS

Symptoms

- Irritation, light sensitivity, and redness occur.
- Pain is mild or does not occur.

Signs

- In 98% of cases the disorder is unilateral.
- Mild conjunctival injection is present.
- Epithelial dendrites are observed with fluorescein staining (Fig. 5-7).
- With advanced disease, stromal scarring and vascularization are possible (Fig. 5-8), and patients may have decreased corneal sensation.

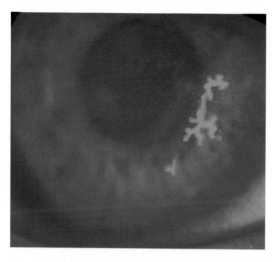

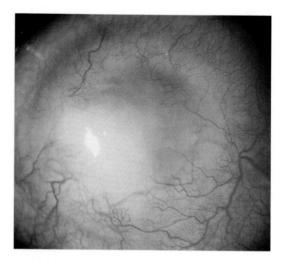

Fig. 5-7 In this case of herpes simplex keratitis an epithelial dendrite stains green with fluorescein dye.

Fig. 5-8 Corneal scarring and corneal vascularization are present in this patient with herpes simplex keratitis.

Treatment

- Urgent referral to an ophthalmologist is necessary for confirmation and treatment.
- Topical antiviral medications are usually applied. NOTE: Topical corticosteroids used indiscriminately to treat herpes simplex keratitis can result in tissue loss and ocular perforation. Therefore the treatment of herpes simplex keratitis should be performed by an ophthalmologist familiar with the diagnosis and treatment of this disorder.

HERPES ZOSTER OPHTHALMICUS

Symptoms

- Pain, headache, and photophobia occur.

Signs

- A vesicular rash is seen in the distribution of the first division of the fifth cranial nerve. If the tip of the nose is involved (Hutchinson's sign), ocular involvement is likely, since both regions are supplied by the nasociliary branch of the first division of the fifth cranial nerve (Fig. 5-9).
- Ocular findings include conjunctivitis, corneal involvement (Fig. 5-10), uveitis (Fig. 5-11), glaucoma, and scleritis (Fig. 5-12).
- Corneal involvement, uveitis, and glaucoma can develop into a chronic disorder possibly refractory to treatment.
- Rare ocular complications include optic neuritis with resultant visual loss and cranial nerve palsies with resultant diplopia.

Differential Diagnosis

- The vesicular rash of herpes simplex virus does not follow a dermatomal distribution, although characteristics of the disorder may otherwise be identical to those of herpes simplex infection.

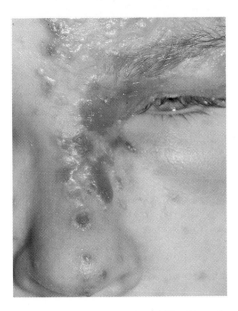

Fig. 5-9 A vesicular rash and Hutchinson's sign are present in herpes zoster ophthalmicus.

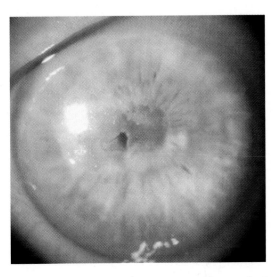

Fig. 5-10 Severe scarring in the cornea has resulted from repeated corneal inflammation from herpes zoster ophthalmicus.

Fig. 5-11 Uveitis has resulted from herpes zoster ophthalmicus. Multiple white keratic precipitates have formed on the posterior cornea from repeated inflammation. Many patients also have elevated intraocular pressure, which can lead to severe glaucoma.

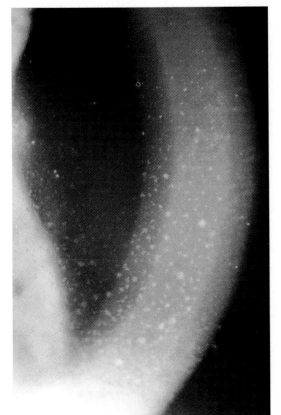

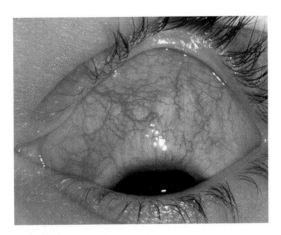

Fig. 5-12 Injection of the conjunctiva and deep episcleral blood vessels with severe pain are present in this example of herpes zoster ophthalmicus with scleritis.

Treatment

- Oral acyclovir (800 mg) is administered 5 times a day for 7 to 10 days. Immunocompromised patients may require intravenous therapy. Newer treatment alternatives include famciclovir (Famvir), with an oral dosage of 500 mg 3 times a day for 7 days, and valacyclovir (Valtrex), with an oral dosage of 1 g 3 times a day for 7 days. The use of valacyclovir is contraindicated in immunocompromised patients. Some immunocompromised patients have developed thrombotic thrombocytopenic purpura/hemolytic uremic syndrome while on this regimen. These new agents have greater bioavailability than oral acyclovir.

- Patients with ocular involvement should be referred to an ophthalmologist within 24 hours. Treatment usually involves administration of topical corticosteroids. Some patients have a protracted clinical course with keratitis, uveitis, and glaucoma.

INFECTIOUS CORNEAL ULCER

Symptoms

- Pain, redness, decreased vision, and photophobia occur.

Signs

- A dense corneal infiltrate with an overlying defect in the epithelium is observed (Fig. 5-13).

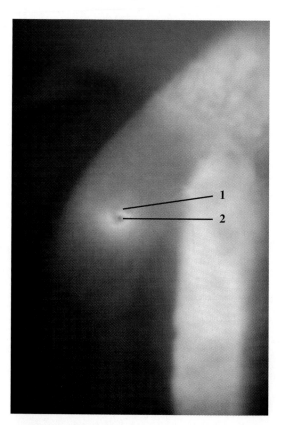

Fig. 5-13   A dense corneal infiltrate *(1)* with an overlying defect in the epithelium *(2)* has resulted from a bacterial corneal ulcer.

- A layering of white cells in the anterior chamber (hypopyon) may be evident (Fig. 5-14).
- Severe corneal ulcers, particularly those resulting from infective gram-negative species, can lead to rapid corneal destruction and ocular perforation (Fig. 5-15).
- Fungal ulcers may have a feathery border (Fig. 5-16).

Associated Factors and Diseases

- The disorder is usually associated with a history of trauma, poor lid apposition, or contact lens wear.
- Fungal ulcers are usually associated with a history of trauma involving vegetable matter or chronic topical corticosteroid use.

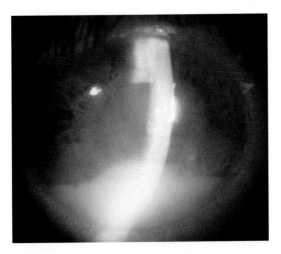

Fig. 5-14   In this example of bacterial corneal ulcer a dense corneal infiltrate and hypopyon are seen.

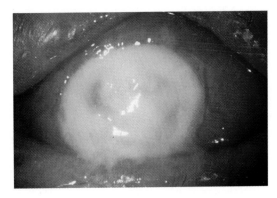

Fig. 5-15   Severe bacterial corneal ulcer has resulted from *Pseudomonas* infection. The entire cornea is white and necrotic. Corneal perforation is imminent.

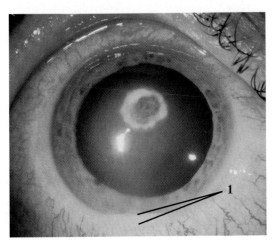

Fig. 5-16   In this fungal corneal ulcer the infiltrate has a feathery margin. Hypopyon *(1)* is also evident.

Treatment

■ Immediate referral to an ophthalmologist is necessary for corneal scraping for Gram's stain and culture.

■ Bacterial ulcers are often treated with fortified antibiotics (e.g., gentamicin, cefazolin).

PTERYGIUM

Symptoms

■ Patients are usually symptom free.

■ Intermittent irritation, redness, and a mild disturbance in visual acuity may occur.

Signs

■ Fibrovascular growth extending from the conjunctiva onto the cornea is present (Fig. 5-17).

Treatment

■ Surgical resection is performed for pterygia that interfere with vision or are actively growing.

RECURRENT EROSION SYNDROME

Symptoms

■ A sudden onset of severe eye pain, blurred vision, and redness occur in the middle of the night or on awakening.

Signs

■ In the acute stage of the disorder the epithelial defect stains with fluorescein (Fig. 5-18).

■ After the epithelial defect heals, diffuse irregularity to the corneal epithelium occurs.

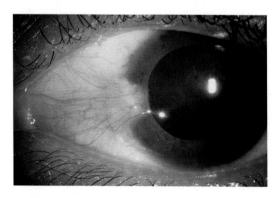

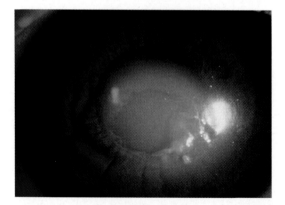

Fig. 5-17 Fibrovascular growth extending from the conjunctiva onto the cornea is evident in this case of pterygium.

Fig. 5-18 In this example of recurrent corneal erosion a defect in the epithelium is evident. The adjacent epithelium is irregular and loose, and the entire area stains lightly with fluorescein dye.

Etiology

■ Poor epithelial adhesion to Bowman's membrane and the underlying corneal stroma causes the disorder.

Associated Factors and Diseases

■ The disorder is usually associated with a previous episode of trauma that resulted in a corneal abrasion.

Treatment

■ In the acute stage the patient is referred to an ophthalmologist within 24 hours for confirmation and treatment.

■ In chronic cases, hypertonic saline ointment (e.g., Muro #128 ointment) is used at night. The hypertonic ointment dehydrates the epithelium, preventing loosening during sleep and a sudden shearing of the epithelium after opening of the lids. The ointment also provides a lubricating function that prevents the lid from adhering to the epithelium. Therapy may be needed for many months.

■ In advanced cases, surgical treatments with stromal puncture or laser treatment to the underlying stroma may be required.

CALCIFIC BAND KERATOPATHY

Symptoms

■ A mild foreign body sensation or severe pain resulting from calcium accumulation on the cornea occurs.

Signs

■ A white accumulation of calcium is seen on the central cornea (Fig. 5-19).

■ "Swiss cheese" holes are usually present in calcium deposits.

Associated Factors and Diseases

■ The disorder is usually associated with chronic ocular inflammation.

■ The disorder may be associated with systemic diseases causing hypercalcemia (e.g., renal failure, sarcoidosis, primary hyperparathyroidism).

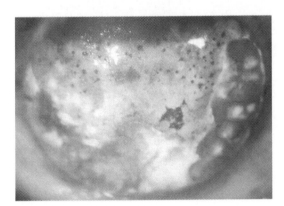

Fig. 5-19 A white, chalky material is deposited across the cornea in this patient with band keratopathy. Small Swiss cheese holes are also seen.

Treatment

■ For calcium deposits that cause discomfort or limit vision, a superficial scraping of the cornea using disodium EDTA is performed.

CORNEAL SURGERY

Corneal Transplantation

Corneal transplantations (penetrating keratoplasty) are performed to restore vision in patients with corneal scarring, corneal edema, or abnormal corneal shape. Donor corneas are harvested postmortem and kept in storage media for up to a week. The central area of corneal malformation is replaced with a circular piece of donor tissue and sutured into place with fine nylon sutures (Fig. 5-20).

Refractive Surgery

Three techniques are currently used to correct myopia. All three flatten the central cornea, thereby correcting nearsightedness (myopia):

■ In radial keratotomy, deep radial incisions are made in the peripheral cornea, which results in central flattening (Fig. 5-21).

■ In photorefractive keratectomy (PRK) an excimer laser is used to flatten the central cornea. This procedure usually results in a mild amount of anterior corneal scarring (Fig. 5-22).

■ In laser in situ keratomileusis (LASIK) a corneal flap is dissected with a microkeratome. The flap is retracted, and an excimer laser is used on the stromal bed, which results in central corneal flattening. Unlike PRK, this procedure does not cause central corneal scarring and is less painful (Fig. 5-23).

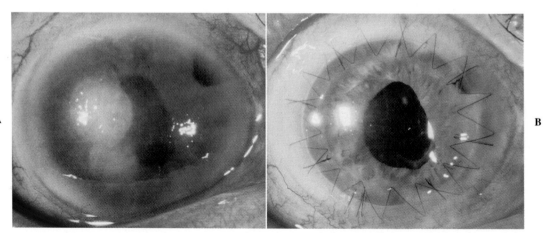

A   B

Fig. 5-20 **A,** Preoperative view of a central corneal scar from a resolved bacterial corneal ulcer. **B,** Same patient 3 weeks after a corneal transplant. Fine nylon sutures hold the transplant in place. The visual axis is clear.

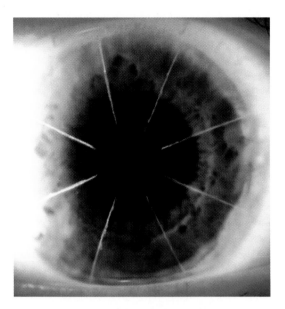

Fig. 5-21 Eight radial incisions in the cornea are made in this example of radial keratotomy.

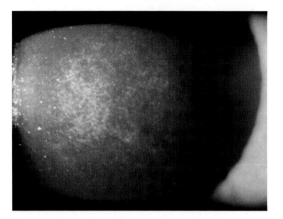

Fig. 5-22 In photorefractive keratectomy the central cornea is flattened with an excimer laser. A central corneal haze is found several months after the procedure.

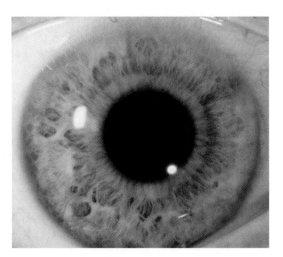

Fig. 5-23 Approximately 2 weeks after laser in situ keratomileusis, no corneal scarring can be detected.

Chapter

6

Scleritis

Michael C. Diesenhouse

ANATOMY

The episclera and sclera are composed of connective tissue, and together they provide a protective coat for the eye (Fig. 6-1). The episclera is a fascial sheath that encases the eye. It has a superficial layer, Tenon's capsule, which acts as a synovial membrane to allow smooth movements of the eye. A deeper layer of the episclera contains a network of vessels. The episclera overlies the primarily avascular sclera and is partly responsible for scleral nutrition. The sclera is composed of collagen and elastic fibers arranged randomly. Its rigid structure is necessary for vision to remain stable during eye movements. The thickness of the sclera varies from approximately 0.3 mm behind the insertion of the rectus muscles to 1.2 mm posteriorly.

INFLAMMATORY CONDITIONS

Inflammation of the episclera and sclera is not common in clinical practice. However, confusion with more common causes of a red eye may lead to a delay in diagnosis. Conjunctivitis usually involves the entire conjunctiva (not just a section), is usually not associated with pain, and generally has a discharge. Episcleritis and scleritis usually involve a section of the eye (although sometimes the entire eye is involved), are associated with mild pain (episcleritis) or severe pain (scleritis), and are not associated with a discharge. On the patient's initial visit, distinguishing between episcleral and scleral inflammation is essential because the management of these two diseases varies considerably. In addition, scleritis is more likely to be associated with exacerbation of a potentially serious systemic disease. (A useful classification is presented in Box 6-1 on pp. 82-83.)

EPISCLERITIS

Symptoms

- Acute onset of redness occurs.
- If pain is present, it is often described as a dull ache localized to the eye.
- Visual acuity is usually normal.
- The patient may report a history of recurrent episodes.

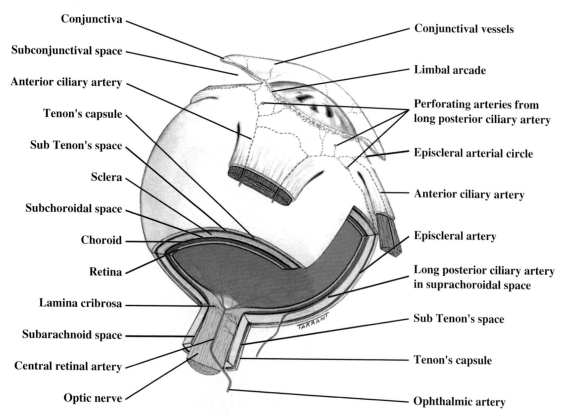

Fig. 6-1   Anteriorly, the episclera lies between the conjunctiva and underlying sclera, to which it is attached by fibrous bands. Posteriorly, it is continuous with the muscular sheath, extends backward to cover the whole of the globe, and merges with the optic nerve sheath behind the eye. It is perforated by the ciliary vessels and nerves and the vortex veins.

Signs

- Sectoral or diffuse redness of one or both eyes is evident.
- Episcleral vessels are engorged, but the vascular pattern is not disturbed.
- If a nodule is present, it is mobile over the underlying sclera.
- Neither discharge nor corneal involvement is present.

Associated Factors and Diseases

- In 75% of cases the origin is idiopathic.
- Other disorders include the following:
  - Collagen vascular diseases
  - Rosacea
  - Gout
  - Herpes zoster virus
  - Syphilis
- The disorder is more prevalent in young adults.

Box 6-1
Classification of episcleritis and scleritis

Episcleritis
- Simple
- Nodular (Fig. 6-2)

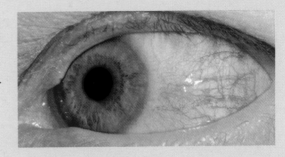

Fig. 6-2 Nodular episcleritis in a patient with gout.

Scleritis
Diffuse anterior
- Diffuse anterior scleritis is the most common but least destructive type (Fig. 6-3).
- Widespread involvement of the sclera is characteristic, but localized changes are also seen.

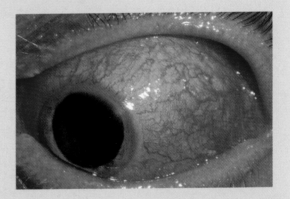

Fig. 6-3 In diffuse anterior scleritis, widespread injection of the conjunctival and deep episcleral vessels occurs.

Nodular anterior
- This form is distinguished by a painful localized elevation of the sclera, which may develop into a nodule (Fig. 6-4).
- Nodular anterior scleritis differs from nodular episcleritis in that the nodule is immobile.
- Approximately 20% of patients progress to necrotizing scleritis.

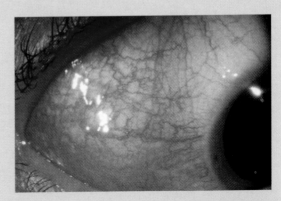

Fig. 6-4 An elevated mass within the area of inflammation occurs in nodular anterior scleritis. Unlike the nodule in episcleritis, this nodule is immobile.

Box 6-1

Classification of episcleritis and scleritis—cont'd

Scleritis—cont'd

Necrotizing

- Necrotizing scleritis is the least common but most destructive form (Fig. 6-5).
- Ocular and systemic complications are seen in 60% of patients.
- Progressive scleral necrosis can lead to scleral thinning and perforation of the globe.
- The disorder is usually associated with a potentially serious systemic disease.

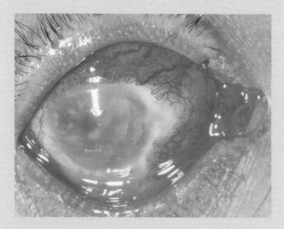

Fig. 6-5 In this patient with rheumatoid arthritis and necrotizing scleritis, avascular areas with tissue loss are adjacent to areas of active inflammation. Prompt and aggressive immunosuppressive treatment is necessary.

Scleromalacia perforans

- Scleromalacia perforans is the only form of scleritis without pain (Fig. 6-6).
- A lack of symptoms is characteristic. Some patients may note decreased vision or a change in the color of the sclera.
- Scleral necrosis and thinning are observed in the absence of inflammation.
- Perforation of the globe may occur with minor trauma.
- The disorder is predominantly bilateral and seen almost exclusively in patients with rheumatoid arthritis.

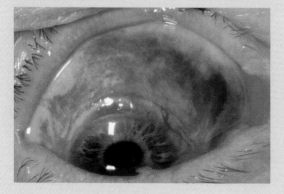

Fig. 6-6 Marked scleral thinning, a characteristic of scleromalacia perforans, allows exposure of the underlying choroid. This gives the eye a bluish hue, a discoloration best seen in daylight.

Workup

- The phenylephrine test involves instillation of a drop of phenylephrine 2.5% in the eye, which helps distinguish between dilated episcleral and scleral vessels. Unlike the deeper scleral vessels, episcleral vessels blanch when topical phenylephrine is applied.

Treatment

- Referral to an ophthalmologist is necessary for confirmation and treatment.
- Most cases are self-limited and resolve without treatment.
- Initially, cold compresses and/or a topical vasoconstrictor are used. Topical corticosteroids may be administered by an ophthalmologist.
- If topical medications do not provide relief, a course of an oral nonsteroidal anti-inflammatory drug is instituted.
- Resistance to treatment may signify the presence of an associated systemic disease.

SCLERITIS

Several types of scleritis exist (see Box 6-1). Although each type has distinct characteristics, these entities have many of the same symptoms and signs.

Symptoms

- The onset of the disorder is gradual.
- The hallmark symptom is severe pain that may radiate to the temple or jaw. Often the pain awakens the patient at night.
- Photophobia is present.
- Tearing occurs.
- Vision is normal or mildly decreased.
- Episodes may recur.

Signs

- The globe is tender to palpation.
- Sectoral or diffuse edema of the sclera occurs with engorgement of the overlying episcleral vessels.
- Nodules and scleral necrosis may be present.
- Corneal and intraocular inflammation may coexist.

Associated Factors and Diseases

- The origin is usually idiopathic, but almost half of the patients have an associated systemic disease. The inflammation of the eye may serve as a clue to an underlying disease or warn of increased severity in a known condition.

- Disorders that may coexist with scleritis include the following:
  - Rheumatoid arthritis
  - Systemic lupus erythematosus
  - Polyarteritis nodosa
  - Wegener's granulomatosis
  - Relapsing polychondritis
  - Ankylosing spondylitis
  - Giant cell arteritis
  - Gout
  - Herpes zoster
  - Syphilis
  - Tuberculosis

Workup

- In the phenylephrine test, deep episcleral and scleral vessels do not blanch when topical 2.5% phenylephrine is applied.
- The patient's eye is viewed with normal lighting. An eye with scleritis may have a bluish hue when seen in daylight, which can signify thinning of the sclera. This discoloration can be easily overlooked in a darkened room.

Treatment

- Referral to an ophthalmologist is necessary for confirmation and treatment.
- Because scleritis may be the presenting sign of a systemic disease, a thorough systemic evaluation is warranted. The management of scleritis necessitates the use of systemic medications. If an associated systemic disease is identified, therapy is appropriately modified.
- Initial treatment involves administration of nonsteroidal antiinflammatory drugs or systemic corticosteroids.
- In advanced cases, cytotoxic agents may be prescribed. These medications have side effects and contraindications, so the treatment protocol must be individualized for each patient.
- Treatment guidelines are based on the persistence of inflammation, with the degree of resolution of pain used to gauge disease control.
- For management of patients with scleritis a team approach between the ophthalmologist and primary care physician is essential.

Lens Abnormalities

Andrew R. Harrison and Jay H. Krachmer

ANATOMY

The lens is a biconvex and grossly transparent structure located directly behind the iris. In adults, it is approximately 9 mm in diameter and 4 mm thick. The lens consists of 65% water and 35% protein (which is the highest protein content of any body tissue). No pain fibers, blood vessels, or nerves are found in the lens. The lens has three layers: the capsule, cortex, and nucleus (Fig. 7-1). The lens capsule is a thin, semipermeable membrane that envelops the entire lens. The anterior capsule is markedly thicker than the posterior capsule. The lens cortex is composed of lens cells, or fibers, that are produced continuously throughout life. The old lens fibers migrate centrally as new fibers are produced. The oldest lens fibers, which are those that have lost their nuclei, comprise the nucleus. The lens is held in place by ligaments known as *zonules,* which are composed of numerous fibrils that arise in the ciliary body and insert into the lens capsule. Contraction of the ciliary body causes relaxation of zonules with resultant thickening of the lens, thereby allowing the eye to focus on near objects. This is known as *accommodation.*

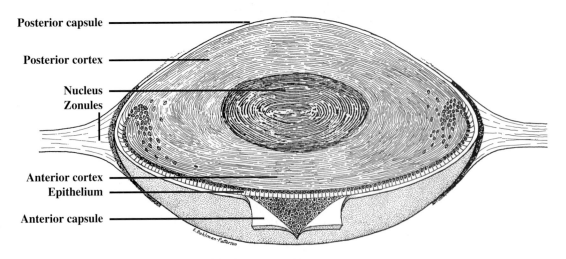

Posterior capsule
Posterior cortex
Nucleus
Zonules
Anterior cortex
Epithelium
Anterior capsule

Fig. 7-1 Normal lens anatomy.

PRESBYOPIA

Symptoms

- Reading is difficult.
- Reading material is held farther from the eyes.
- Distance vision is blurry after the patient reads.

Signs

- Only near vision decreases; the ability (or inability) to see distant objects remains the same.

Etiology

- With age the lens becomes increasingly inelastic and can no longer "thicken" to focus on near objects (Fig. 7-2). This disorder, also called "old sight," usually becomes clinically significant at 40 to 45 years of age.

Treatment

- For patients with normal distance vision, simple reading glasses may be purchased without a prescription over the counter at pharmacies.

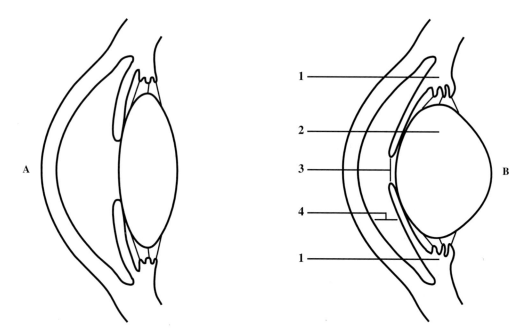

Fig. 7-2   A, Cross-section of the eye in the nonaccommodative state. **B,** During accommodation to focus on a near object, the ciliary body *(1)* moves forward, relaxing the zonules, which allows the lens *(2)* to thicken in the anteroposterior axis. The iris *(3)* constricts and the space between the cornea and iris, the anterior chamber *(4),* decreases.

■ For patients with distance vision requiring correction, the following apply:
  • Spectacle correction with bifocal (distance and near) or trifocal (distance, intermediate, and near) lenses
  • Monovision contact lenses in which one eye is corrected for distance vision and the other eye for near vision
  • Contact lens correction of distance vision and simple reading glasses for near vision

SENILE CATARACT

A cataract is any opacity in the crystalline lens. Senile cataract is an age-related disorder, and four types occur (Box 7-1).

Symptoms

■ A slowly progressing visual loss or blurring occurs over months to years.
■ Glare is a problem, particularly from oncoming headlights during night driving.
■ Double vision in one eye (monocular diplopia) occurs.
■ Fixed spots in the visual field are present.
■ Color perception is reduced.
■ With a nuclear cataract, near vision may improve ("second sight").
■ With a posterior subcapsular cataract, near vision decreases.

Signs

■ Opacification of the lens is evident.

Workup

■ Cataracts are best seen after dilation of the pupil. The examiner looks through the +5 lens of a direct ophthalmoscope held about 6 inches from the patient's eye.

Treatment

■ For early nuclear cataracts, a change in spectacle prescription may improve vision.
■ For small central opacities, pupillary dilation may improve vision.
■ Surgical removal of the lens and placement of an intraocular lens implant is performed.
■ Cataract surgery is not performed with lasers. However, a laser may be used if an after-cataract is present (see p. 93).

CATARACT SURGERY

Cataract surgery is one of the most frequently performed surgical operations. Over 1.5 million cataract surgeries are performed annually in the United States. An estimated 5 to 10 million individuals in the United States become visually disabled each year because of cataracts.

Indications

Cataract surgery is indicated in the following instances:
■ To improve a patient's lifestyle, which depends on an individual's visual needs
■ To prevent a secondary glaucoma or uveitis

Box 7-1
Types of senile cataract

Nuclear

- A yellow-brown discoloration of the central part of the lens is observed (Fig. 7-3).
- The nuclear type of cataract becomes evident at 50 years of age and progresses slowly until the entire nucleus is opaque.

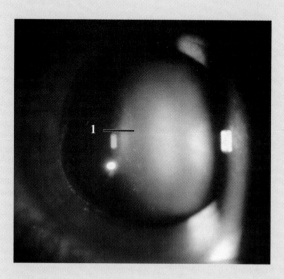

Fig. 7-3 In cases of nuclear cataract the yellow-brown color of the central nucleus *(1)* is evident.

Cortical

- Radial or spokelike opacities in the periphery of the lens extend to involve the anterior or posterior lens (Fig. 7-4).
- Patients are often symptom free until the lens changes involve the central lens.

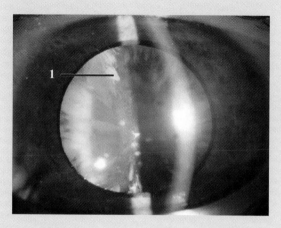

Fig. 7-4 Peripheral spokelike opacities *(1)* in the cortex are visible in this patient with cortical cataract.

Continued

Ophthalmology for the Primary Care Physician

Box 7-1

Types of senile cataract—cont'd

Posterior subcapsular
- Opacities appear in the most posterior portion of the lens adjacent to the posterior capsule, often forming a plaque (Fig. 7-5).
- Posterior subcapsular cataract is most commonly associated with systemic or topical corticosteroid use.
- Because the visual axis is involved, this type causes a disproportionate number of symptoms for its size.

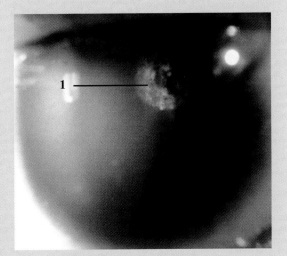

Fig. 7-5 The central location of a posterior sub-capsular cataract *(1)*.

Dense white
- A white discoloration of the central part of the lens is observed.
- A dense white cataract is often seen in combination with cortical cataracts in older patients (Fig. 7-6).
- This type may be severely disabling because of the marked visual loss it produces.

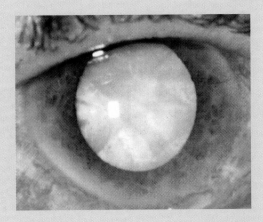

Fig. 7-6 Advanced central (nuclear) and peripheral (cortical) opacification is seen in this patient with a dense white cataract.

- To permit visualization of the fundus to monitor patients with diseases of the optic nerve (e.g., glaucoma) or retina (e.g., diabetic retinopathy)
- To permit visualization of the fundus before retinal surgery or laser treatment

Preoperative Considerations

Every patient undergoing cataract surgery needs a complete ophthalmic examination to rule out an underlying ophthalmic pathologic condition that may contribute to the patient's visual symptoms. Evaluation of the retina is especially important in patients with diabetes because diabetic retinopathy can be exacerbated after cataract surgery.

The necessity of a preoperative medical evaluation for cataract surgery is undergoing review. Most patients are referred to their primary care provider for a complete history, physical examination, and appropriate laboratory testing. This may include an electrocardiogram, a chest radiograph, a hematocrit value, and a potassium level depending on the patient's medical status. With newer surgical techniques, minimal sedation is necessary, so the need for a complete medical evaluation is in question.

The use of anticoagulants (including aspirin) in patients who are undergoing cataract surgery is also being studied. The risk of intraoperative and postoperative bleeding may not be significantly increased when anticoagulants are not discontinued before surgery. Using newer surgical techniques, a surgeon may not need to perform injections or incisions in areas containing blood vessels; therefore the risk of bleeding is markedly reduced. Consultation with the ophthalmic surgeon performing the operation is recommended before the primary care physician changes a patient's anticoagulation regimen.

Prognosis and Risks

The prognosis for cataract surgery using current techniques is excellent. Approximately 95% of patients obtain improved vision after cataract surgery.

The risks of cataract surgery, as with any ocular surgery, include infection and bleeding that can lead to blindness. The risk of infection is approximately 0.02%. The risk of retrobulbar hemorrhage is 0.1% with retrobulbar anesthesia. The risk of intraocular hemorrhage during cataract surgery is 0.06%. Late-onset risks include retinal detachment and the development of glaucoma.

Anesthesia

Most cataract surgery is performed using local anesthesia with monitored anesthesia care. Anesthesia and akinesia of the eyelid and eye are obtained using local block techniques. Some surgeons inject short-acting intravenous anesthetics before performing the block. A recent development in cataract surgery is the use of topical anesthesia, in which topical anesthetic drops provide the anesthesia. This type of anesthesia is not indicated in certain patients and is currently performed by a minority of ophthalmic surgeons. General anesthesia is relatively rare in cataract surgery today. It may still be used for patients who are unable to lie still or who have language or hearing problems that may compromise a surgeon's ability to perform the operation safely.

Procedure

Cataract surgery is performed primarily as an outpatient procedure. The surgery takes approximately 20 to 45 minutes to perform. The two most commonly performed surgical

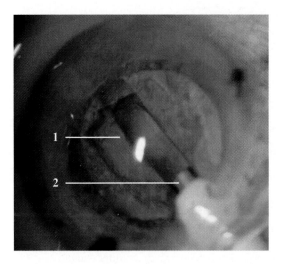

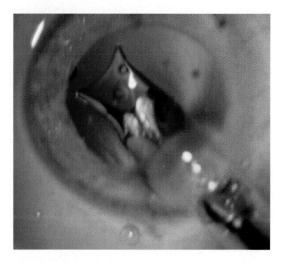

Fig. 7-7   Removal of the nucleus *(1)* with the phaco-emulsification handpiece *(2)*.

Fig. 7-8   Placement of a foldable lens implant into the remaining capsular bag.

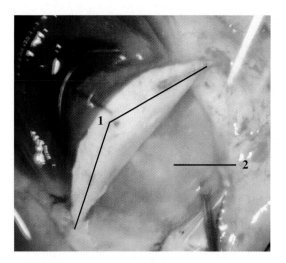

Fig. 7-9   Removal of the nucleus by extracapsular cataract extraction. Note the larger incision size *(1)* and removal of the nucleus in one piece *(2)*.

techniques to remove the lens are phacoemulsification and extracapsular cataract extraction. Phacoemulsification is the preferred procedure because of the smaller incision size and faster visual rehabilitation.

Phacoemulsification. In phacoemulsification the surgeon makes a 2- to 6-mm incision and removes the anterior portion of the lens capsule. A phacoemulsification instrument emits ultrasonic vibrations and provides suction for break up and extraction of the hard nuclear lens material (Fig. 7-7). The surgeon uses a mechanical irrigation and suction instrument to remove the lens cortex and then places the lens implant in the remaining capsular bag. Flexible lens implants are now available that can be folded and introduced through a small incision into the eye, where they are unfolded (Fig. 7-8). The smaller wounds may be self-sealing or require only a few sutures.

Extracapsular cataract extraction. In extracapsular cataract extraction the surgeon makes a 10- to 11-mm superior sclerocorneal incision and removes the anterior portion of the lens capsule. The entire nucleus is extracted through the incision (Fig. 7-9). The surgeon uses a mechanical irrigation and suction instrument to remove the lens cortex, places the implant in the remaining capsular bag, and sutures the incision.

Postoperative Care

If cataract removal is performed under local anesthesia, most patients can go home 2 to 3 hours after the surgery. The patient is usually ambulatory on the day of the procedure. The eye may be bandaged overnight, and the patient usually returns the following day. The patient is typically given an antibiotic and steroid drops for the first few weeks after surgery. Protection of the operated eye with glasses or a metal shield is required for several weeks. Permanent glasses are usually prescribed 3 to 8 weeks after surgery .

After-Cataract (Secondary Membrane)

In 10% to 30% of patients undergoing cataract surgery, the posterior capsule opacifies, producing significant visual distortion. This usually occurs several months to years after cataract surgery. Treatment involves a noninvasive technique using the neodymium:YAG laser to create a small hole in the opacified posterior capsule in the visual axis. A complication of this procedure is a transient rise in intraocular pressure, which may require medical treatment. The most serious complication is retinal detachment, which may occur weeks to months after the procedure in up to 1% of patients.

Uveitis

Terry Kim

ANATOMY

The uveal tract is a heavily pigmented and highly vascular structure composed of three distinct anatomic components: the iris, ciliary body, and choroid (Fig. 8-1). The iris represents the most anterior portion of the uveal tract and is the only portion that is directly visible by external or slip lamp examination. It is located behind the cornea (with the space between the cornea and iris known as the *anterior chamber*) and is responsible for giving the eye its color. The central opening of the iris is the pupil, which constricts or dilates depending on the amount of light entering the eye. The ciliary body is contiguous with the iris and has numerous functions, including aqueous humor production and accommodation. The choroid has a posterior location and lies between the retina and sclera. Its main role is to provide a blood supply to the outer retina. These three components together form a continuous uveal lining that can be affected by inflammatory conditions within the eye.

Uveitis is a general term used to describe any inflammatory condition involving the uveal tract. Different classifications and terminology are used to denote the specific sites of the uveal tract primarily involved. For the anterior segment of the eye the terms *iritis* and *iridocyclitis* describe inflammation of the iris and iris–ciliary body complex, respectively. The terms *vitritis, retinitis,* and *choroiditis* designate inflammation in various parts of the posterior segment of the eye. In this text the term *anterior uveitis* means any inflammation of the iris and/or ciliary body and the term *posterior uveitis* denotes any inflammation of the vitreous, retina, and/or choroid. Distinguishing the segment primarily affected by a uveitis guides formulation of a differential diagnosis, workup, and treatment. Some disorders appear exclusively as an anterior or a posterior uveitis, although a few (e.g., sarcoidosis, Behçet's syndrome, syphilis, tuberculosis) can be either anterior or posterior. Because of the close anatomic and functional relationships of the vitreous, retina, and choroid, pinpointing the principal site of involvement, especially in the posterior segment, is often difficult. Classification of a uveitis as anterior or posterior may be difficult because both segments may be involved. A severe anterior uveitis may result in anterior vitreous changes, whereas a vitritis may manifest with signs in the anterior chamber. When both segments of the uveal tract are definitely involved, the condition is called *panuveitis*. The term *endophthalmitis* is reserved for cases in which the inflammation is predominantly centered within the vitreous, a special type of posterior uveitis because of its severity and need for prompt diagnostic workup and treatment (see Chapter 9).

Iris + Ciliary body   +   Choroid = Uveal tract

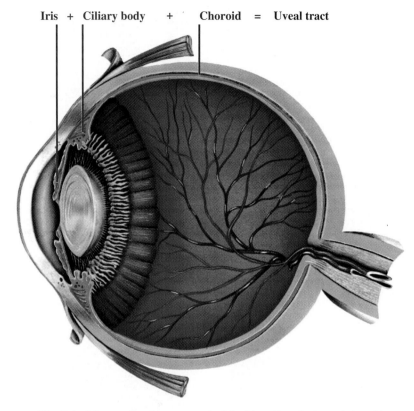

Fig. 8-1   The uveal tract, composed of the iris, ciliary body, and choroid.

ANTERIOR UVEITIS

Symptoms

- Redness, photophobia, and pain occur.
- Vision is normal or decreased.
- The onset of symptoms is acute or insidious.
- Possible nonocular symptoms (e.g., back pain, joint stiffness, dysuria) are caused by various systemic disorders associated with uveitis.

Signs

- The disorder is unilateral or bilateral.
- Conjunctival injection occurs, primarily surrounding the cornea (ciliary injection) (Fig. 8-2).
- Deposits on the posterior surface of the cornea (keratic precipitates) vary in size and appearance (fine and whitish precipitates in nongranulomatous uveitis and large, grayish, "mutton-fat" precipitates in granulomatous uveitis) (Figs. 8-3 and 8-4).
- Floating inflammatory cells and protein (flare) in the anterior chamber are detectable only with the aid of a slit lamp biomicroscope. If severe enough, these inflammatory cells can layer in the anterior chamber (hypopyon) (Fig. 8-5).

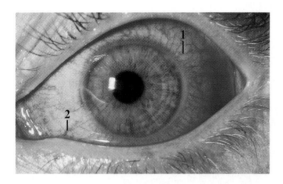

Fig. 8-2 Marked ciliary injection *(1)* in addition to generalized conjunctival injection *(2)* in this patient with ankylosing spondylitis.

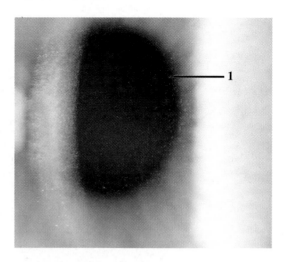

Fig. 8-3 Fine keratic precipitate *(1)* of a nongranulomatous anterior uveitis.

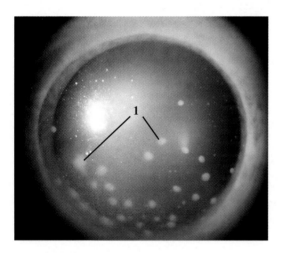

Fig. 8-4 Mutton-fat keratic precipitates *(1)* are diffusely scattered on the posterior surface of the cornea.

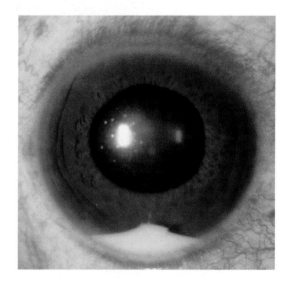

Fig. 8-5 Accumulation of inflammatory cells forming a hypopyon in the anterior chamber.

- Adhesions of the iris to the front surface of the lens (posterior synechiae) occur, which may cause a small or an irregularly shaped pupil (Fig. 8-6).
- A constricted pupil is evident, even without posterior synechiae.
- Nodules of inflammatory cells are found on the iris surface. These are termed *Koeppe nodules* if they are located at the pupillary margin and *Busacca nodules* if located on the remainder of the iris surface (Fig. 8-7).

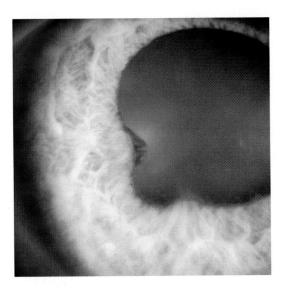

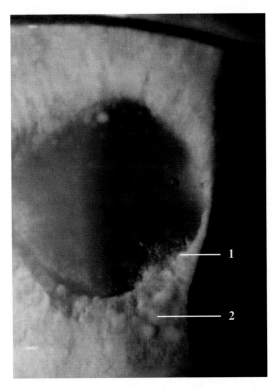

Fig. 8-6 Posterior synechiae causing iris pigment deposition on the anterior lens surface and an irregularly shaped pupil.

Fig. 8-7 Koeppe *(1)* and Busacca *(2)* nodules of sarcoid uveitis.

Etiology

- Most cases have an idiopathic origin.
- Many local and systemic associations can occur (Box 8-1).

Associated Factors and Diseases

- Cataract and glaucoma are associated with anterior uveitis.
- Low intraocular pressure (hypotony) may be present.

Differential Diagnosis

- Differential diagnoses include the following:
  - Conjunctivitis (injected conjunctiva but *no* cells or flare in the anterior chamber)
  - Sclerouveitis (uveitis secondary to an inflammation of the sclera)
  - Intraocular malignancy (e.g., leukemia)

Workup

- A careful history and complete ocular examination are necessary.
- The general physical examination is directed at possible systemic findings of the various conditions associated with an anterior uveitis.

- For patients with unilateral, nongranulomatous, first-episode disease and unremarkable histories and examinations, no systemic workup is needed.
- For patients with bilateral, granulomatous, recurrent episode disease and unremarkable histories and examinations, the followings steps are taken:
  - A nonspecific diagnostic workup is initiated, including CBC, ESR (preferably Westergren), ANA, RPR or VDRL, FTA-ABS or MHA-TP, PPD with anergy panel, CXR, and Lyme titer (if in endemic area and indicated).
  - The diagnostic workup is supplemented with other tests and subspecialty consults if the need for this is strongly indicated by symptoms, history, or physical findings (e.g., angiotensin-converting enzyme for ruling out sarcoidosis, sacroiliac spine x-ray examination for ruling out ankylosing spondylitis, consultation with a rheumatologist for ruling out psoriatic arthritis).

Treatment

- Patients should be referred to an ophthalmologist within 24 hours.
- A topical cycloplegic agent (e.g., homatropine hydrobromide 5%, atropine sulfate 1%) is administered 2 to 3 times a day.
- A topical corticosteroid (e.g., Pred-Forte 1%, Flarex 0.1%) is administered 4 to 6 times a day. An ophthalmologist initiates this prescription.

Box 8-1
Classification of anterior uveitis

Autoimmune disorders
- HLA-B27–positive anterior uveitis
  - Ankylosing spondylitis
  - Reiter's syndrome
  - Inflammatory bowel disease (ulcerative colitis and Crohn's disease)
  - Psoriatic arthritis
- Juvenile rheumatoid arthritis

Infections
- Syphilis
- Tuberculosis
- Lyme disease
- Herpes simplex
- Herpes zoster

Malignancies*
- Lymphoma
- Leukemia

Other conditions
- Idiopathic disease
- Trauma
- Postoperative complication
- Sarcoidosis
- Behçet's syndrome

*Noninflammatory conditions that can mimic the clinical findings of an anterior uveitis.

Prognosis

- Overall, the prognosis is excellent for patients with a first-time, nongranulomatous anterior uveitis and less favorable for patients with a recurrent, granulomatous type.

POSTERIOR UVEITIS

Symptoms

- Vision is commonly decreased or blurred. Floaters occur.
- Occasionally redness, pain, and photophobia occur.
- The onset is acute or insidious.

Signs

- The disease can be unilateral or bilateral.
- Inflammatory cells within the vitreous cause a hazy view of the fundus of the eye (Fig. 8-8).
- Optic disc swelling and edema are observed.
- Retinal and choroid hemorrhages, exudates, infiltrates, and vascular sheathing are seen (Fig. 8-9). These abnormalities can be difficult to discern without indirect ophthalmoscopy; the view may also be lessened by a constricted pupil and interference from overlying inflammatory cells.

Etiology

- Toxoplasmosis is the most common cause of posterior uveitis (Fig. 8-10).
- In AIDS patients with symptoms of a posterior uveitis, cytomegalovirus retinitis should be ruled out or confirmed (see Chapter 9).
- Many local and systemic associations can occur (Box 8-2).

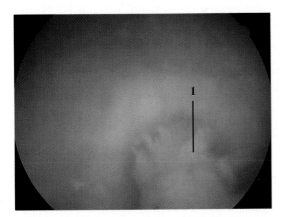

Fig. 8-8 Inflammatory vitreous cells causing a hazy view of the fundus in this case of lens-induced posterior uveitis. Note the large lens fragment *(1)*.

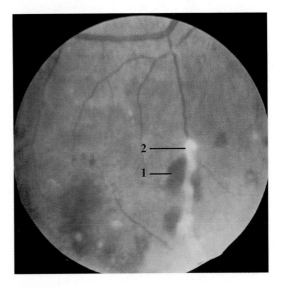

Fig. 8-9 Sarcoid posterior uveitis showing retinal hemorrhage *(1)* and vascular sheathing *(2)*.

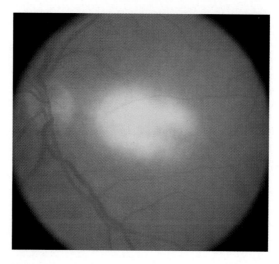

Fig. 8-10 Toxoplasmosis lesion located near the optic disc.

Box 8-2
Classification of posterior uveitis

Autoimmune disorders
- Vogt-Koyanagi-Harada syndrome (uveoencephalitis)
- Polyarteritis nodosa
- Lens-induced posterior uveitis

Infections
- Toxoplasmosis
- Toxocariasis
- Ocular candidiasis (see Chapter 9)
- Ocular histoplasmosis
- Cytomegalovirus
- Acute retinal necrosis (herpes zoster)
- Tuberculosis
- Syphilis

Malignancies*
- Retinoblastoma (see Chapter 12)
- Malignant melanoma
- Lymphoma
- Leukemia

Other conditions
- Idiopathic disease
- Sarcoidosis
- Behçet's syndrome

*Noninflammatory conditions that can mimic the clinical findings of a posterior uveitis.

Associated Factors and Diseases

■ Associated disorders include the following:
  • Chorioretinal scars
  • Exudative retinal detachment
  • Macular edema
  • Epiretinal membrane

Differential Diagnosis

■ Differential diagnoses include the following:
  • Retinal detachment
  • Intraocular malignancy (e.g., retinoblastoma)
  • Intraocular foreign body

Workup

■ A careful history and complete ocular examination are essential.
■ The general physical examination is directed at the possible systemic findings of the conditions associated with a posterior uveitis.
■ A nonspecific diagnostic workup and other tests and subspecialty consults may be initiated if the need for this is strongly indicated by symptoms, history, or physical findings.

Treatment

■ Patients should be referred to an ophthalmologist within 24 hours.
■ Topical cycloplegic and topical corticosteroid agents are administered if anterior inflammation is present.
■ Decisions on further treatment (e.g., periocular corticosteroid injections, intravitreal antibiotic injections, systemic medications, potential intraocular surgery) need to be made by an ophthalmologist.

Prognosis

■ The prognosis varies greatly depending on the etiology, severity of inflammation, and promptness of appropriate therapy.

Retina

Timothy W. Olsen

THE retina is a highly specialized sensory tissue that forms as a direct extension of the central nervous system in embryologic development. It translates light energy focused by the anterior ocular structures into a complex series of impulses that the brain perceives as vision. Because clarity of the ocular media is required for vision, the examination of the retina offers a unique opportunity to examine neurologic tissue and the vasculature directly. The retinal vasculature may be viewed directly, photographed, or imaged using fluorescein angiography. Vascular changes seen in the retina are often representative of the systemic vasculature. This chapter discusses retinal findings that will serve as a useful guide for primary care physicians in diagnosing systemic disease and common retinal disorders.

ANATOMY

A useful landmark during direct ophthalmoscopy is the optic nerve. It lies in the nasal portion of the retina and is easily viewed as the examiner approaches the eye from a slightly temporal aspect. Once a retinal vessel is evident, the vascular branching pattern always "points" toward the optic nerve (Fig. 9-1). After visualizing the optic nerve, the clinician focuses the direct ophthalmoscope on the retinal vasculature. The optic nerve is approximately 1.5 mm in diameter, and a retinal vein on the surface of the nerve is approximately 125 μm. The arteries appear thinner and more orange-red, whereas the veins are larger and more crimson. The normal arterial-to-venous ratio (A:V ratio) is approximately 2:3. As a rule, veins do not cross veins, arteries do not cross arteries, and veins and arteries travel together and frequently cross over or under each other (arteriole-venule crossings).

When the patient looks directly into the light of the direct ophthalmoscope, the area with a slightly darker orange pigmentation and an absence of retinal vasculature is the fovea, located 4 mm temporal and 0.8 mm inferior to the optic nerve. The small yellow reflex in the center of this area is the foveolar light reflex; it is present during most normal examinations. The macula is a circular area 5.5 mm in diameter centered on the fovea (generally the area within the temporal blood vessel arcades adjacent to the optic nerve). Peripheral retinal structures and pathologic conditions located anterior to the equator of the eye require indirect ophthalmoscopic techniques.

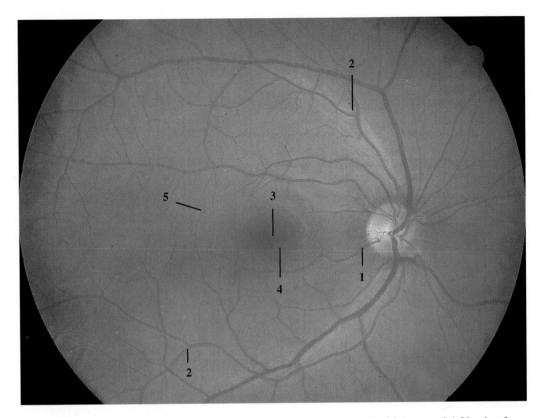

Fig. 9-1 Normal fundus. A normal, pink optic nerve, cup-to-disc ratio of 0.1, normal A:V ratio of 2:3, and a cilioretinal artery *(1)* extending from the optic nerve and inferior to the fovea. Note the branching points of the blood vessels "point" *(2)* toward the optic nerve. The foveolar reflex *(3)*, fovea *(4)*, and macula *(5)* are seen.

The normal retina and blood vessel walls are mostly transparent tissues. The ophthalmoscopically visible retinal vessel is actually an arterial or a venous "blood column." The normal orange color of the red reflex is produced by the vasculature of the choroid, retinal pigment epithelium, and choroidal melanocytes. The retina has two separate blood supplies. The central retinal artery supplies the "inner retina," or the retinal layers toward the center of the eye. The "outer retina," or the retinal layers toward the outer wall of the eye, is supplied by the highly vascular choroid. The high oxygen demand of the photoreceptors located in the outer retina is provided by the choroid. The fundus of lightly pigmented patients has a "blonde" appearance with readily visible choroidal vessels (Fig. 9-2). The fundus of darkly pigmented patients has a "brunette" appearance with less apparent choroidal vasculature. Examiners can easily differentiate choroidal blood vessels from retinal vessels because the retinal vasculature follows a typical branching pattern centered on the optic nerve; the choroidal pattern demonstrates an irregular branching pattern of larger-caliber, poorly defined vessels. Retinal vessels pass anterior to choroidal vessels. A blood vessel that supplies the retinal circulation frequently arises from the choroidal circulation at the optic nerve; this is called a *cilioretinal vessel* (see Fig. 9-1).

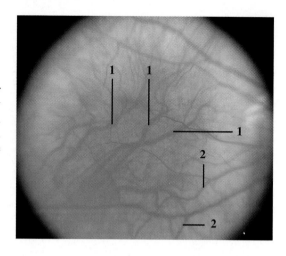

Fig. 9-2 Fundus of an albino with the absence of ocular pigmentation. The choroidal blood vessels *(1)* are readily visible. These are differentiated from the normal retinal vessels *(2)* by their size and branching pattern. Normal retinal vessels are seen emanating from the optic nerve and crossing over the choroidal vessels.

Fig. 9-3 Cross-sectional anatomy of the retina and choroid.

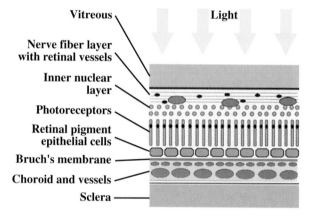

A basic understanding of the cross-sectional anatomy of the retina helps identify important pathologic states of this structure (Fig. 9-3). The inner retina contains the nerve fiber layer and ganglion cell nuclei, which extend their axons through the optic nerve and chiasm and synapse primarily in the lateral geniculate nucleus of the brain, with some fibers extending to the midbrain to subserve the pupillary light reflex. The inner retinal layer also contains the retinal vasculature. Conditions that cause ischemia of the retinal vasculature are manifest primarily in the nerve fiber layer and seen clinically as opacification of the inner retina. Axoplasmic stasis of the nerve fiber layer results in the clinically evident lesion known as a *cotton-wool spot* (Fig. 9-4). These whitish lesions follow the distribution of the nerve fiber layer and have hazy or fluffy borders. They used to be described as "soft exudates," a misnomer because a cotton-wool spot is an infarction rather than an exudation. Flame-shaped hemorrhages also occur in the nerve fiber layer. If a retinal vessel bleeds into the inner retinal layer, the blood intercalates with the nerve fibers like

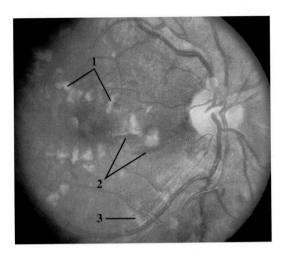

Fig. 9-4 Multiple cotton-wool spots *(1)* in the perifoveal region in a young male with disseminated microemboli after bone marrow transplantation. Ischemia of the perifoveal capillaries is responsible for the cotton-wool spots. Multiple frame-shaped hemorrhages *(2)* in the nerve fiber layer are also present. The arcuate, radiating striae extending from the optic nerve *(3)* represent the light reflex from the normal nerve fiber layer.

paint spilled on the fibers of split wood. Pathologic conditions located in the deeper layers of the retina appear more localized. For example, "dot and blot" hemorrhages commonly seen in patients with diabetes mellitus and localized lipid exudates, or "hard exudates," occur in the deeper layers of the retina and remain more circular and well localized.

Clinicians often use fluorescein angiography in the diagnosis and treatment of retinal disorders. Fluorescein is an extremely safe, water-soluble dye that appears white or hyperfluorescent in photographs as it circulates through the retinal and choroidal vasculature. Detailed examination at the capillary level is possible using this technique. A breakdown of the "blood-retina" barrier results in leakage of the dye into the retina and appears as a fuzzy region in the later phase of the angiogram. In addition, areas of nonperfusion or ischemia appear dark or hypofluorescent on the angiogram.

DIABETIC RETINOPATHY

Diabetes represents the leading cause of blindness in the Western world in people under the age of 50 years. The current standard of care is for all patients with diabetes to be evaluated by an ophthalmologist. Patients with newly diagnosed diabetes should be scheduled for a baseline evaluation and establish a relationship with an ophthalmologist for annual examinations. Patients with type I diabetes are unlikely to have retinopathy at the time of diagnosis. Primary care providers should consult an ophthalmologist within the first 6 months to 1 year of diagnosis of these patients. Those with type II diabetes may have retinopathy at the time of diagnosis. Therefore prompt referral for a baseline examination is recommended for those patients with newly diagnosed type II diabetes. The progress of diabetic retinopathy may accelerate during periods of strong hormonal influence such as pregnancy and puberty, so clinicians should closely follow and monitor patients during such periods.

Other than cataracts, patients with diabetes lose vision as a result of injury to the retinal vasculature. The three basic forms of diabetic retinopathy that may result in a loss of vision are proliferative diabetic retinopathy, diabetic macular edema, and ischemia of the macula.

PROLIFERATIVE DIABETIC RETINOPATHY

Proliferative diabetic retinopathy results from retinal ischemia. As perfusion to the retina is compromised, ischemic retinal tissue releases angiogenic factors (e.g., vascular endothelial growth factor) that stimulate abnormal new vessel growth, or neovascularization. Global retinal ischemia results in neovascularization emanating from the optic nerve, a high-risk condition (Fig. 9-5). Neovascularization may also occur at any location in the retina but typically occurs along the vascular arcades. It may also occur on the surface of the iris and impart a red-brown color known as *rubeosis iridis* that may lead to neovascular glaucoma, a severe form of glaucoma (Fig. 9-6). Neovascularization is also dangerous because the vessels grow into the vitreous gel instead of the retina. Movement or traction of the vitreous gel may shear these fragile vessels, leading to vitreous hemorrhage. Recurrent vitreous hemorrhage then leads to the formation of contractile, fibrous scar tissue that may pull the retina toward the center of the eye, producing tractional retinal detachments (Fig. 9-7).

Symptoms

- Some patients with severe proliferative retinopathy may have 20/20 visual acuity and be unaware of any symptoms. Therefore all patients with diabetes should be screened.
- Vision may decrease slowly or suddenly.
- Floaters, possibly indicating vitreous hemorrhage, are usually described as a "shower."
- Blind spots in the vision (scotomata) are reported.

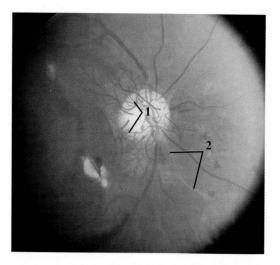

Fig. 9-5 Fronds of neovascularization *(1)* on the disc are present in this right eye. Temporally, two cotton-wool spots have adjacent intraretinal hemorrhage and preretinal hemorrhage. Native retinal arteries are narrowed and show evidence of sclerosis *(2)*.

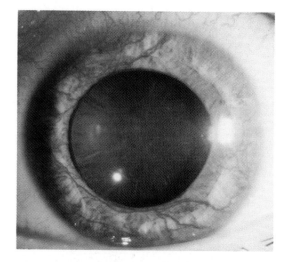

Fig. 9-6 Dilated pupil of a patient with poorly controlled diabetes displaying advanced rubeosis iridis, or neovascularization of the iris. These vessels are on the surface of the iris, may occlude the normal drainage of aqueous fluid from the eye, and lead to a severe form of glaucoma.

Signs

- Neovascularization, or fine lacy blood vessels, are seen on the optic nerve, retina (see Fig. 9-5), or iris surface (see Fig. 9-6).
- Preretinal hemorrhages are boat-shaped hemorrhages that may be located anterior to the retinal vessels and block the view of these structures (Fig. 9-8).
- Cotton-wool spots are often present.
- Venous beading, dilation, or engorgement is present.
- Dot and blot intraretinal hemorrhages usually occur.
- Loss of the red reflex and resulting inability to view the fundus are possible with a vitreous hemorrhage.
- Areas of tractional retinal detachment may be observed (see Fig. 9-7).
- Whitish fibrovascular tissue on the retinal surface may occur in a pattern along the vascular arcades and above the optic nerve.

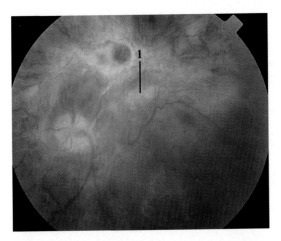

Fig. 9-7 A large white sheet of fibrovascular tissue is present on the surface of the retina in this patient with diabetes. Contraction of the tissue distorts the retinal vessels and tractionally detaches the retina. The yellow substance deep to the fibrovascular tissue *(1)* is lipid, which results from chronic exudation of incompetent vessels. Surgical intervention (vitrectomy) is needed to remove the fibro-vascular tissue and reattach the retina.

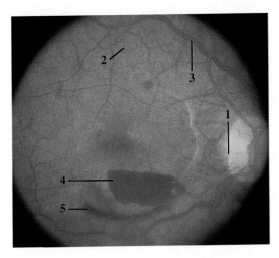

Fig. 9-8 Proliferative diabetic retinopathy with high-risk characteristics. Neovascularization is present at the optic nerve *(1)* and along the vascular arcades *(2)*. Retinal veins are engorged *(3)*, and a preretinal hemorrhage *(4)* is present inferior to the fovea. This boat-shaped hemorrhage blocks the view of the retinal vessels. A more diffuse hemorrhage *(5)* is present in an arcuate pattern just inferior to the preretinal hemorrhage that represents a mild vitreous hemorrhage.

Differential Diagnosis

■ Differential diagnoses include the following:
   • Diabetes
   • Vascular occlusions—central or branch retinal vein or artery occlusions
   • Radiation retinopathy, which may appear identical to diabetic retinopathy
   • Blood dyscrasias—sickle cell retinopathy (especially in patients with SC disease), anemias, leukemias, thalassemias, and hyperviscosity syndromes
   • Retinal emboli
   • Carotid disease, aortic arch syndrome, and carotid-cavernous fistula
   • Uveitis (e.g., sarcoidosis)

Workup

■ Laboratory tests include fasting blood glucose level, oral glucose tolerance test, hemoglobin A_{1C}, CBC with differential count, hemoglobin electrophoresis, serum protein electrophoresis, and angiotensin-converting enzyme titer.

■ Clinically, carotid ultrasound or chest x-ray imaging is performed as indicated.

Treatment

NOTE: The Diabetes Control and Complications Trial (DCCT) has shown that "tight" glycemic control decreases the progression of diabetic retinopathy, nephropathy, and neuropathy. The primary care physician's role is therefore *essential* in decreasing the incidence of vision loss from diabetic retinopathy in cases of both proliferative retinopathy and diabetic macular edema.

■ Diabetic patients with neovascularization should be promptly referred to an ophthalmologist.

■ Retinal laser photocoagulation destroys the peripheral retina and decreases the release of vasoproliferative growth factors from the ischemic retinal tissue. Photocoagulation also creates multiple choroid-to-retina adhesions that limit the progression of a tractional retinal detachment.

Follow-Up

■ To address the risk of anticoagulation, the clinician does the following:
   • The guidelines for anticoagulation regimens in patients at risk for coronary artery disease, stroke, or other conditions are *not* altered because of the presence of proliferative diabetic retinopathy. Although the risk for vitreous hemorrhage is no greater during anticoagulation therapy, if such hemorrhage occurs, it may be more severe. Most hemorrhages clear with time, but some eventually require vitrectomy surgery. *No* ophthalmic complications should compromise a life-threatening condition requiring anticoagulation medication.
   • Ophthalmologic consultation is indicated to monitor the diabetic retinopathy when the patient is medically stable. For example, a patient with diabetes taking anticoagulants for unstable angina is best seen by an ophthalmic consultant after appropriate cardiac care rather than being seen first by the ophthalmologist to rule out proliferative diabetic retinopathy while anticoagulation therapy is delayed. Even if proliferative diabetic retinopathy were present, laser photocoagulation is not performed until the patient is medically stable. Improvement in the proliferative retinopathy may require several weeks or months and involve multiple treatment sessions.

DIABETIC MACULAR EDEMA

The earliest detectable clinical alteration in the vasculature of a patient with diabetes is the formation of microaneurysms (Fig. 9-9). Generally, the retinal vascular endothelium has "tight junctions" that form the inner blood-retina barrier, analogous to the blood-brain barrier. The microaneurysms have an increased permeability because of an incompetent blood-retina barrier and leak intravascular fluid into the retinal tissue. The fluid may accumulate in the foveal area, leading to decreased visual acuity. Alternatively, decreased visual acuity may result from ischemia or lack of perfusion to the fovea.

Symptoms

- No symptoms may be noted. Diabetic patients may have normal vision and edema requiring laser treatment; therefore all need ophthalmologic screening.
- Vision may be decreased unilaterally or bilaterally.

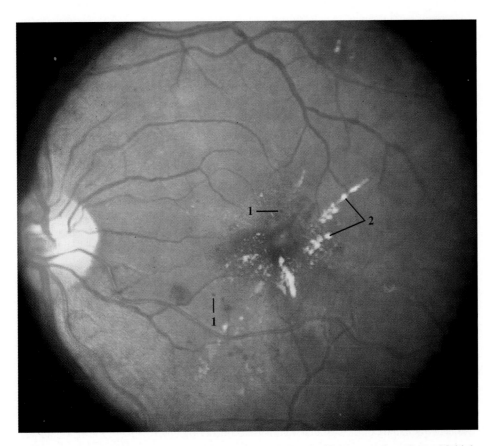

Fig. 9-9 Insulin-dependent diabetic patient with clinically significant macular edema. Multiple small red dots (microaneurysms) *(1)* are present throughout the macular area. Linear streaks of yellow deposits or hard exudates *(2)* are accumulations of lipid material from chronic leakage of the microaneurysms. Loss of the normal foveal light reflex suggests the presence of macular edema.

Signs

- Graying or a slight opacification of the retina results from edema in the macula.
- Microaneurysms are usually adjacent to retinal veins but may be found at any location in the retina.
- Dot and blot intraretinal hemorrhages occur.
- Cystoid changes in the fovea may be seen.
- Hard exudates are yellowish lesions with discrete borders that may be isolated, linear, or stellate or form a "circinate ring" around leakage sites.

Differential Diagnosis

- Differential diagnoses include the following:
  - Diabetes
  - Vascular occlusions—central or branch retinal vein occlusions
  - Hypertensive retinopathy
  - Radiation retinopathy
  - Choroidal neovascularization (subretinal neovascularization usually associated with age-related macular degeneration)
  - Macroaneurysms (larger retinal aneurysms associated with systemic hypertension)

Treatment

NOTE: As mentioned previously, the DCCT has shown that tight glycemic control decreases the progression of diabetic retinopathy. Therefore the actions of the primary care physician are critical in decreasing the incidence of vision loss from diabetic macular edema.

- Patients should be referred to an ophthalmologist.
- Laser photocoagulation (based on Early Treatment of Diabetic Retinopathy Study [ETDRS] findings) is performed to decrease the further decline in visual acuity by reducing the amount of macular edema.

HYPERTENSIVE RETINOPATHY

Systemic hypertension may affect the retinal vasculature in several ways. The traditional classification systems of hypertensive retinopathy were designed in the 1930s to 1950s and predate the more focused antihypertensive efforts currently used to manage patients with systemic hypertension. For this reason the retinal vascular changes described in the classification systems are important to understand, but the classification system itself is rarely used today. Autoregulatory mechanisms in the retinal vasculature limit the ability of a clinician using an ophthalmoscopic examination to detect mild to moderate elevations in systemic blood pressure.

Useful information may be obtained from the ophthalmoscopic examination. Chronicity of the hypertension may be evident by the hallmark of hypertensive retinopathy, which is diffuse arteriolar narrowing. As stated, the blood vessel walls are virtually invisible in the normal retina, and the examiner actually sees the blood column. Chronic hypertension results in thickening of the vascular wall with a concomitant narrowing of the vessel lumen. The normal A:V ratio of 2:3 may change to 1:3 or 1:4 in patients with chronic hypertension. A "copper-wire vessel" is a dated term used to describe the yellowing of the linear light reflex seen on the surface of a narrowed arteriolar vessel affected by chronic hypertension. However, with the brighter, halogen-light sources, this color change is not easily

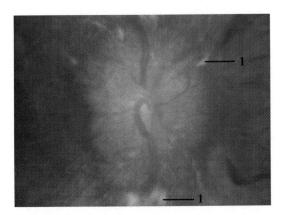

Fig. 9-10 Swollen optic nerve (bilateral) caused by acute renal failure and accelerated systemic hypertension (blood pressure of 220/140 mm hg). The optic disc margins are fuzzy with a loss of detail of the vessels as they pass over the disc. Multiple small cotton-wool spots *(1)* are present. Veins are dilated and tortuous.

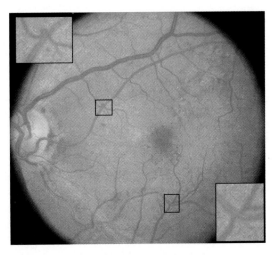

Fig. 9-11 In this patient with diabetes and chronic hypertension, the A:V ratio is approximately 1:3 or 1:4 with significant arteriolar narrowing. Note the deviation or "humping" of the venules *(top inset)* as they cross over the arterioles. The artery crosses over the vein and causes "nicking" or attenuation of the venule *(bottom inset)* immediately under the crossing point.

appreciated. "Silver wire" was used to describe a white retinal vessel without a visible blood column. These terms are currently referred to as *arteriolar narrowing* (copper wire) and *sclerosis of the vessels* (silver wire). Patients with acute or accelerated hypertension may exhibit papilledema (Fig. 9-10) with or without a stellate macular exudation sometimes referred to as a *macular star*.

Symptoms
- Vision may be normal, slightly blurred, or suddenly decreased.
- A blind spot in the vision (scotoma) may be reported.
- Double vision may occur.

Signs
- Arteriolar narrowing is diffuse in cases of chronic hypertension (Fig. 9-11) or a focal spasm in patients with acute hypertension.
- A:V crossing changes result from constriction of the common adventitial sheath at the crossing of an arteriole and a venule.
- Sclerotic vessels may be observed.
- Cotton-wool spots may be evident.
- Microaneurysms may be noted.
- Lipid exudation may occur and have a macular star configuration.
- Retinal edema may be present.
- Branch retinal vein or artery occlusion may occur.

- Macroaneurysm may cause exudation or rupture, producing acute vision loss from hemorrhage (subretinal, intraretinal, preretinal, or vitreous).
- Bilateral disc edema and swelling indicates accelerated hypertension or renal failure.
- Exudative retinal detachments indicate preeclampsia in pregnant patients.

Differential Diagnosis

- Differential diagnoses include the following:
  - Diabetic retinopathy
  - Atherosclerosis (e.g., carotid disease)
  - Arteriosclerosis
  - Accelerated hypertension ("malignant hypertension")
  - Renal failure
  - Radiation retinopathy
  - Papilledema from increased intracranial pressure
  - Pseudotumor cerebri
  - Preeclampsia/eclampsia
  - Systemic lupus erythematosus and other collagen vascular diseases
  - Pheochromocytoma
  - Adrenal disease
  - Anemia
  - Coarctation of the aorta
  - Other causes of systemic hypertension

Treatment

- Treatment is directed toward the underlying hypertension and systemic vascular or renal disorders. Chronic hypertensive retinopathy does not require specific ophthalmic treatment. Acute hypertensive retinopathy with papilledema is also treated by prompt control of the systemic blood pressure and usually requires inpatient management with imaging studies to rule out an intracranial lesion.
- Patients with decreased vision, retinal macroaneurysm, branch retinal artery or vein occlusion, and an exudative maculopathy should be referred to an ophthalmologist for possible laser evaluation.
- For preeclampsia or eclampsia the infant is delivered and exudative detachments usually resolve postpartum. Permanent visual loss from pregnancy-associated complications is rare and may result from retinal or occipital lobe ischemia.

RETINAL ARTERY OCCLUSION

Retinal artery occlusions may involve the central retinal artery (CRAO) or a branch of the central retinal artery (BRAO). Unilateral involvement may be obvious or noticeable only after the patient closes the uninvolved eye. Cilioretinal arteries supply a portion of the macula in up to 20% of eyes (see Fig. 9-1). Perfusion of the macula by a cilioretinal artery, which arises from the choroidal blood supply, may result in macular sparing despite a retinal artery occlusion (Fig. 9-12). Retinal whitening may fade with time (Fig. 9-13). Alternatively, CRAO may cause ischemia to the macula with subsequent vision loss. A soft, glistening, yellow embolus conforming to the blood vessel lumen or forming a Y-shaped obstruction (Fig. 9-14)

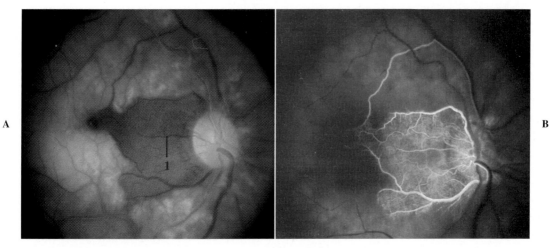

Fig. 9-12 A, Central retinal artery obstruction with a patent cilioretinal artery *(1)* sparing the fovea. Diffuse retinal whitening from the retinal ischemia appears several hours after the arterial occlusion. The normal-appearing retina between the optic nerve and fovea is perfused by the centrally located cilioretinal arteriole. **B,** Fluorescein angiogram of the same patient. Note the dark appearance of the fundus that occurs from lack of retinal artery perfusion. The cilioretinal arteriole is present in the center of the hyperfluorescent area.

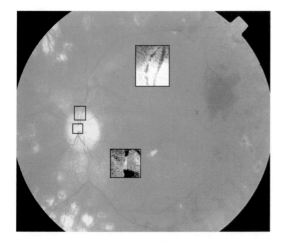

Fig. 9-13 This 1-week-old central retinal artery obstruction has a fading central cherry-red spot (composed of adjacent lipid from diabetic macular edema). Note the segmentation or "boxcarring" effect of vascular stasis within the retinal arterioles and venules *(top inset).* An embolus is present at the level of the optic nerve *(bottom inset).* Hypopigmented panretinal photocoagulation spots are present outside the vascular arcades.

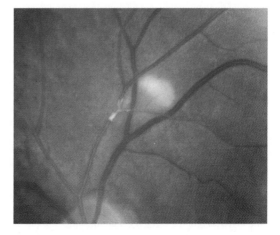

Fig. 9-14 A Y-shaped embolus probably representing a cholesterol embolus from carotid disease. Note the cotton-wool spot peripheral to the arteriolar occlusion.

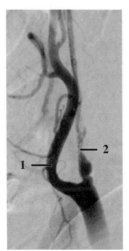

Fig. 9-15 Carotid angiography of the carotid bifurcation. The external carotid artery is patent *(1)*, whereas the internal carotid is severely obstructed *(2)*.

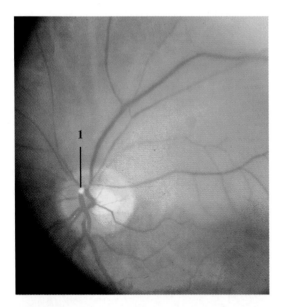

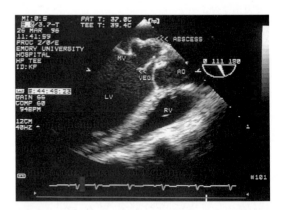

Fig. 9-16 A highly refractile calcific embolus *(1)* is present on the optic nerve. A wedge-shaped area of retinal whitening corresponds to the distribution of the branch retinal artery occluded by the embolus.

Fig. 9-17 Transesophageal echography of the aortic valve reveals a dense vegetation *(Veg)* and an abscess.

at a branch point usually is a cholesterol embolus (Hollenhorst plaque) that arises from the carotid arteries (Fig. 9-15). A hard, whitish plaque (Fig. 9-16) may represent a calcific embolus from an abnormal heart valve (Fig. 9-17).

Symptoms

- A sudden, painless unilateral loss in vision and visual field occurs in patients with CRAO.
- A sudden, painless visual field loss corresponds to a horizontal hemifield in cases of BRAO. For example, a superior BRAO causes an inferior visual field defect.
- In cases of amaurosis fugax a transient loss of vision implies an impending CRAO or BRAO. Classically, patients describe a curtain descending over their vision that clears over several minutes.

Signs

- A relative afferent pupillary defect is present.
- If a patient with retinal artery occlusion is seen within the first few hours of the onset of the disorder, retinal edema may not yet be present.
- An embolus may be seen at the level of the optic nerve in cases of CRAO.
- An embolus may be seen at a branch point of an arteriole in cases of BRAO.
- A cherry-red spot represents ischemia and edema of the entire posterior retina and occurs within several hours of occlusion. The red color at the center fovea results from perfusion of the choroid through the thinner retinal tissue and contrasts with the surrounding, relatively thick, white perifoveal retina.
- Arcuate retinal whitening corresponds to the retinal distribution of the occluded vessel.
- Segmentation, or "boxcarring," of the retinal vessels may be present.
- Cilioretinal sparing, or a pattern of normal retina surrounding a cilioretinal artery, may be observed.

Etiology

- Possible disorders include the following:
  - Carotid atherosclerotic disease
  - Cardiac valvular disease
  - Giant cell arteritis—jaw claudication, scalp tenderness, tongue pain, or polymyalgia rheumatica and its associated symptoms possibly present in older patients.
  - Thrombosis from hypercoagulative states, including pregnancy, oral contraceptive use, lupus anticoagulant, resistance to activated protein C (factor V Leiden mutation), antithrombin III, homocysteinuria, and protein C or protein S deficiency
  - Cardiac myxoma
  - Intravenous drug abuse and talc retinopathy (Fig. 9-18)
  - Lipid emboli resulting from trauma
  - Disseminated intravascular coagulopathies (DICs) such as pancreatitis, amniotic fluid emboli, trauma, and sepsis
  - Sickle cell anemia
  - Polyarteritis nodosa
  - Corticosteroid injections around the head and neck

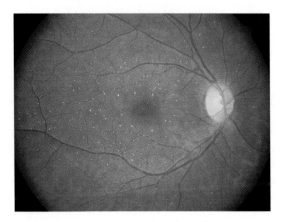

Fig. 9-18 Multiple talc emboli from intravenous drug use.

- Retinal migraine
- Syphilis
- Cat-scratch disease (*Bartonella henselae* infection)
- Trauma
- Ophthalmic artery occlusion (involving the retinal and choroidal circulation)—a similar disorder in which vision is usually worse (patients usually lacking any light perception) and total whitening of the retina occurs

Workup
- Evaluation is directed by the clinical examination, the age of the patient, and any known systemic medical associations.
- The examiner auscultates the carotid arteries and heart, listening for the carotid bruits or murmurs (e.g., aortic stenosis).
- If the patient is over the age of 55 years, the clinician should inquire about giant cell arteritis symptoms.
- A neurologic history and examination is performed.
- Carotid ultrasonography or angiography is performed.
- Cardiac echography is performed.
- Laboratory evaluation is modified for each patient and may include ESR, CBC with differential count, PT/PTT, and hypercoagulation workup if indicated (antithrombin III, protein S, protein C, resistance to activated protein C [factor V Leiden mutation], lupus anticoagulant panel, homocysteinuria testing, serum protein electrophoresis, and hemoglobin electrophoresis).

Treatment
NOTE: Emergency ophthalmologic consultation is indicated to confirm or rule out a retinal artery obstruction. Despite the poor visual prognosis associated with this disorder, efforts are directed toward dislodging an embolus and moving it "downstream" to minimize the amount of retinal involvement. Several immediate maneuvers to dilate the retinal vascular

system or decrease the intraocular pressure to dislodge the embolus are within the scope of the primary care provider. The following apply to the acute management of retinal artery occlusion:

- An immediate ophthalmologic consultation is necessary.
- For ocular massage the clinician uses gentle but firm digital pressure on the globe with the patient's eyelids closed for 10 to 15 seconds. A rapid release of the pressure creates a transient decrease in intraocular pressure that may lead to dislodgment of the embolus. The clinician can repeat this procedure several times. If the patient has undergone recent ophthalmic surgery (within 1 month) or trauma with a hyphema or an open globe, massage is contraindicated.
- In carbogen treatment the patient rebreathes a mixture of 95% oxygen and 5% carbon dioxide, which may dilate the retinal vasculature. The patient rebreathes the mixture for 10 minutes every 2 hours in most cases. If no improvement occurs after two or three treatments, the treatment is discontinued.
- Intravenous or oral Diamox (500 mg) is administered. In patients with a sulfa allergy, alternative drugs are used.
- A topical β blocker (e.g., timolol 0.5%) is administered.
- Sublingual administration of nitroglycerin may also cause some vascular dilation.
- Anterior chamber paracentesis is performed at the slit lamp. The ophthalmologist passes a 30-gauge needle on a tuberculin syringe through the cornea near the limbus into the anterior chamber. Removal of aqueous fluid immediately lowers the intraocular pressure. This may be the most effective method to dislodge an embolus. Potential complications include cataract formation from inadvertent lens touch, hyphema, and endophthalmitis.
- For patients in whom an anticoagulation regimen is indicated, medical consultation is recommended. Treatment of embolic arterial occlusions should be similar to the protocol used for patients with stroke.

Follow-Up

- All patients with artery occlusions require monthly ophthalmologic examinations for approximately 6 months after the initial event. The ophthalmologist determines the subsequent need for follow-up.
- Neovascularization of the retina or iris may occur and should be promptly treated with retinal laser photocoagulation by an ophthalmologist.

RETINAL VEIN OCCLUSION

As with retinal artery occlusion, retinal vein occlusion (RVO) may involve either the central retinal vein (CRVO) or a branch of the central retinal vein (BRVO). CRVOs involve all four quadrants of the retina (Fig. 9-19), whereas BRVOs involve one quadrant and have an arcuate pattern corresponding to the vein's area of drainage (Fig. 9-20). Venous occlusive events are relatively common in the older population. As with artery occlusions, vein occlusions may only be noticed by the patient when the uninvolved eye is covered. The mechanism of a CRVO is probably a thrombus that occurs in the venule at the exit site from the eye within the optic nerve. BRVOs usually occur at the site of an arteriole-venule crossing. Chronic hypertensive changes of the vessel wall and constriction of the common

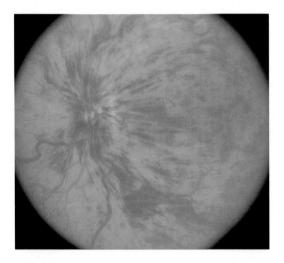

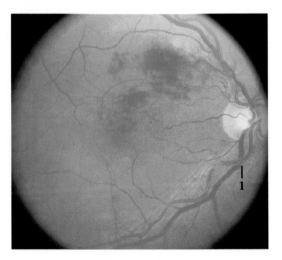

Fig. 9-19 Central retinal vein occlusion in a patient with 20/400 visual acuity. Note the dramatic retinal hemorrhages in all four quadrants. Significant venous dilation and tortuosity are present. Mild to moderate ischemia are seen with diffuse cotton-wool spots. The optic disc is blurred with peripapillary hemorrhage.

Fig. 9-20 Branch retinal vein obstruction involving the superotemporal venule that drains in an arcuate, quadrantic distribution in the area of retinal hemorrhage. The A:V crossing change of the inferotemporal venule *(1)* is representative of A:V nicking. Both the BRVO and the A:V nicking are associated with chronic systemic hypertension.

adventitial sheath around both vessels at the crossing point are responsible for the venous occlusion. BRVOs are associated with systemic hypertension. The venous occlusion impedes the flow of blood from the retinal circulation. A severe obstruction is termed an *ischemic RVO,* whereas a partial obstruction is a *nonischemic RVO.*

Symptoms

- Sudden or gradual, unilateral, painless blurry vision or loss of vision occurs.
- Severe unilateral pain, redness, and loss of vision are reported. This may represent the neovascular glaucoma associated with RVOs (informally called "90-day glaucoma" because it usually occurs 3 months after an RVO).
- Unilateral visual field loss corresponds to a horizontal hemifield in cases of BRVO.

Signs

- A relative afferent pupillary defect most commonly occurs in cases of ischemic CRVO.
- A "blood-and-thunder" fundus is seen.
- Dilated and tortuous veins are noted.
- A flame-shaped hemorrhage is evident.
- Vitreous hemorrhage may occur.
- Cotton-wool spots are present.
- Macular edema is noted.
- Exudates are common.
- Neovascularization of the retina or iris can occur and is usually associated with glaucoma.

Workup

- The examiner evaluates the patient for systemic hypertension.
- Especially for patients under 50 years of age, systemic evaluation may be needed.
- A pregnancy test is performed.
- Information about oral contraceptive use is elicited.
- Other thrombotic events, including deep vein thrombosis, pulmonary emboli, frequent miscarriages, and a family history of thrombosis are addressed.
- Laboratory evaluation is modified for each patient and may include β-HCG, ESR, CBC with differential count, PT/PTT, and hypercoagulation workup if indicated (antithrombin III, protein S, protein C, resistance to activated protein C [factor V Leiden mutation], lupus anticoagulant panel, homocysteinuria testing, serum protein electrophoresis, and hemoglobin electrophoresis).
- Testing is performed for thyroid eye disease and tumors, which cause compression of the central retinal vein as it exits the eye.

Treatment

- Ophthalmologic evaluation is mandatory. Patients should be seen by the ophthalmologist within 48 to 72 hours of diagnosis.
- A BRVO with macular edema may result in decreased vision. Laser photocoagulation helps correct macular edema and the neovascular complication seen in patients with BRVO.

Follow-Up

- Patients with CRVO should be assessed every month for the first 6 months by the ophthalmologist to lower the risk of neovascular complications.
- Visual prognosis depends on the severity of the venous occlusion, level of retinal ischemia, and rate at which collateralization occurs. Neovascularization implies a worse prognosis, especially the development of neovascular glaucoma. Some patients experience resolution of the venous occlusion with good visual acuity, whereas others suffer a significant loss of vision.

SICKLE CELL RETINOPATHY

Paradoxically, the patients with the most severe retinal involvement are those with milder systemic involvement, such as those with hemoglobin SC (sickle cell and hemoglobin C) or S-Thal (sickle cell and thalassemia). These patients generally appear otherwise healthy, may have a negative sickle-cell test result, and are less likely to have "sickle-crisis." Approximate percentages of sickle patterns in African-Americans are as follows: AS (sickle trait), 8.5%; SS (sickle cell anemia), 0.4%; SC (SC-disease), 0.2%; and S-Thal, 0.03%.

Symptoms

- Vision may be normal or slightly blurred.
- A sudden or progressive, painless loss of vision may occur.
- Floaters are reported if vitreous hemorrhage exists.
- Flashes occur.
- A blind spot in vision (scotoma) may be present.

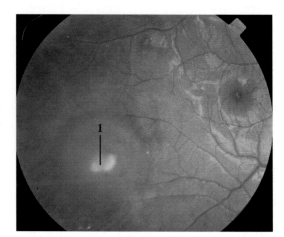

Fig. 9-21 The right eye of an African-American man with sickle cell disease. Note the normal fovea to the right with a salmon-patch hemorrhage *(1)* inferotemporal to the fovea.

Signs

- Intraretinal and subretinal hemorrhage, or "salmon-patch," occurs at the sites of vessel-wall blowout from a sickle obstruction of the arteriole (Fig. 9-21).
- A healed hemorrhage displays spiculated pigment migration, or a "black-sun burst."
- Iridescent spots are refractile deposits of hemosiderin from a previous intraretinal hemorrhage.
- Vitreous hemorrhage may be seen.
- Retinal detachment occurs in rare cases.
- "Sea fans," or peripheral neovascularization, is extremely difficult to see with direct ophthalmoscopy.
- Dilated vessels result from peripheral arteriovenous shunts.
- Peripheral neovascularization, gliosis, tractional retinal detachments, and ridges of proliferative tissue are possible. The examiner looks at the peripheral red reflex of both eyes (dilated) while standing several feet away from the patient using a direct ophthalmoscope. An asymmetric red reflex is abnormal, and a white reflex in one eye strongly suggests peripheral retinal pathology.
- Comma-shaped capillaries of the conjunctiva may be observed.
- CRAOs or BRAOs can occur.

Etiology

- Lower oxygen tension in the peripheral retina causes sickling with vascular occlusion and peripheral retinal ischemia. Vasoproliferative factors are released from the ischemic retina and may result in peripheral retinal neovascularization and subsequent vitreous hemorrhages.

Differential Diagnosis

- Differential diagnoses are the same as those for proliferative diabetic retinopathy (see p. 108).

Associated Factors and Diseases

■ Patients with African or Mediterranean heritage have a higher incidence of sickle cell retinopathy.

■ Sickle-cell patients may have painful sickle crises.

Treatment

■ Referral to an ophthalmologist is needed for a baseline peripheral retinal examination and annual examination. Patients with visual symptoms, vitreous hemorrhage, or retinal detachment require more urgent and frequent ophthalmologic evaluation.

■ Use of laser photocoagulation is controversial but may be beneficial in some circumstances.

■ Retinal detachment requires prompt ophthalmologic evaluation for possible surgical repair.

RETINITIS PIGMENTOSA*

Retinitis pigmentosa is a large group of retinal degenerations, most of which are inherited. Many cases are sporadic without any obvious inheritance pattern. Genetic defects affect genes that code for the photoreceptor proteins rhodopsin and peripherin and other retina-specific genes. Advancements in molecular biology hold promise for future treatments of these conditions.

Symptoms

■ Vision is normal or decreased.

■ Night blindness (nyctalopia) occurs. Patients may report difficulty adapting to the dark (as in finding a seat in a darkened movie theater).

■ Photophobia is present.

■ Shimmering or tiny blinking lights (photopsias) are noted.

■ Blind spots in vision (scotomata) occur.

■ A peripheral visual field loss occurs.

■ Color vision is disturbed.

■ Affected relatives experience similar symptoms.

Signs

■ The fundus may appear normal.

■ "Bone-spicule" pigmentary retinopathy is observed (Fig. 9-22).

■ Optic nerve pallor is evident.

■ Arteriolar narrowing results in severely attenuated vasculature.

■ A cataract may be seen.

■ Visual fields are constricted.

■ The "golden-ring" sign is a yellowish-white halo surrounding the optic disc that is eventually replaced with pigmentation or atrophy.

---

*Patient information on this subject may be obtained through the Retinitis Pigmentosa Foundation, Inc. (Baltimore, Md).

Workup

- The retinal response to a light stimulus is measured (electroretinography).
- Formal visual field testing is performed.
- A family history is obtained. The severity of disease and prognosis may be similar to those of affected family members. In general, autosomal recessive cases are more severe, whereas autosomal dominant cases are less severe.
- Genetic studies and examination of family members are performed. Genetic consultation is encouraged.

Differential Diagnosis

- Differential diagnoses include the following:
  - Drug use (especially chloroquine, Mellaril, and chlorpromazine)
  - Maternal infections such as syphilis, rubella, and toxoplasmosis, which may cause pigmentary retinal changes similar to those of retinitis pigmentosa
  - Vitamin A deficiency (identical signs and symptoms)

Associated Factors and Diseases

- Patients with Usher's syndrome (retinitis pigmentosa and deafness) may constitute up to 50% of those who are both deaf and blind (Fig. 9-22).
- Most patients (90% to 100%) with Bardet-Biedl syndrome have retinitis pigmentosa in addition to polydactyly, obesity, hypogonadism, and mental retardation.
- Kearns-Sayre syndrome involves retinitis pigmentosa, ptosis, chronic progressive external ophthalmoplegia, cardiac arrhythmia, heart block, defective mitochondria, and "ragged red" fibers on muscle biopsy.
- Patients with Alström syndrome have retinitis pigmentosa, diabetes mellitus, obesity, deafness, renal failure, acanthosis nigricans, baldness, hypogenitalism, and hypertriglyceridemia.
- Many other genetic diseases are associated with retinitis pigmentosa.

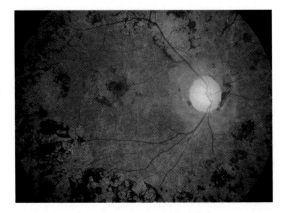

Fig. 9-22 A 50-year-old African-American woman with Usher's syndrome (type II). She is deaf and has severe loss of vision (20/400). The peripheral retina displays the typical bone-spicule pattern seen with retinitis pigmentosa. A central "bull's-eye" maculopathy is also present.

Treatment

■ The following apply to cases of treatable or "pseudo–retinitis pigmentosa":
  • Patients with vitamin A deficiency may initially be seen as having pseudo–retinitis pigmentosa and have malabsorption conditions or malnutrition. Treatment consists of vitamin A supplementation.
  • Patients with Bassen-Kornzweig syndrome have abetalipoproteinemia, acanthocytosis, ataxia, and neuropathy. The indicated treatment consists of vitamin A and E supplementation.
  • Refsum's syndrome is a phytanic acid storage disease (elevated levels of serum phytanic acid). Treatment involves phytanic acid restriction (decreased ingestion of dairy products, meat, and fish oil).
  • Gyrate atrophy results from ornithine transferase deficiency. Treatment includes supplementation of pyridoxine with an arginine-restricted diet.
■ For other common forms of retinitis pigmentosa, use of supplemental vitamin A palmitate (15,000 IU daily) is controversial. This treatment should be avoided in sexually active young women not using contraception because of the teratogenic effects of vitamin A treatment. If patients are taking vitamin A supplementation, the clinician needs to order and monitor liver function studies.

AGE-RELATED MACULAR DEGENERATION

Age-related macular degeneration (AMD) is the most common cause of legal blindness in the Western world and commonly affects individuals over the age of 65 years. The cause of AMD is unknown; however, risk factors include older age, female gender, lighter pigmentation, and smoking and the disease may have a genetic component.

Degeneration of the supporting structures of the outer retina and photoreceptors is responsible for the deterioration of vision. The most common abnormality seen in AMD is the presence of drusen, or yellowish deposits deep to the retina. Drusen may be small, yellowish crystals (Fig. 9-23) or larger, soft-yellow deposits (Fig. 9-24). Drusen may also be localized to the foveal area or more peripherally located along the arcades. Deposits are usually multicentric and may be mild or extensive, giving the fundus a "bumpy" appearance. Drusen limit the nutritional and metabolic support available to the outer retina.

The two common types of AMD are exudative and atrophic, with the atrophic variety appearing more often. Areas of atrophy of the retinal pigment epithelium impart a geographic area of pallor to the macular area. Exudative macular degeneration occurs as neovascularization originating from the choroidal vasculature grows under the retina, leaks fluid and lipid, and may bleed. The end-stage of this process is a large subretinal scarring process (disciform scar) that destroys the overlying retina.

Symptoms

■ The onset of blurry vision may be gradual or acute.
■ Wavy or distorted vision (metamorphopsia) may occur.
■ Intermittent shimmering lights (photopsias) may be noted.
■ A central blind spot (scotoma) may occur.

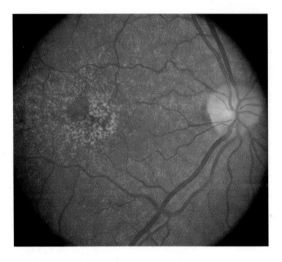

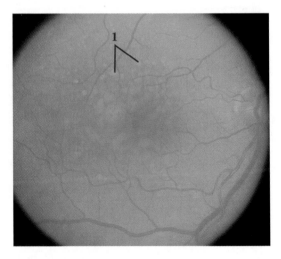

Fig. 9-23 Extensive small or cuticular drusen in a 56-year-old African-American man.

Fig. 9-24 Multiple soft drusen *(1)* in a 75-year-old white woman with age-related macular degeneration.

Fig. 9-25 Patient with extensive soft drusen *(1)* temporal to the fovea of the right eye. Note the circular greenish lesion with radiating exudate *(2)*. This lesion is typical for choroidal neovascularization or "wet" AMD.

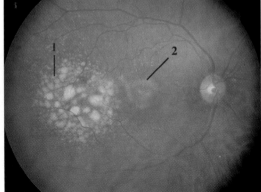

Signs

- Visual acuity may be decreased.
- Amsler grid distortion may occur. (An Amsler grid is a chart with horizontal and vertical lines that is used to detect distortion or blind spots within the central 10 degrees of the visual field [see Fig. 1-12].)
- Multiple, large, soft drusen with pigment mottling indicate a worse prognosis.
- A loss of normal pigmentation, with a yellow-white geographic area of atrophy, may occur.
- Subretinal or intraretinal blood or serous fluid may be present.
- Subretinal blood may appear greenish or gray (Fig. 9-25).
- Serous (clear fluid) or hemorrhagic (dark red, black, or yellow) retinal detachment may occur.

Workup

- Amsler grid testing is performed.
- Fluorescein or indocyanine green angiography is performed.
- Family members are evaluated if an inherited pattern is suspected.

Treatment

- For acute vision changes, the patient should be referred to an ophthalmologist within 24 hours.
- Laser photocoagulation may be performed.
- Subretinal surgery is currently an experimental option.
- Low vision aids, specifically various forms of image magnification, are often used.

Prognosis

A large multicentered prospective randomized clinical trial (Macular Photocoagulation Study) has clearly shown the benefit of laser photocoagulation in selected cases of exudative AMD. The complications are destruction of the macula by the laser and a high rate of disease recurrence. Bilateral involvement is common, and surgical treatment is limited. Based on current clinical studies, definitive recommendations regarding treatment with antioxidant vitamins or special "eye formulations" cannot be made with any degree of certainty. Further clinical trials should help clarify those therapeutic options that are effective.

ROTH SPOTS

Roth spots are retinal hemorrhages with a white center and may be caused by various systemic and ocular conditions (Fig. 9-26). The most likely source of the white center is a fibrin plug. Other suggested causes are infected foci and leukemic infiltrate. Treatment is directed at the underlying etiologic process. Vision is often normal.

Differential Diagnosis

- Differential diagnoses include the following:
  - Septic emboli, possibly secondary to subacute bacterial endocarditis
  - Diabetes with a resolving intraretinal hemorrhage
  - Leukemic retinopathy
  - Purtscher's retinopathy, which is associated with trauma, pancreatitis, and disseminated intravascular coagulation disorders
  - CRVO or BRVO
  - Pernicious anemia
  - Sickle-cell disease
  - Systemic lupus erythematosus
  - Collagen vascular disease
  - Anoxia (altitude sickness)
  - Carbon monoxide poisoning
  - Hypertensive retinopathy
  - Birth trauma, with similar changes possibly occurring in the mother after delivery
  - Physical abuse
  - Intracranial hemorrhage

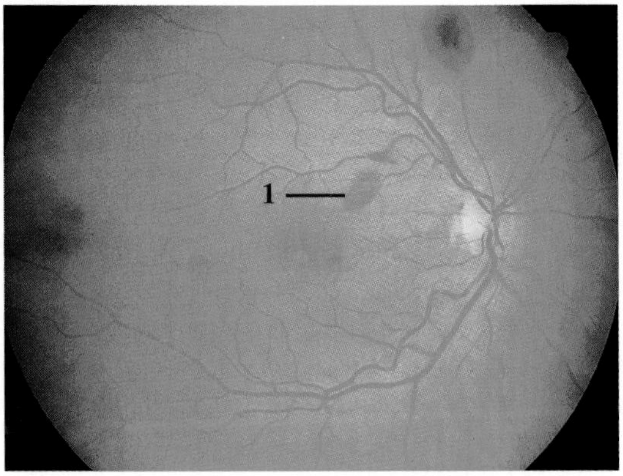

Fig. 9-26 Patient with subacute bacterial endocarditis. A classic Roth spot, or white-centered hemorrhage, is present within the superotemporal arcade *(1)*.

CYTOMEGALOVIRUS RETINITIS

Currently, approximately 30% to 40% of patients infected with the human immunodeficiency virus (HIV) develop cytomegalovirus (CMV) retinitis at some point, usually after the T-cell lymphocyte count has dropped below 50/mm^3. These patients require periodic dilated ophthalmoscopic examination. Retinal detachment affects approximately 25% to 40% of those with CMV retinitis. Therefore CMV represents a major source of morbidity in patients affected by HIV. CMV retinitis may also occur in immunosuppressed individuals, such as those receiving transplants and patients with lymphoma or leukemia.

Symptoms

- Many patients have no symptoms.
- Floaters can occur.
- Vision may be blurred or decreased.
- Blind spots in vision (scotomata) occur.
- Flashes (photopsias) may indicate retinal detachment.

NOTE: The appearance of any new visual symptoms in an HIV-positive individual requires a dilated ophthalmologic examination.

Signs

- Keratic precipitates are stellate shaped on the corneal endothelium.
- Vitreous cells are present.
- Patchy areas of retinal whitening have accompanying areas of hemorrhage. This may occur posteriorly or peripherally (Fig. 9-27).
- The leading edge of retinal whitening often has punctate areas of retinal whitening.
- The disorder progresses slowly.

Differential Diagnosis

- Differential diagnoses include the following:
  - Acute retinal necrosis, or progressive outer retinal necrosis, a rapidly progressive retinitis with a poor prognosis that requires immediate treatment and that has varicella-zoster virus as the presumed etiologic agent

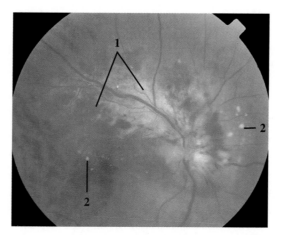

Fig. 9-27 Sight-threatening CMV retinitis involves the macula and optic nerve of this HIV-positive young man. White, infected retina with intraretinal hemorrhage is present in the arcuate distribution of the nerve fiber layer *(1)*. A small amount of lipid exudation near the fovea and nasal to the optic nerve is also seen *(2)*.

- Toxoplasmosis, a more active vitritis, usually associated with an old chorioretinal scar
- HIV retinopathy, including cotton-wool spots and retinal hemorrhages
- Infectious causes such as tuberculosis, syphilis, *Pneumocystis carinii, Mycobacterium avium-intracellulare,* histoplasmosis, blastomycosis, coccidioidomycosis, and Candida and *Aspergillus* infections

Treatment

- For intravenous ganciclovir the induction dosage is 5 mg/kg 2 times a day for 2 to 3 weeks followed by intravenous maintenance therapy of 5 mg/kg daily. The primary side effect is neutropenia.
- For intravenous foscarnet the induction dosage of 90 mg/kg 2 times a day for 2 to 3 weeks followed by intravenous maintenance therapy of 90 to 120 mg/kg daily. Adequate hydration is essential to minimize the primary toxicity (nephrotoxicity). Nausea is common.
- For intravenous cidofovir the dosage is 5 mg/kg weekly combined with oral probenecid (2 g 3 hours preinjection and 2 and 8 hours postinjection). Dosages are modified if a change in renal functioning occurs.
- Reinduction may be required with progression of disease while the patient is receiving maintenance therapy.
- The combination therapy of ganciclovir and foscarnet is used when CMV disease is unresponsive to monotherapy or resistance is suspected.

- For oral ganciclovir the dosage is 1 g 3 times a day. Patients using oral ganciclovir for maintenance therapy may have a greater risk of disease progression.
- Intravitreal administration of ganciclovir or foscarnet is delivered weekly by an ophthalmologist.
- An intravitreal ganciclovir implant necessitates surgery and does not provide a prophylactic effect against systemic or fellow eye CMV involvement. The implant must be replaced every 8 months. Intraocular levels are 5 times higher than with intravenous treatment.
- Many newer agents are currently being investigated.

Follow-Up

- If the retinitis can be controlled with medication, vision may remain normal. Sight-threatening disease occurs when the optic nerve or macula is involved.
- Retinal detachment may also cause sudden vision loss; surgical management must be considered in these cases.
- The risk of contralateral eye involvement with CMV retinitis while the patient is being treated with intravenous ganciclovir is approximately 20%.
- Primary care physicians should keep in mind that all antiviral therapy is virostatic only; if the patient discontinues treatment, CMV retinitis will recur.

TOXOPLASMOSIS

Toxoplasma gondii is an obligate intracellular parasite common among humans and animals (e.g., cats). Ocular toxoplasmosis is a potentially blinding, necrotizing retinitis that may recur.

Symptoms

- Vision is blurred or decreased.
- Wavy or distorted vision (metamorphopsia) may occur.
- Floaters may be seen.
- Pain is variable.

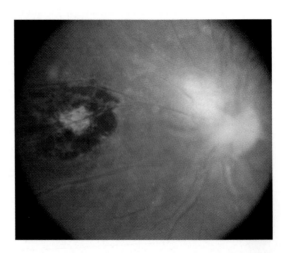

Fig. 9-28 Left eye of a young man with elevated toxoplasmosis titers. Note the old, healed toxoplasmosis lesion *(black)* nasal to the optic nerve. The optic nerve has an area of whitening with overlying vitreous cells that obscure the disc margin.

Signs

- Vitreous debris is seen.
- Iritis or cells are present in the anterior chamber.
- Yellow-white areas of retinitis are observed.
- The optic nerve is yellow-white and swollen (Fig. 9-28).
- Retinal vascular infiltrates (periarteritis) can occur.
- Old chorioretinal scars are found in the affected or fellow eye.
- Macular edema can occur.

Differential Diagnosis

- Differential diagnoses include the following:
  - Uveitis
  - Sarcoidosis
  - Acute retinal necrosis, with herpes zoster infection the presumed etiologic process
  - *Toxocara canis* infection, syphilis, and HIV infection

Treatment

- Treatment of sight-threatening lesions, that is, those involving the macula and optic nerve or those with significant intraocular inflammation, is as follows:
  - "Triple therapy" for 4 to 6 weeks:
    - Pyramethamine and folate
    - Sulfadiazine, sulfisoxazole, or Triple Sulfa
    - Clindamycin
  - Alternatively, trimethoprim and sulfamethoxazole (Bactrim DS)
  - Oral prednisone—40 to 60 mg every day for 3 to 4 weeks, then tapering: used to limit the inflammation-mediated retinal destruction

POSTSURGICAL ENDOPHTHALMITIS

Any invasive ophthalmologic procedure may result in endophthalmitis and should be ruled out or confirmed as the cause in all cases of significant postoperative pain or inflammation.

Symptoms

- Pain is not always present.
- Redness occurs.
- Vision is decreased.
- Floaters are seen.

Signs

- Hypopyon, or cells in the anterior chamber, are observed (Fig. 9-29).
- Conjunctival injection is present.
- Hazy vitreous or obscuration of the posterior pole (vitritis) occurs.

Treatment

- The current standard of care involves either a vitreous culture with an intraocular injection of antibiotics or vitreous surgery with intravitreal injection of antibiotics.
- Immediate ophthalmologic referral is essential when endophthalmitis is suspected.

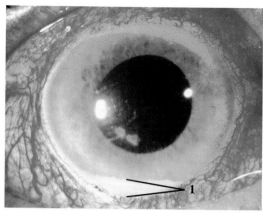

Fig. 9-29 Endophthalmitis. Acute postoperative hypopyon layering in the inferior portion of the anterior chamber *(1)*. Note the conjunctival injection in this painful, infected eye.

TRAUMA-ASSOCIATED ENDOPHTHALMITIS

Any full-thickness wound into the eye (an open globe by definition) requires emergency ophthalmologic evaluation. Posttraumatic endophthalmitis should be suspected in all cases, particularly with trauma involving an intraocular foreign body or a dirty wound. Any patient history suggestive of an intraocular foreign body necessitates radiologic imaging to rule out this injury. Many open globe injuries are treated with intravitreal and/or systemic intravenous antibiotics.

ENDOGENOUS ENDOPHTHALMITIS

Endogenous endophthalmitis results from septic emboli to the retinal or choroidal circulation. Patients are usually sick from the underlying sepsis and manifest with vitritis, focal areas of retinitis, and anterior chamber reaction, ranging from a few cells to a layering of cells in the anterior chamber (hypopyon). Intravenous drug abusers, immunocompromised patients, and hospitalized patients with chronic indwelling catheters or central lines are at risk for endogenous endophthalmitis. *Candida* endophthalmitis usually appears as a small area of focal retinitis that enlarges into a fluffy-white vitreous opacity. Infection may progress to complete opacification of the vitreous. Intravitreal amphotericin and treatment of the systemic infection are indicated. Vitreous surgery may be required in severe cases. Vitreous cultures are helpful and may reveal the causative organism.

POSTERIOR VITREOUS DETACHMENT

Posterior vitreous detachment occurs in most individuals with time. This usually occurs in the fifth to seventh decades of life. Highly myopic (nearsighted) individuals are likely to develop a posterior vitreous detachment at an earlier age because of the larger size of the eye. The vitreous is firmly adherent in the peripheral retina, less firmly adherent at the optic nerve and along the major retinal vessels, and weakly adherent along the surface of the retina. As the vitreous separates from the posterior retina, traction is transferred to the peripheral retina, where tears or breaks may occur.

Symptoms

■ Patients report flashing lights.

■ Floaters are seen.

Treatment

■ Because the symptoms of a posterior vitreous detachment may herald a retinal detachment, indirect ophthalmoscopy by an ophthalmologist is required and should be performed within 24 hours of diagnosis.

■ No treatment is indicated.

■ Laser photocoagulation or cryotherapy may be used for any new retinal tears associated with symptoms.

RETINAL DETACHMENT

A retinal detachment occurs when fluid separates the retina from the underlying retinal pigment epithelium; causes of this condition vary. A rhegmatogenous (from the Greek *rhegma,* meaning "breakage") retinal detachment typically occurs when the vitreous separates from the retina (posterior vitreous detachment) and causes a tear or break (Fig. 9-30). Liquefied vitreous fluid then dissects between the retina and retinal pigment epithelium, resulting in a detached retina. Serous or exudative retinal detachments occur from a leakage of fluid caused by a process occurring under the retina without a tear or break in the retina. A tractional retinal detachment results from scar tissue formation in the vitreous gel, leading to centripetal traction forces on the retina toward the center of the eye. Tractional retinal detachments commonly occur with proliferative diabetic retinopathy as the result of repeated vitreous hemorrhage.

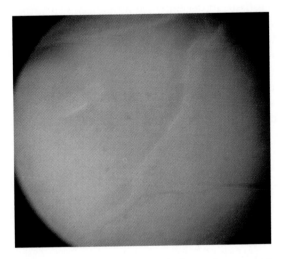

Fig. 9-30 Horseshoe-shaped retinal tear that occurred after a posterior vitreous detachment and led to a retinal detachment.

Symptoms

- Flashes occur.
- Floaters are seen.
- A visual field loss occurs, which patients often describe as a curtain, shadow, or bubble of fluid.
- Vision is wavy or distorted (metamorphopsia).
- Vision is decreased.

Signs

- A relative afferent pupillary defect is observed.
- The visual field loss is unilateral and may be sectoral, quadrantic, hemifield, or total.
- Retinal hydration lines, or rugae, have an appearance similar to ripples on a pond.

Workup

- Retinal detachments are difficult to diagnose with a direct ophthalmoscope. A simple technique using a direct ophthalmoscope allows the clinician to compare the red reflexes of the two eyes from a distance of several feet. Any differences in the quality of the reflex should be evaluated. An eye with a retinal detachment may have a lighter-colored reflex (yellow or orange) in the affected eye.

Treatment

- Patients should be referred for immediate ophthalmologic evaluation.
- Surgical intervention is necessary because untreated retinal detachments may lead to blindness in the affected eye.

EPIRETINAL MEMBRANE

A thin sheet of fibrous tissue, or an epiretinal membrane, may form on the surface of the retina, often after a posterior vitreous retinal detachment. Contraction of the membrane wrinkles and distorts the retina.

Symptoms

- Vision is decreased.
- Vision is wavy or distorted (metamorphopsia).
- Patients report difficulty reading with the affected eye.

Signs

- Amsler grid distortion is seen.
- A whitish, folded membrane is evident on the retinal surface (Fig. 9-31).
- The retinal vasculature is distorted.
- Macular edema may be present.

Treatment

- Ophthalmologic referral is indicated.
- Occasionally an epiretinal membrane breaks free from the retina and vision spontaneously improves. If the patient's vision is minimally affected, no treatment is required.

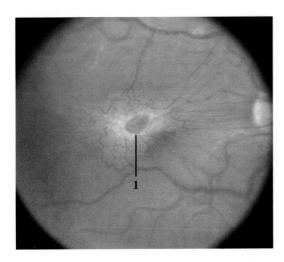

Fig. 9-31 Epiretinal membrane *(1)* that is contracting and pulling the retinal elements centrally with accompanying wrinkles, folds, and vascular distortions.

■ If vision is significantly affected (usually 20/50 to 20/70 or worse), surgical removal of the membrane is necessary to improve the vision and distortion.

Follow-Up
■ The overall visual prognosis is good.

VITREOUS HEMORRHAGE

Vitreous hemorrhage is the result of an underlying vascular process and occurs in many disorders. Because visualization of the retina may be impossible, ophthalmic echography may be needed to determine the presence of an accompanying retinal detachment. Treatment is directed at the underlying etiologic process.

Differential Diagnosis
■ Differential diagnoses include the following:
  • Proliferative diabetic retinopathy
  • Posterior vitreous detachment with an avulsed retinal vessel
  • Retinal tear through a vessel (with or without a retinal detachment)
  • Macroaneurysm
  • Trauma
  • Subarachnoid or subdural hematoma (Terson's syndrome)
  • Any retinal vascular lesion

RETINAL SURGERY

Advancements in retinal surgery over the last 20 to 30 years have been dramatic because of the development of microsurgical techniques and a better understanding of complex biologic processes. Many formerly blinding conditions such as diabetic retinopathy and

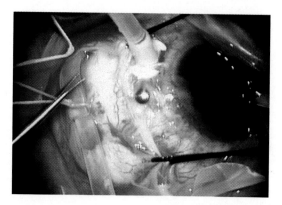

Fig. 9-32 The external placement of a silicone scleral buckle. The element is sewn to the scleral surface. Note that black silk sutures are supporting the rectus muscles. The white infusion tubing and gold plug represent sclerotomy entry sites into the eye for vitreous dissection instrumentation.

recurrent retinal detachments can now be managed more effectively. The two primary forms of retinal surgery are scleral buckling and vitrectomy surgery. The primary indication for surgery is a retinal detachment.

Standard scleral buckling surgery usually involves the placement of a solid silicone band around the equator of the eye to relieve the internal traction and support the eye wall under the retinal tear (Fig. 9-32). The scleral buckle alters the internal fluid dynamics and decreases the rate of subretinal fluid accumulation. Either laser treatment or cryotherapy is used to form an adhesion of the retina to the underlying choroid in the area of the tear. A buckle and the chorioretinal adhesion reattach most rhegmatogenous retinal detachments. In certain situations an intraocular gas bubble may be used to reattach the retina (pneumatic retinopexy).

The surgeon begins a vitrectomy by making three small incisions in the sclera (sclerotomies) of the eye. One sclerotomy accommodates an infusion line; the other two are used for instrumentation of the posterior segment of the eye. The surgeon views the inside of the eye through a surgical microscope that contains various contact lenses and prisms and uses illuminated picks, scissors, and forceps to perform delicate dissections of scar or proliferative tissue from the retinal surface. Heavy liquids, air, gas, or silicone oil may be used to reattach the retina. Laser photocoagulation seals the retinal tear and may be used to treat ischemic retina (panretinal photocoagulation).

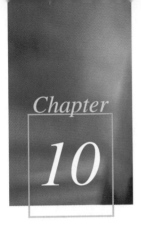

Glaucoma

Allen D. Beck

ANATOMY

Aqueous humor is produced by the epithelium of the ciliary body (Fig. 10-1). The aqueous flows past the lens, around the iris, into Schlemm's canal via the trabecular meshwork, and then into aqueous and episcleral veins. The trabecular meshwork is the site of the greatest resistance to aqueous outflow and is located at the junction between the cornea and iris. This region of the eye is referred to as the *anterior chamber angle.* The entire volume of aqueous is turned over approximately every 100 minutes. Intraocular pressure (IOP) is determined by the balance between the production and outflow of aqueous humor. The range of normal IOP is 10 to 21 mm Hg. An intraocular pressure of 22 mm Hg or greater is considered abnormal. Diurnal variations in IOP are well documented for both normal and glaucomatous individuals. These IOP swings mean that the IOP may be in the normal

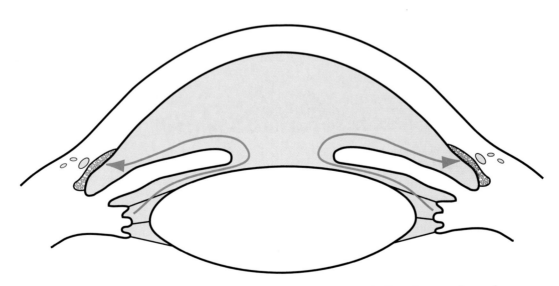

Fig. 10-1 Anatomy of the anterior portion of the eye demonstrating the flow of aqueous humor from the ciliary body to the trabecular meshwork.

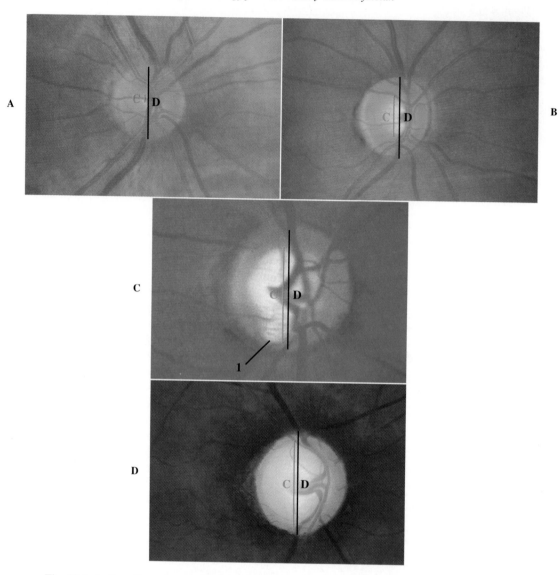

Fig. 10-2 A, Cup-disc ratio of 0.1. **B,** Cup-disc ratio of 0.5. **C,** Cup-disc ratio of 0.8 vertically with inferior notching *(1)* of the nerve. **D,** Cup-disc ratio of 0.90 vertically. *C,* Cup; *D,* disc.

range at certain times of the day in patients with glaucoma. Damage from glaucoma is manifested by optic nerve cupping (Fig. 10-2). Loss of neurons and glial tissue causes glaucomatous cupping secondary to mechanical and ischemic mechanisms. The damage to the optic nerve results in characteristic patterns of visual field loss (Fig. 10-3). Visual field loss in glaucoma classically respects the horizontal meridian. Visual acuity and the central visual field usually remain normal until late in the disease process.

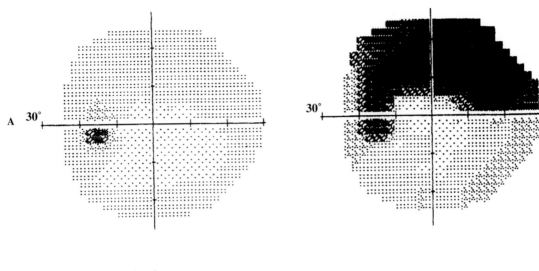

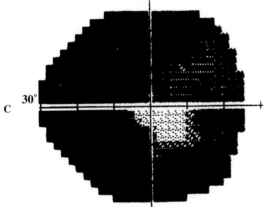

Fig. 10-3 A, Normal automated visual field. Light areas mean the test object is seen normally. Dark areas in the field mean the test object is seen poorly or not at all. The one dark area in the field represents the physiologic blind spot created by the optic nerve. **B,** Glaucomatous visual field demonstrating dense loss of the superior field with respect to the horizontal meridian. **C,** Advanced glaucomatous visual field loss demonstrating preservation of the central visual field. The visual acuity is near normal (20/25) despite advanced visual field loss.

DEFINITIONS AND EPIDEMIOLOGY

The term *glaucoma* refers to a group of diseases with progressive optic nerve damage and visual field loss. In most cases of glaucoma the IOP is consistently above the normal range, although in some cases the IOP may always be within the normal range. The prevalence of glaucoma is approximately 0.5% of the total population. Elevated IOP without signs of optic nerve or visual field damage (ocular hypertension) occurs in approximately 1.5% of the total population. Glaucoma can be broadly categorized into open-angle glaucoma and angle-closure glaucoma. Most cases of glaucoma are open angle, which means that the eye has a structurally normal outflow pathway (see Fig. 10-1). In angle-closure glaucoma, blockage of aqueous flow between the lens and iris causes a forward shifting of the iris and closure of the anterior chamber angle (Fig. 10-4). Patients with angle-closure glaucoma may experience acute symptoms of severe pain and blurred vision, and those with a chronic form of angle-closure glaucoma have slow elevation of IOP and no symptoms.

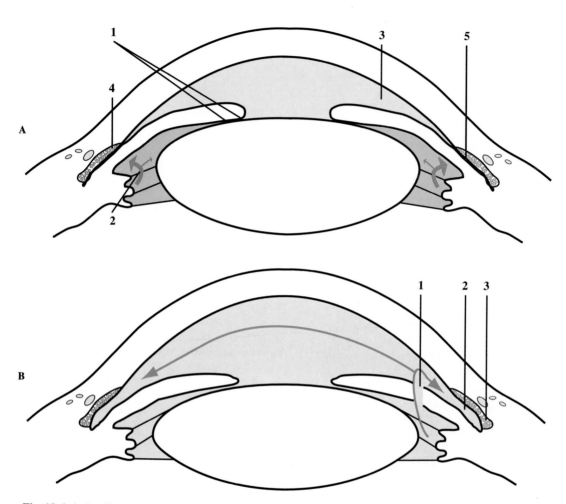

Fig. 10-4 A, Pupillary block prevents flow of aqueous into the anterior chamber. The iris is pressed firmly against the lens *(1),* blocking aqueous flow *(2)* into the anterior chamber *(3).* Instead, the iris is pushed against the trabecular meshwork *(4).* The peripheral anterior chamber angle is thus closed *(5),* blocking aqueous outflow and raising the IOP. **B,** A small hole in the peripheral iris *(1)* is made with a laser (laser iridectomy) and allows aqueous to enter the anterior chamber of the eye. This opens the anterior chamber angle *(2)* and allows aqueous to drain normally through the trabecular meshwork *(3).*

OPEN-ANGLE GLAUCOMA

Symptoms

- Patients usually have no symptoms although decreased vision may be noted late in the disease course.

Signs

- IOP is elevated.
- Optic nerve cupping occurs (see Fig. 10-2).

Associated Factors and Diseases

- Increasing patient age is associated with a progressive increase in the prevalence of glaucoma.
- Glaucoma is more prevalent, develops at an ealier age, and is more severe in African-Americans as compared with white individuals.
- A family history of open-angle glaucoma is associated with a fivefold to sixfold increase in the risk of glaucoma development.
- The prevalence of ocular hypertension in patients with diabetes mellitus is 2 to 3 times higher than in the general population. The possibility of an increased risk of ocular hypertension in patients with systemic hypertension has not been determined definitively.

Workup

- *Measurement of IOP* (see Chapter 1): The gold standard is Goldmann applanation tonometry. IOP is determined by measurement of the force required to flatten the central cornea. Fluorescein dye and a topical anesthetic are required, as is skill in interpretation of the fluorescent semicircles to determine the IOP directly by a scale associated with this device.

  A relatively new device, the Tono-Pen, can be used more easily to measure IOP. Multiple applanation measurements are averaged by this instrument, which displays the IOP as a digital readout. Greater cost is one drawback to the Tono-Pen.
- *Pupillary examination:* A relative afferent pupillary defect may be present in asymmetric cases of glaucoma.
- *Ophthalmoscopy:* Evaluation with a direct ophthalmoscope provides important diagnostic clues. Because the IOP may be in the normal range in a patient with glaucoma, the clinician who measures IOP and examines the optic nerve will more likely diagnose glaucoma correctly. A cup-disc ratio of 0.6 or greater is one sign of glaucoma. Asymmetry of 0.2 or greater in the cup-disc ratio and focal asymmetry in the neuroretinal rim are also highly suggestive. Dilation of the pupil with tropicamide 1% and phenylephrine 2.5% ophthalmic solutions greatly facilitates optic nerve evaluation.
- Eyes with a narrow chamber angle should not be dilated. (A simple penlight test for this condition is shown in Fig. 10-5.)

Treatment

- Any patient with abnormal findings on optic nerve examination, an afferent pupillary deficit, or an elevated IOP should be referred to an ophthalmologist for evaluation and possible treatment.

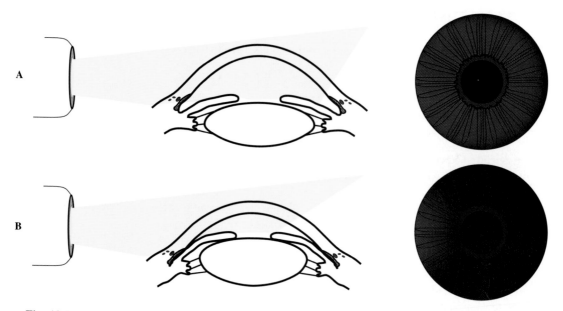

Fig. 10-5 Use of the penlight to demonstrate a shallow anterior chamber. **A,** A penlight aimed obliquely to the eye will illuminate nearly the entire iris with a deep anterior chamber. **B,** With a shallow anterior chamber, only a portion of the iris is illuminated, with shadowing over the remainder.

Fig. 10-6 The whitish, elevated area on the superior portion of the eye is a filtering bleb in a patient with open-angle glaucoma.

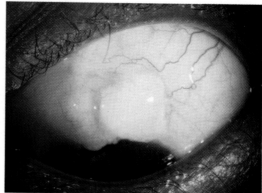

- Treatment usually begins with medication:
  - Medications work by one of two methods to lower IOP: decreasing the production of aqueous or increasing the outflow of aqueous. Medications that decrease aqueous production include topical β-blockers (Timoptic, Betagan, Betoptic, Ocupress, Optipranolol, and Betimol), oral carbonic anhydrase inhibitors (Diamox and Neptazane), a topical carbonic anhydrase inhibitor (Trusopt), and alpha-2 agonists (Iopidine and Alphagan). Medications that improve aqueous outflow include topical miotic agents (Pilocar, Pilostat, Pilagan, Isopto Carpine, Isopto carbachol, and Phospholine Iodide), a prostaglandin analog (Xalatan), and epinephrine preparations (Epifrin, Epitrate, Glaucon, and Propine).

- Eyedrops gain access to the systemic circulation via the nasal mucosa of the naso-lacrimal system, and systemic side effects can be noted with these medications (see Chapter 16).
- Surgical options include the following:
  - Open-angle glaucoma not responsive to medical treatment can be treated with laser and incisional surgery.
  - Laser trabeculoplasty involves placement of multiple, low-energy burns to the trabecular meshwork, decreasing the IOP significantly in approximately 80% of cases.
  - Trabeculectomy bypasses the normal outflow pathway by the creation of a surgical fistula. An elevation of the conjunctiva known as a *filtering bleb* is a sign of a successful trabeculectomy (Fig. 10-6).
  - Conjunctivitis associated with a filtering bleb should prompt immediate referral to an ophthalmologist because of the risk of infection spreading inside the eye (endophthalmitis).

ACUTE ANGLE-CLOSURE GLAUCOMA

Symptoms

- Vision is blurred, usually in one eye.
- Halos are seen around light fixtures (almost always uniocular).
- Intense ocular pain and photophobia occur.
- Vasovagal symptoms such as diaphoresis, nausea, and vomiting are possible.

Signs

- A middilated pupil is seen (Fig. 10-7).
- Conjunctival injection and lid edema are present.
- Corneal edema with blurring of the light reflex occurs.
- IOP is markedly elevated, often 60 to 80 mm Hg.

Associated Factors and Diseases

- Women are affected 3 to 4 times more commonly than men.
- The peak age range for occurrence of angle-closure glaucoma is between the ages of 55 and 70 years.
- The disorder occurs in shorter, smaller, far-sighted eyes with narrow chamber angles (see Fig. 10-5).
- Stress, a darkened room, and drugs that can dilate the pupil may precipitate an acute angle-closure attack. Many systemic medications with anticholinergic or sympathomimetic action carry a warning against use in persons with glaucoma. This applies to patients with a narrow chamber angle only, not to patients with open-angle glaucoma. Because most glaucoma cases are open angle, these medications are rarely contraindicated in medical practice. Consultation with the patient's ophthalmologist is recommended for the primary care physician if a question arises over a possible medication contraindication.

Treatment

- Acute angle-closure glaucoma is an ophthalmic emergency and requires *immediate* referral to an ophthalmologist.

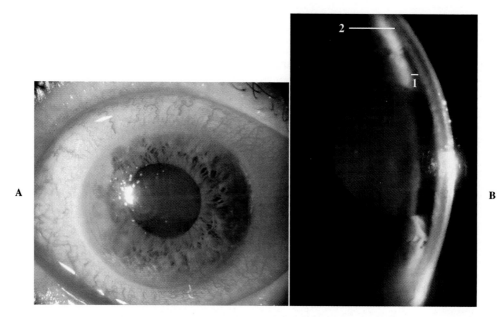

Fig. 10-7 Acute angle-closure glaucoma. **A,** Acutely elevated pressure produces an inflamed eye with corneal edema (note fragmented light reflex) and a middilated pupil. **B,** Slit-lamp examination shows a very shallow central anterior chamber (space between cornea and iris) *(1)* and no peripheral chamber *(2).*

- Initial medical treatment to lower the IOP involves a topical β-blocker (e.g., timolol 0.5%—1 drop), carbonic anhydrase inhibitors (e.g., Diamox 500 mg intravenously or 250 mg orally 2 times), and osmotic agents (e.g., oral isosorbide 50 to 100 g or intravenous mannitol 1 to 2 g/kg given over 45 minutes—500 ml of mannitol 20% contains 100 g of mannitol).
- In most cases, laser iridectomy (creating a full-thickness opening in the peripheral iris) reopens at least a portion of the angle with marked lowering of the IOP (see Fig. 10-4).

Follow-Up

- After an acute angle-closure event, a portion of the angle may remain closed because of scarring of peripheral iris tissue to the cornea, causing chronic angle-closure glaucoma. Chronic angle-closure glaucoma may also occur without any symptoms, just like open-angle glaucoma. Treatment involves medications and incisional surgery such as trabeculectomy. Laser trabeculoplasty is not effective. Laser iridectomy may be recommended for individuals with very narrow angles who are at significant risk for the development of either acute or chronic angle-closure glaucoma.

Neuroophthalmology

Timothy J. Martin

ANATOMY

The visual pathways extend from the front of the cranium (the eyes) to the most posterior aspect of the brain (the occipital cortex). As a result of this structural intracranial arrangement, patients with pathologic conditions frequently are first seen because of vision loss.

Nerve Fiber Layer and the Optic Nerve

Over 120 million photoreceptors in the retina receive the image focused by the cornea and lens. Initial processsing takes place in the retina, with approximately 1 million ganglion cells sending axons to the brain forming the optic nerve. These axons traverse the innermost layer of the retina in a peculiar pattern; they arch above and below the sensitive fovea to form the optic nerve. The pattern of visual field loss in optic nerve disease reflects the course and organization of these nerve fibers, producing visual field defects that generally respect the horizontal meridian.

Chiasm and Posterior Visual Pathways

Axons from ganglion cells representing right visual space are routed through the chiasm (with nasal retinal axons from the right eye crossing in the chiasm and joining temporal retina axons from the left) to form the left optic tract, synapsing in the left lateral geniculate body (and vice versa for left visual space) (Fig. 11-1). Thus lesions posterior to the chiasm produce homonymous visual field defects (field loss on the same side in both eyes) that respect the vertical meridian. From the lateral geniculate body, superior fibers representing the inferior visual field travel directly through the parietal lobe to the occipital cortex to synapse in the superior occipital lobe. Inferior fibers take a more indirect route, sweeping around the temporal horn of the ventricular system (Meyer's loop) and through the temporal lobe to neurons in the inferior occipital cortex. From the chiasm posteriorly, corresponding axons from the right and left eyes that represent the same point in visual space move closer together as they converge on a common point in the occipital cortex. Thus the more posterior a lesion is, the more congruous the resultant visual field defects become: homonymous visual defects in each eye look more alike in shape.

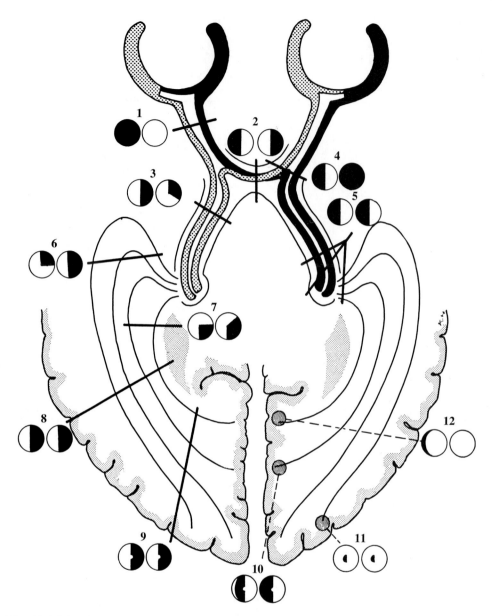

Fig. 11-1 The visual system and visual field defects resulting from lesions at various points in the visual pathway. An optic nerve lesion only affects the visual field of one eye *(1)*. However, bilateral optic nerve lesions are not uncommon. Lesions of the body of the chiasm tend to produce bilateral temporal visual field defects *(2)* (see also Fig. 11-9). Optic tract lesions (and all lesions posterior) produce defects that are homonymous on the same side in both eyes *(3)*. Lesions at the junction of the optic nerve and chiasm severely affect vision in the ipsilateral eye but produce an often asymptomatic temporal peripheral visual field defect in the contralateral eye *(4)*. Complete homonymous hemianopic visual field defects are nonlocalizing; that is, they can occur anywhere from the optic tract to the occipital lobe *(5* and *8)*. A unilateral homonymous hemianopia does not decrease visual acuity. Lesions in the temporal lobe produce superior homonymous defects *(6)*. Parietal lesions cause inferior homonymous defects *(7)*. Occipital lobe lesions are highly congruous *(9* to *11)*. Bilateral occipital infarctions can profoundly affect visual acuity and visual fields bilaterally, with normal-appearing fundi and normal pupillary responses.

OPTIC NERVE DISORDERS

The optic disc is the proximal end of the optic nerve and can be observed with the ophthalmoscope. Optic nerve lesions may produce visible disc edema (swelling), infiltration, pallor, or pathologic cupping (from glaucoma). Lesions of the nerve more distant from the disc may not cause any observable optic disc abnormality acutely (such as retrobulbar optic neuritis), but with time the normal pink color of the neural rim turns pale.

NONARTERITIC ANTERIOR ISCHEMIC OPTIC NEUROPATHY

Symptoms

■ A sudden, painless loss of vision occurs, frequently noted on arising in the morning.

Signs

■ Patients are usually older than 40 years.
■ The unilateral swollen optic disc, often segmental and containing flame-shaped hemorrhages, results in optic disc pallor as the edema resolves over 4 to 6 weeks (Fig. 11-2, *A* and *B*).

A

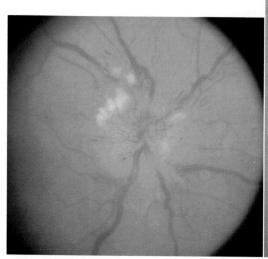

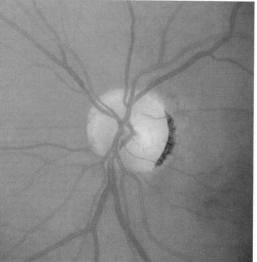

B

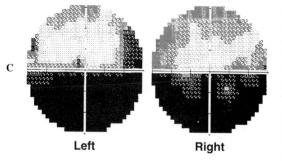

C

Left   **Right**

Fig. 11-2 Nonarteritic anterior ischemic optic neuropathy in a 49-year-old man with diabetes. This patient was initially seen with sudden, painless vision loss in his right eye. Approximately 2 years before, he had a similar event in his left eye. **A,** Right optic disc shows optic disc edema, flame-shaped hemorrhage, and cotton-wool spot concentrated on upper half of the disc. **B,** Left, previously affected disc shows pallor of upper disc (sectoral pallor), with some pink still present inferiorly. **C,** Bilateral inferior altitudinal visual field defects were present (corresponding to superior optic disc events).

■ An altitudinal (upper or lower quadrants) visual field defect is common (Fig. 11-2, *C*).
■ A relative afferent pupillary defect is present if the fellow eye is normal.

Etiology and Associated Factors and Diseases
■ Vision loss results from atherosclerotic or thrombotic occlusion of arteries supplying the optic disc.
■ Hemodynamic compromise is a potential cause, occurring in patients with severe hypotension or blood loss.
■ The disorder is associated with hypertension, diabetes, coronary artery disease, and other vasculopathic conditions.

Differential Diagnosis
■ Differential diagnoses include the following:
  • Arteritic anterior ischemic optic neuropathy (giant cell arteritis)
  • Optic neuritis
  • Infiltrative optic neuropathy
  • Asymmetric papilledema
  • Compressive optic neuropathy

Workup
■ Westergren erythrocyte sedimentation rate testing should be performed to look for evidence of vasculitis.
■ Medical evaluation for hypertension, diabetes, and anemia is indicated.
■ Neuroimaging may be required in uncertain or progressive cases.

Treatment
■ No treatment has been proved effective; intravenous and oral steroids are of uncertain help.
■ Daily aspirin may reduce the incidence of an episode in the fellow eye.

Follow-Up
■ Visual field testing should be performed at 2 weeks and 2 months.
■ Progression of visual deficits may require more extensive investigation such as neuroimaging.
■ Mild improvement in the central vision may occur in about 50% of patients. Simultaneous or rapidly sequential anterior ischemic optic neuropathy (both eyes within a few months) suggests arteritis.

GIANT CELL ARTERITIS: ARTERITIC ANTERIOR ISCHEMIC OPTIC NEUROPATHY
Symptoms
■ A sudden vision loss occurs in one or both eyes.
■ Vision loss is frequently extreme.
■ Systemic symptoms include headache, scalp and temple tenderness, myalgia, arthralgia, low-grade fever, anemia, malaise, weight loss, anorexia, and jaw claudication.

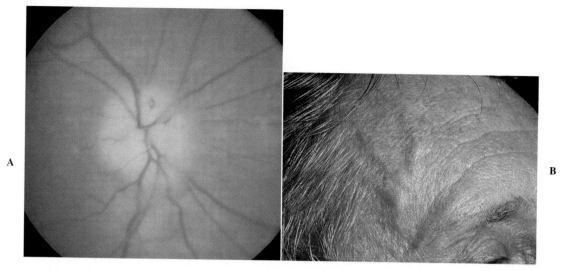

Fig. 11-3 Arteritic anterior ischemic optic neuropathy (giant cell arteritis). A 73-year-old man noted the progressive decline of vision in his right eye to no light perception over 2 days. He experienced headaches and malaise over several weeks. Although his erythrocyte sedimentation rate was only 33, he was immediately admitted for high-dose intravenous corticosteroids for suspected giant cell arteritis. **A,** Pale swelling of the right optic disc, characteristic of arteritic anterior ischemic optic neuropathy. The left optic disc (not shown) is normal. **B,** The temporal artery was firm, pulseless, and tender. A temporal artery biopsy confirmed the diagnosis of giant cell arteritis.

Signs

- The frequency of the disorder increases with each successive decade of life: younger than 50 years of age, it is very rare; at ages 50 to 59 years, it occurs occasionally. Most cases occur in patients 60 years of age or older.
- Pale optic disc swelling or only minimal optic disc changes occur that seem out of proportion to vision loss (Fig. 11-3, *A*).
- Temporal arteries are often firm, tender, or pulseless (Fig. 11-3, *B*).
- The erythrocyte sedimentation rate is generally greater than 50 but can occasionally be normal.
- Mild anemia commonly occurs.
- A third, fourth, or sixth cranial nerve palsy may also occur, as can vision loss from a central retinal artery occlusion.
- A relative afferent pupillary defect is present in unilateral cases.

Etiology

- Vision loss is caused by vasculitic occlusion of arteries to the optic disc.

Differential Diagnosis

- Differential diagnoses include the following:
  - Nonarteritic anterior ischemic optic neuropathy (when disc edema present)
  - Compressive optic neuropathy (especially with minimal disc signs)

Workup

- Measurement of the erythrocyte sedimentation rate should be performed immediately.
- A temporal artery biopsy should be performed within days of corticosteroid administration.
- Neuroimaging may be needed if the diagnosis is uncertain.
- An ophthalmology consultation should be obtained to aid in the diagnosis and management of vision loss.
- Chest x-ray imaging, electrolyte levels, and blood glucose level are needed to evaluate existing medical problems that may be exacerbated by corticosteroid administration, such as tuberculosis, diabetes, and hypertension. If the patient has a history of a positive tuberculin test, empiric isoniazid therapy should be considered.

Treatment

- Corticosteroids are administered immediately: intravenous methylprednisolone 250 mg every 6 hours for 3 days with acute vision loss (followed by oral, daily prednisone) or prednisone 80 to 100 mg orally if giant cell arteritis is suspected but no vision loss has occurred.

Follow-Up

- A second biopsy of the contralateral temporal artery or other tender scalp artery is recommended if the first biopsy results are negative but a strong clinical suspicion remains.
- Long-term corticosteroid use (with slow taper, following erythrocyte sedimentation rate at intervals) requires careful medical support to monitor the potentially serious side effects.

OPTIC NEURITIS

Symptoms

- A unilateral vision loss occurs over several days.
- Pain with eye movement is common.
- Patients may relate a history of transient neurologic disturbances.
- Spontaneous recovery occurs over weeks.

Signs

- The age of patients is usually 15 to 45 years.
- Two thirds of patients initially have normal-appearing discs; one third have optic disc edema.
- Central visual field loss is common, but any disc-related visual field defect (such as altitudinal) may be present (Fig. 11-4).
- A relative afferent pupillary defect is usually present in the affected eye but may be absent if a previous event occurred in the fellow eye.
- Spontaneous, near complete recovery of visual deficit occurs within months in most cases.

Etiology

- The disorder results from demyelination of the optic nerve, with either an idiopathic origin or in association with multiple sclerosis.
- In some cases the disorder is presumed to have a postviral origin.

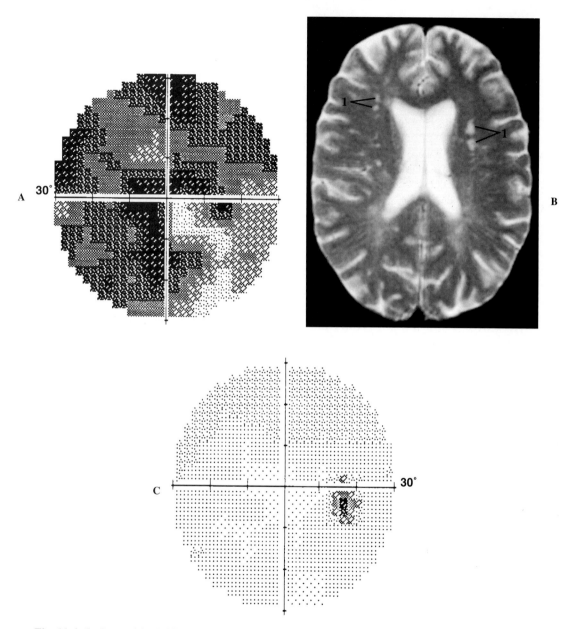

Fig. 11-4 Optic neuritis. A 32-year-old woman noted progressive decline in the vision of her right eye over 5 days, as well as pain with eye movement. The optic discs and fundus were normal, but a large relative afferent pupillary defect was present in the right eye. **A,** Initial visual field testing, with significant visual field loss and a visual acuity of counting fingers only. **B,** MRI revealed periventricular white matter plaques *(1)* characteristic of multiple sclerosis. **C,** Visual field testing 3 months later was normal, and the visual acuity had improved to 20/20. Although the patient received high-dose intravenous corticosteroids initially, she developed other neurologic dysfunction within a year.

Differential Diagnosis

- In patients with poor vision but normal optic discs initially, the following apply:
  - Compressive optic neuropathy
  - Vasculitis
  - Carcinomatous meningitis
  - Trauma
  - Radiation-induced optic neuropathy
  - Toxic or nutritional optic neuropathy (bilateral)
- In patients with swollen discs, the following apply:
  - Anterior ischemic optic neuropathy
  - Leber's optic neuropathy
  - Hypertensive optic neuropathy
  - Infiltrative or compressive optic neuropathy

Workup

- Ophthalmic evaluation is required to rule out other ocular disease and to perform formal visual field testing.
- Magnetic resonance imaging (MRI) of the brain and orbits with contrast is needed to assess treatment options (see Fig. 11-4, *B*).
- CBC, electrolytes, and chest x-ray imaging should be performed if corticosteroid treatment is anticipated.

Treatment

- For patients with white matter plaques found on MRI, intravenous methyl-prednisolone (250 mg) is administered every 6 hours for 3 days, with an optional 10-day oral corticosteroid taper. This treament reduces future multiple sclerosis–related neurologic events and hastens visual recovery but does not affect final visual outcome.
- For patients without white matter changes found on MRI, intravenous corticosteroid treatment has no proven long-term advantage, but this treatment is often used to hasten recovery in "one-eyed" patients or those with severe vision loss. Oral cortico-steroids must *not* be used alone, since they increase the incidence of recurrence of optic neuritis.

Follow-Up

- Neurologic evaluation is needed for evidence of multiple sclerosis.
- Visual field testing is repeated at intervals to ensure the course of the disease is consistent with optic neuritis. Failure of the patient to improve as expected necessitates additional workup.

PAPILLEDEMA

The term *papilledema* refers to bilateral optic disc edema from elevated intracranial pressure but does not identify the underlying etiologic process. Both brain tumors and pseudo-tumor cerebri (idiopathic intracranial hypertension) produce papilledema in affected patients.

Symptoms

- Headache, nausea, and vomiting occur.
- Brief, transient episodes of vision loss often occur with postural changes.
- Pulsatile tinnitus may occur.
- Horizontal diplopia results from paresis of the sixth cranial nerve.
- Other neurologic dysfunction may be present with an intracranial mass.

Signs

- Optic disc edema is present in both eyes (Fig. 11-5, *A* and *B*).
- Visual loss is not acute, except for enlargement of the blind spot. Chronic papilledema can cause visual field loss (Fig. 11-5, *C*).
- Patients with pseudotumor cerebri are often obese females aged 12 to 40 years.
- Unilateral or bilateral sixth cranial nerve paresis may occur.

Etiology

- Elevated intracranial pressure is caused by the following:
  - Intracranial mass
  - Impediment of cerebrospinal fluid flow—dural sinus thrombosis, arteriovenous malformation, aqueductal stenosis, meningitis, and trauma (e.g., intracranial hematoma, subarachnoid hemorrhage)
  - Idiopathic intracranial hypertension (pseudotumor cerebri) associated with obesity and some medications (vitamin A, some antibiotics such as tetracycline, and corticosteroids)

Differential diagnosis

- Differential diagnoses include the following:
  - Pseudopapilledema (anomalous optic discs)
  - Bilateral optic neuritis
  - Bilateral anterior ischemic optic neuropathy
  - Bilateral infiltrative optic neuropathy (e.g., sarcoidosis, tuberculosis, metastatic cancer)
  - Hypertensive retinopathy ("malignant" hypertension)

Workup

- Blood pressure is measured.
- Neuroimaging (MRI with contrast preferred) is performed immediately to look for a mass or dural sinus thrombosis.
- A lumbar puncture is needed to measure the opening pressure and examine the spinal fluid if neuroimaging is normal.
- Neurosurgery and neurology consultation are necessary for identified causes.
- Ophthalmology and neurology consultation are needed to confirm and follow pseudotumor cerebri and perform formal visual field testing.

Treatment

- For idiopathic intracranial hypertension (pseudotumor cerebri), the following apply:
  - Weight loss (very effective)
  - Acetazolamide (effective)

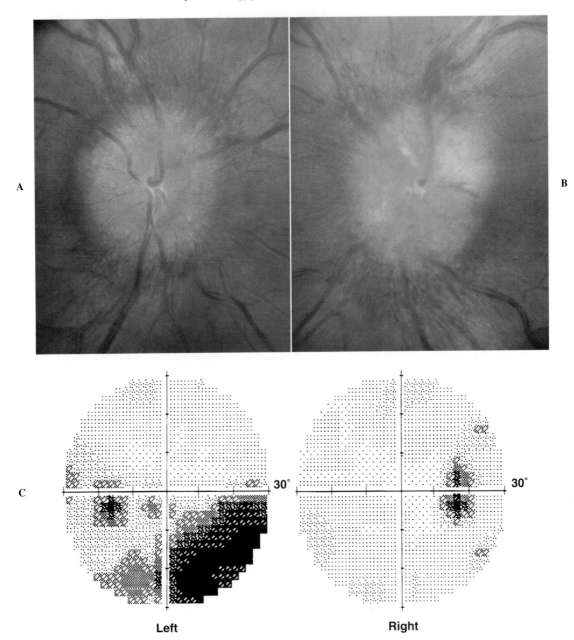

Fig. 11-5 Idiopathic intracranial hypertension (pseudotumor cerebri). A 39-year-old woman had brief episodes of vision loss in both eyes lasting seconds and headache. MRI was normal, and lumbar puncture revealed an opening pressure of 400 mm H_2O. Right eye (**A**) and left eye (**B**) show papilledema (bilateral optic disc swelling from elevated intracranial pressure). **C,** Visual acuity was 20/20 in each eye, with visual field testing demonstrating enlargement of the blind spots bilaterally, and a visual field defect was seen in the left eye. This type of visual field defect ("nasal step") is characteristic of optic disc disease, following the nerve fiber layer pattern and respecting the horizontal meridian.

- Administration of furosemide (less effective)
- Neurosurgical shunt or optic nerve sheath fenestration possibly needed in cases of visual field deterioration despite medical therapy
■ For other conditions such as a mass and dural sinus thrombosis, the etiologic process determines the treatment.

Follow-Up

■ Frequent, formal visual field testing is required in patients with chronic papilledema because their visual acuity may remain 20/20 despite progressive peripheral visual field loss.

OTHER OPTIC NEUROPATHIES

Infiltrative Disorders

■ Lymphoproliferative cells (e.g., lymphoma, leukemia), infectious agents (tuberculosis), or inflammatory (sarcoidosis) granulomas may invade the optic nerve, resulting in an elevated, swollen appearance.
■ Leukemic infiltration of the optic disc with visual loss is a true radiation oncologic emergency; prompt treatment may preserve vision.

Toxic and Nutritional Disorders

■ A slow, bilateral loss of central vision occurs, with mild pallor of the temporal aspect of the optic nerve.
■ Alcohol abuse and a poor diet are common causes, suggesting nutritional and substance abuse consultation; folic acid and thiamine supplementation may improve vision.
■ Other causes include pernicious anemia and heavy metal (lead) toxicity.
■ Medications (e.g., ethambutol, isoniazid, streptomycin, digitalis) are sometimes implicated.

Leber's Optic Neuropathy

■ A rapid, sequential bilateral loss of central vision occurs in young men and occasionally women.
■ Mild disc swelling may occur in acute cases, with disc pallor developing with time.
■ Mitochondrial DNA mutations are passed from often asymptomatic women to their children; however, usually the disorder manifests in males.

Optic Nerve Trauma

■ Traumatic optic nerve injury may be caused by direct trauma from foreign bodies or bony fragments or indirect trauma from a blunt injury to the brow or cranium, even without fractures.
■ The optic disc may appear normal at first, but pallor develops in 4 to 8 weeks.
■ High-dose intravenous corticosteroids may be of benefit during the acute phase.
■ Decompression of the bony optic canal has been advocated by some clinicians.
■ In all cases the presence of associated ocular trauma (e.g., retinal detachment, penetrating injuries) must be determined.

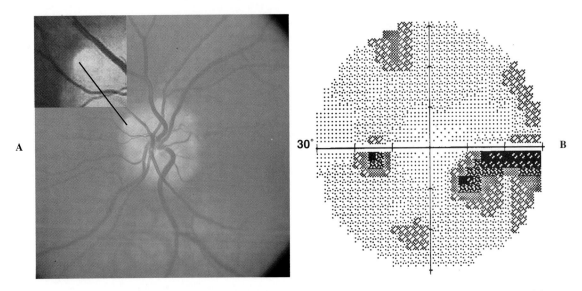

Fig. 11-6 Optic disc drusen in an adult. **A,** Drusen can be seen in this left eye as yellowish-white lumps, giving the disc margin a bumpy, scalloped appearance. **B,** Visual acuity is 20/20, but peripheral visual field loss (nasal step) is present.

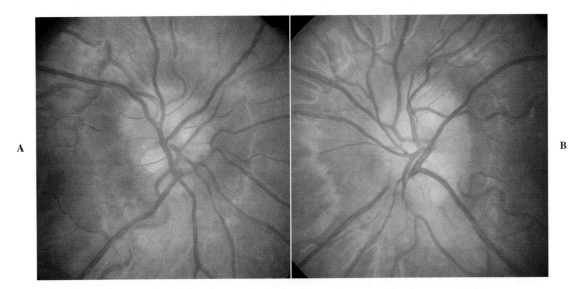

Fig. 11-7 Buried optic disc drusen in a 7-year-old girl. In young people, drusen may be buried deep in the substance of an optic disc. The resulting disc elevation is difficult to distinguish from papilledema. **A,** Right eye. **B,** Left eye.

Optic Nerve Pallor

- Optic nerve pallor is the final common pathway of almost all optic nerve insults.
- If the etiologic process is unknown, neuroimaging is required to look for compressive etiology (e.g., tumor).

Optic Nerve Head Drusen

- Hyaline material is present in the substance of the optic disc (in 1% of population).
- This rocklike, irregular, yellow material may be exposed on the disc surface in older patients (Fig. 11-6, *A*).
- Peripheral visual field defects may occur; however, visual acuity is almost never affected (Fig. 11-6, *B*).
- The occurrence is bilateral in 70% of patients.
- The drusen are often "buried" in young patients, making it difficult for clinicians to distinguish these elevated discs from discs with true edema (Fig. 11-7).

OPTIC NERVE TUMORS

Symptoms

- Vision loss is slow and progressive.
- Proptosis (eye pushed forward) or double vision is possible.

Signs

- Gradual pallor of the optic disc occurs, although it may appear normal early in the disease (Fig. 11-8, *C*).
- Disc edema is possible in anterior lesions.
- Vascular shunt vessels are possible on the optic disc.
- Optic nerve–related visual field defects demonstrate a slow, relentless progression (Fig. 11-8, *B*).
- Nystagmus may be present in children.

Etiology

- In children, optic nerve glioma is most common; 90% are diagnosed before 20 years of age and 25% have neurofibromatosis. The course of the disease is slow in children. In adults, it is very aggressive, resulting in blindness and death.
- Optic nerve meningiomas are more common in adults and originate from the optic nerve sheath or adjacent dural structures.
- Metastatic disease to the orbit may cause compression of the optic nerve.

Differential Diagnosis

- Differential diagnoses include the following:
  - Optic neuritis (especially with vision loss and normal fundus)
  - Other optic neuropathic conditions, including glaucoma
  - Thyroid eye disease, which can cause optic nerve compression, proptosis, and diplopia

Workup

- Neuroimaging (computed tomography or MRI of both brain and orbits with contrast) is needed (Fig. 11-8, *A*).

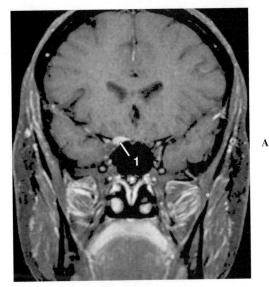

Fig. 11-8 Optic nerve compression. A 32-year-old woman reported gradual loss of vision in her right eye. **A,** MRI showed an enhancing mass *(1)* abutting the right optic nerve, consistent with a meningioma. **B,** Resultant visual field loss in the right eye. **C,** Optic disc pallor in the right eye. **D,** Normal left optic disc.

A

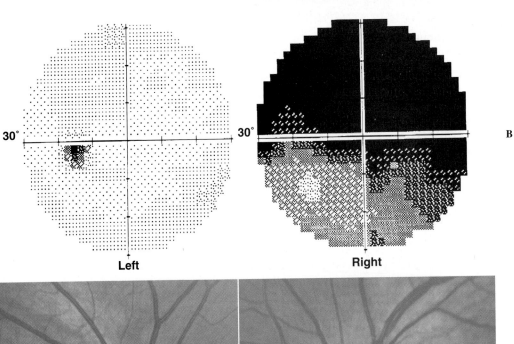

30°   30°   B

Left   Right

C   D

Treatment

■ Consultation with ophthalmology and neurosurgery is required for definitive diagnosis and management.

CHIASMAL COMPRESSION

At the chiasm, axons arising from the nasal and temporal retina begin to separate from each other. The nasal retina fibers cross through the middle of the chiasm into the opposite optic tract; the temporal retinal fibers course along the lateral aspect of the chiasm into the optic tract on the same side. A chiasmal lesion typically interrupts the crossing nasal retinal fibers to produce a bitemporal visual field defect (see Fig. 11-1).

Symptoms

■ Slow, progressive vision loss may occur in one or both eyes.
■ Headache sometimes occurs.
■ Symptoms related to the pituitary dysfunction may be identified.

Signs

■ Insidious optic disc pallor develops over time.
■ Bilateral temporal visual field defects occur with chiasmal compression (Fig. 11-9, *B*).
■ The third through sixth cranial nerves may be affected by tumors that invade the cavernous sinus.

Etiology

■ The disorder may result from pituitary macroadenoma or apoplexy, meningioma, craniopharyngioma, and other sellar masses.

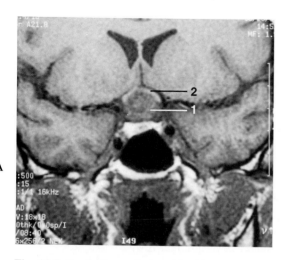

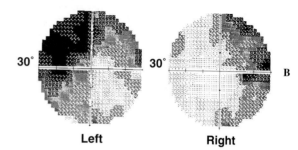

Fig. 11-9 Craniopharyngioma with chiasmal compression. **A,** MRI shows a mass *(1)* elevating and compressing the chiasm *(2).* **B,** Bilateral temporal visual field defects are present.

Differential Diagnosis

- Differential diagnoses include the following:
  - Bilateral optic neuropathies, especially those affecting central vision and enlarging the (temporal) blind spot, such as Leber's and other hereditary optic neuropathies and toxic or nutritional optic neuropathies
  - Anomalous optic discs, in which abnormalities of the retina around the blind spot can produce temporal visual field defects
  - Trauma

Workup

- Neuroimaging (MRI with contrast preferred) is performed with attention to the sella (see Fig. 11-9, *A*).

Treatment

- Neurosurgical consultation is necessary.
- Ophthalmic consultation is necessary for formal visual field testing to follow the progress of the disease, regardless of the therapeutic course.

ANISOCORIA

To evaluate anisocoria, the examiner first determines which pupil is abnormal by noting pupil size in darkness and in light. When the larger pupil is abnormal (does not constrict well), the anisocoria is greatest in bright light (as the normal pupil becomes small). When the smaller pupil is abnormal (does not dilate well), the anisocoria is greatest in darkness (as the normal pupil dilates). As a general rule, the pupil that reacts poorly to direct light is the abnormal pupil. Essential, or physiologic, anisocoria is common, with a small difference in pupillary size (generally less than 1 mm) remaining constant in light and dark. Previous trauma and eye surgery are common causes for different pupil sizes.

LARGER PUPIL ABNORMAL

Etiology, Associated Factors and Diseases, and Differential Diagnosis

- In third nerve palsy, a dilated pupil with ptosis and/or a motility abnormality suggests compression of the third cranial nerve (i.e., an aneurysm). Pupillary dilation in isolation, *without any other sign* of oculomotor nerve dysfunction, is unlikely to result from compression of the third cranial nerve.
- Adie's syndrome results from an often idiopathic insult to the ciliary ganglion in the orbit. Pupillary response is brisk when the patient tries to see a target inches from the nose, but the reaction to light is very poor (Fig. 11-10).
- Pharmacologic causes include instillation of any anticholinergic or sympathomimetic compound into the eye (e.g., dilating drops, contamination from scopolamine patches, jimson weed).
- Because of possible nonneurologic causes such as eye trauma, iritis, angle-closure glaucoma, and eye surgery, patients with anisocoria should have an ophthalmic evaluation.

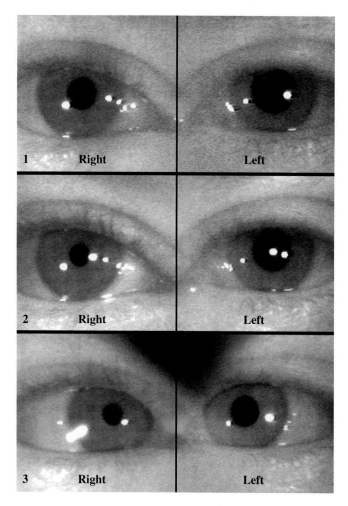

Fig. 11-10 Adie's pupil. In room light the anisocoria is evident *(1)*. In bright light the normal right pupil becomes small, but the affected left eye responds poorly *(2)*. However, with a sustained near focus, the affected pupil does become smaller *(3)*. This finding of a better response to a near stimulus than to a light stimulus is termed *light-near dissociation* and is characteristic of Adie's pupil.

Workup

■ An ophthalmologist may use pharmacologic tests for cholinergic supersensitivity in Adie's pupil, with pilocarpine 0.125% producing marked constriction of the affected pupil and little effect on the normal eye. Pharmacologic dilation with anticholinergic agents can be identified with the use of pilocarpine 1%; this agent does not constrict the affected eye but produces marked constriction in the normal eye.

Treatment

- If a third nerve palsy is suspected as the cause of a dilated pupil, immediate referral to an ophthalmologist (neuroophthalmologist if available), neurologist, and/or neurosurgeon is necessary to evaluate the possibility of an expanding aneurysm.
- If no sign of third nerve dysfunction is present, the patient should be seen again within a week; pharmacologic dilation should have resolved (unless repeated) and the examiner can recheck for any developing signs of third nerve dysfunction.

SMALLER PUPIL ABNORMAL

Etiology, Associated Factors and Diseases, and Differential Diagnosis

- In patients with Horner's syndrome (oculosympathetic paresis), a 1- to 2-mm ptosis is virtually always present. Facial anhydrosis may be more difficult to identify (Fig. 11-11).
- Other causes of a small pupil such as eye trauma, iritis, angle-closure glaucoma, and eye surgery will likely be evident with an ophthalmic evaluation.

Workup

- In a patient with Horner's sydrome an ophthalmologist may use pharmacologic tests to verify an oculosympathetic paresis. Cocaine 10% does not dilate the affected pupil as well as the unaffected eye. Localization of the lesion is also necessary. Hydroxyamphetamine does not dilate the affected pupil well in postganglionic (sympathetic fibers from the superior cervical ganglion in the neck to the eye) lesions. Common etiologic processes for postganglionic lesions include cluster headache, an idiopathic origin, and carotid artery dissection. Preganglionic lesions (affecting fibers from the hypothalamus; through the brainstem, spinal cord, chest cavity, and neck; and to the superior cervical ganglion) are frequently serious (e.g., malignancy, stroke), requiring specialist evaluation and imaging of the brain, neck, and chest.

Treatment

- The underlying etiology determines treatment.

DISORDERS OF THE VISUAL MOTOR SYSTEM

THIRD NERVE PALSY

The third cranial nerve (oculomotor nerve) is complex, innervating all the extraocular muscles (including the levator palpebrae, which elevates the eyelids) except the lateral rectus and superior oblique muscles. It also innervates the pupillary sphincter.

Fig. 11-11 Horner's syndrome. The mild ptosis (1 to 2 mm) and smaller pupil (in room light) can be seen on the affected right side.

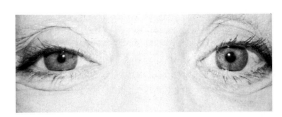

Symptoms

■ A droopy eyelid (ptosis) occurs.

■ Diplopia results if the drooping eyelid does not cover the eye.

■ Headache or periorbital pain is often present, depending on the etiology.

Signs

■ The eye is often turned down and out.

■ The ptosis is total or mild.

■ Deficiencies in raising, lowering, or moving the eye toward the nose may be partial or total (Fig. 11-12).

■ A dilated pupil is more common with compression (aneurysm) than ischemia.

Etiology

■ An ischemic cranial mononeuropathy is a common etiology in patients who are elderly or have vascular risk factors such as hypertension and diabetes.

■ Vasculitis (giant cell arteritis) can cause ischemic cranial neuropathies.

■ Compression by aneurysm, tumor, or uncal herniation can cause third nerve dysfunction.

■ The disorder commonly results from trauma.

Differential Diagnosis

■ Differential diagnoses include the following:
  • Ocular myasthenia gravis
  • Thyroid eye disease
  • Brainstem lesions

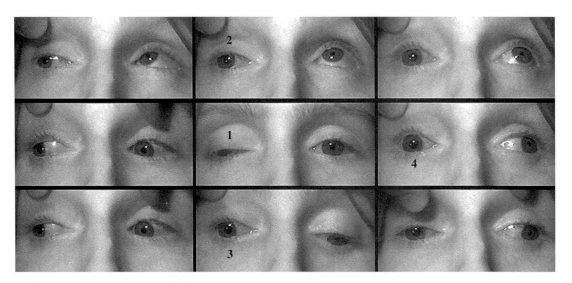

Fig. 11-12 Third cranial neve paresis with pupil involvement. Note the profound right ptosis (lid droop) and the down-and-out position of the right eye *(1)*. Gaze positions demonstrate poor elevation *(2)*, depression *(3)*, and inability to turn the eye inward (adduction) *(4)*. Note the dilated pupil in the affected right eye.

Workup

- MRI of the brain with contrast (and often MR angiography) is required in patients without obvious vascular risk factors.
- Cerebral angiography may be necessary in patients suspected to have an aneurysm, especially younger patients (younger than 45 years of age) and those with pupil involvement.
- An ophthalmologist who is confident in the diagnosis of a pupil-sparing third nerve paresis in a patient with vascular disease (with presumed ischemic mononeuropathy) may elect to simply observe if no evidence of vasculitis exists.

Treatment

- The underlying etiology determines treatment.

Follow-Up

- Patients with presumed ischemic mononeuropathy should return within a week to ensure that progression to pupil involvement has not occurred.
- Patients with ischemic mononeuropathy should recover in 6 to 12 weeks; further investigation is required for those who do not.

FOURTH NERVE PALSY

The fourth cranial (trochlear) nerve innervates only the superior oblique muscle, but this muscle has a complex action. It can tilt, depress, and move the eye away from the nose.

Symptoms

- Vertical or oblique diplopia occurs.
- Objects may appear tilted.

Signs

- Patients may adopt a head tilt to minimize diplopia.
- The eye does not depress well when adducted (toward the nose) (Fig. 11-13).

Etiology

- The disorder commonly results from trauma.
- A congenital origin is very common.
- The disorder results from ischemic cranial mononeuropathy.

Differential Diagnosis

- Differential diagnoses include the following:
  - Ocular myasthenia gravis
  - Skew deviation (vertical misalignment after brainstem stroke)
  - Thyroid eye disease

Workup

- Fourth nerve palsy is difficult to diagnose and follow without careful measurement of the ocular alignment by an ophthalmologist.

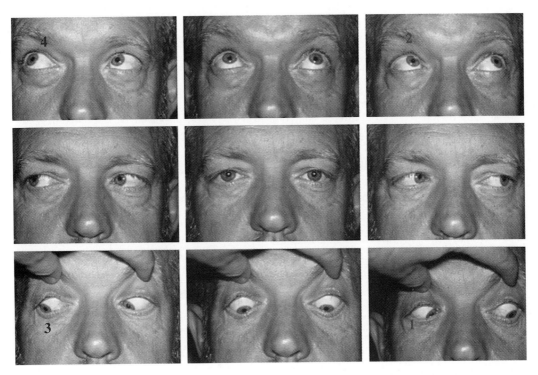

Fig. 11-13 Traumatic right fourth cranial nerve paresis. Note that the right eye does not look as far down when the gaze is directed to the left and down *(1)*. It also "overacts" or looks up too far in upgaze *(2)*. This often subtle finding is best appreciated by comparing it with the normal responses of the opposite side *(3 and 4)*.

- In patients at risk for ischemic events, only minimal workup (determination of the erythrocyte sedimentation rate to look for giant cell arteritis) may be needed.

Treatment

- Treatment is directed toward alleviating symptoms. Prisms (stick-on Fresnel prisms or built-in prisms) are rarely of help because of the torsion and gaze dependence of symptoms. A clip-on occluder (fits on patient's eyeglasses) helps eliminate diplopia by blocking the image from one eye.

SIXTH NERVE PALSY

The sixth cranial (abducens) nerve exits the brainstem at the pontomedullary junction, climbs up the clivus, and travels through the cavernous sinus into the orbit to innervate the lateral rectus muscle.

Symptoms

- Horizontal diplopia is worse in gaze toward the palsied muscle.
- Headache or periorbital pain occurs.

Signs

- Esotropia (eyes turned in) is present.
- An abduction deficit (eye not moving out well) is present (Fig. 11-14).
- Patients may adopt a head turn position to minimize the diplopia.

Etiology and Associated Factors and Diseases

- Brainstem lesions from infarct, demyelination, or tumor (progressive symptoms) may be associated with facial paresis.
- The following apply to peripheral nerve lesions:
  - Ischemic cranial mononeuropathy (most common) in older patients with vascular disease
  - Tumors of the cerebellopontine angle (possibly associated with hearing loss and ataxia)
  - Cavernous sinus disease (e.g., tumor, carotid-cavernous fistula)
  - Trauma
  - Intracranial hypertension (associated papilledema)
  - Idiopathic origin
  - Postviral syndrome in children (with possibility of tumor addressed)

Differential Diagnosis

- Differential diagnoses include the following:
  - Thyroid eye disease
  - Congenital esotropia
  - Ocular myasthenia gravis

Workup

- Ophthalmic evaluation is necessary for measurement of the deficit and evaluation for associated signs such as papilledema.
- Testing for the erythrocyte sedimentation rate is performed to address the possibility of vasculitis in elderly patients.
- Neuroimaging (MRI with contrast) is indicated in patients without obvious vascular risk factors, progression of symptoms, or other cranial nerve involvement.

Treatment

- The underlying cause determines treatment.
- For transient cases, an alternating clip-on occluder can prevent diplopia.
- For long-term cases the ophthalmologist may consider prisms, botulinum injection (of antagonist medial rectus), and eye muscle surgery.

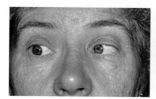 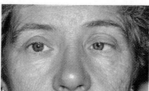 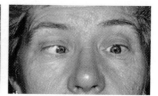

Fig. 11-14 Left sixth cranial nerve paresis. Note the poor movement of the left eye in left gaze.

CAROTID-CAVERNOUS FISTULA

Symptoms

■   A chronic red eye or eyes occur.

■   Double vision is common.

■   Pulsating intracranial noises may be reported.

Signs

■   Dilated, tortuous conjunctival vessels are usually found (Fig. 11-15).

■   Dysfunction of the third, fourth, or sixth cranial nerve may be identified.

■   Proptosis occurs.

■   A cranial bruit may be heard.

■   A dilated superior ophthalmic vein is often seen on neuroimaging.

■   Intraocular pressure is usually elevated.

Etiology

■   The disorder originates from an abnormal communication between the high-pressure arteries and the low-pressure venous cavernous sinus.

■   The disorder can be direct (high flow), between the internal carotid artery and cavernous sinus (e.g., trauma, rupture of intercavernous aneurysm), or indirect (low flow), originating from the smaller vessels of the external or internal carotid arteries (e.g., congenital, spontaneous).

Differential Diagnosis

■   Differential diagnoses include the following:
  • Thyroid eye disease
  • Orbital or cavernous sinus tumor
  • Orbital inflammatory pseudotumor

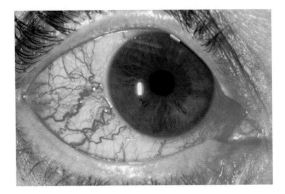

Fig. 11-15 A 64-year-old woman had a red eye, proptosis, and elevated intraocular pressure in her right eye. Diplopia and pulsatile tinnitus were also described. Her examination revealed dilated, tortuous ocular vessels, with subsequent angiography demonstrating a carotid-cavernous fistula.

Workup

- MRI or computed tomography imaging of the brain and orbits with contrast is indicated to demonstrate enlargement of the superior ophthalmic vein and other venous structures connecting to the cavernous sinus.
- Bilateral internal and external carotid angiography will display the source of the fistula, which is often multiple and/or bilateral and can be contralateral to signs, and delineate risks of intracerebral hemorrhage.

Treatment

- Indirect fistulas may spontaneously remit, frequently after diagnostic angiography.
- Therapeutic interventional radiographic procedures (e.g., placement of intravascular coils) may be required.

Follow-Up

- Ophthalmic consultation is needed to follow potential ocular complications of glaucoma or central retinal vein occlusion.

OCULAR MYASTHENIA GRAVIS

Symptoms

- Variable ptosis or diplopia may be the initial reported symptom.
- Symptoms worsen as the day progresses.
- Symptoms improve after the patient naps or rests.
- Generalized myasthenia results in weak chewing, swallowing, or breathing; fatigue of extremities also occurs.

Signs

- Ocular motility measurements vary.
- Ptosis is variable, often with visible fatigue on sustained upgaze (Fig. 11-16).

Etiology

- The disease results from an autoimmune disorder of the neuromuscular junction.

Differential Diagnosis

- Differential diagnoses include the following:
  - Paresis of cranial nerves three (except pupil), four, six, and seven or supranuclear palsy
  - Paraneoplasic (Eaton-Lambert) syndrome
  - Thyroid eye disease
  - Ptosis from other causes (e.g., aging, trauma)
  - Chronic progressive external ophthalmoplegia

Workup

- An acetylcholine receptor antibody titer is specific for the disorder when abnormal.

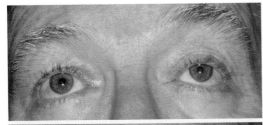

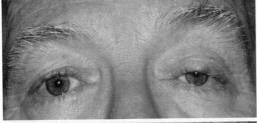

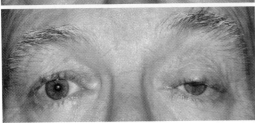

Fig. 11-16 Ocular myasthenia gravis. A 69-year-old man had variable diplopia and a right ptosis. **A,** Eyelid position after resting (with eyes closed) for 5 minutes. **B,** Eyelid position immediately after 20 seconds of sustained upgaze. **C,** Further ptosis after continued fatigue.

- Edrophonium chloride (Tensilon) testing is only helpful if an obvious objective endpoint such as a large degree of ptosis exists. Results of this test may be normal in patients with myasthenia.
- Repetitive nerve stimulation may be abnormal with systemic involvement.
- Single-fiber electromyography (of frontalis or orbicularis muscle) is sensitive and specific but technically difficult.
- Trial of pyridostigmine (Mestinon) may be unremarkable or equivocal.
- Patients with confirmed ocular myasthenia require a neurologic evaluation for systemic disease and a chest computed tomographic study to rule out thymoma.

Treatment

- Alternate occlusion of one eye prevents diplopia.
- Neurology consultant may consider pyridostigmine or low-dose (or alternate-day) prednisone administration.
- Thymectomy, even if the gland is normal in size, may be helpful in controlling the disease in some patients, although the effect may not be seen for 1 to 2 years.

Follow-Up

- Neurologic follow-up is indicated to monitor for the development of generalized disease.

ACQUIRED NYSTAGMUS

Symptoms

■ Oscillopsia ("oscillating" or moving environment) occurs.

■ Vision is blurred.

■ Patients experience vertigo.

Signs

■ Nystagmus ("shakiness") of the eyes is evident and may change with the position of gaze.

Etiology

■ The disorder can result from the following:
  • Blindness from any cause
  • Multiple sclerosis
  • Peripheral vestibular (inner ear) disease
  • Cerebellar or brainstem disease
  • Drug use (e.g., alcohol, lithium, anticonvulsants)

Workup

■ A careful drug history is needed.

■ Evaluation by a neuroophthalmologist or an otolaryngologist is indicated.

■ MRI of the brain with contrast is frequently helpful.

Treatment

■ The underlying etiology determines treatment.

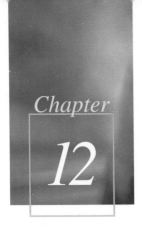

Pediatric Ophthalmology*

Arlene V. Drack

DEVELOPMENT OF THE VISUAL SYSTEM

At birth the macula (the very center of the retina and the only place in which 20/20, detailed vision is possible) is not fully formed. Although infants perceive shape, color, motion, and gross pattern, true central fixation and detailed visual acuity do not develop until 3 to 4 months after term birth (3 to 4 months corrected age for babies born prematurely). This is the reason infants do not follow objects consistently or keep their eyes aligned perfectly. The best stimulus for vision during the first weeks of life is a human face; babies usually follow a face (but not a toy) at about 6 weeks old. During these first months of life as the macula thins and develops the potential for better acuity, the brain is learning to see. These first months are the critical period of vision development; severe disruption of normal vision not corrected before 3 to 4 months of age results in lifelong visual deficit despite later treatment. The visual learning curve of the brain continues at a rapid pace until about 2 years of age, the period which stereopsis (three-dimensional binocular depth perception) develops.

Fusion and stereopsis keep the eyes aligned and working together. The brain's development of vision continues until approximately 9 years of age. After this age, serious vision problems that began early in life can rarely be completely corrected.

At birth a normal term infant is hyperopic, or farsighted, because the eye is relatively short. This means that when the ciliary muscle, which changes the lens shape to focus images, is completely at rest, images are focused behind and not on the retina and the image is blurred. To clear the image, the infant eye focuses (accommodates) to pull the image forward onto the retina (Fig. 12-1). Infants and young children have strong ciliary muscles and can accommodate to see well at distance and near. Near work takes more accommodative effort than far work. As the child grows, the eyes grow, and as the eyes elongate, the hyperopia decreases. Most eye growth occurs before 2 years of age, with slow growth thereafter to about 13 years.

Infants who are more farsighted than normal may have difficulty as they grow older and their accommodative capacities decrease. Usually this is manifest between 2 and 4 years

*The author would like to thank Mary Lopez for expert preparation of this manuscript. This chapter is dedicated to Mary Drack.

A   B   C

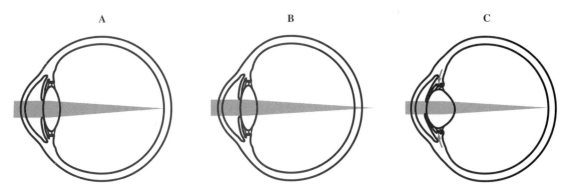

Fig. 12-1 A, The normal eye, after developing full length, focuses on the retina without accommodation. **B,** An infant's eye focuses behind the retina without accommodation. **C,** An infant's eye focuses on the retina when the ciliary body moves forward *(arrows),* relaxing the zonules and thickening the lens (accommodation).

of age as the acute onset of in-turning of the eyes (esotropia). Symptoms may also occur with reading in late adolescence or early adulthood.

Children who are less hyperopic than normal (i.e., those with eyes longer than the norm) may become myopic, or nearsighted, as they grow. A symptomatic decrease in distance vision usually becomes manifest at approximately 9 to 11 years of age in girls and slightly later in boys. Once myopia begins, it usually increases slowly throughout puberty and the early adulthood years.

APPROACH TO THE PEDIATRIC EYE EXAMINATION

Vision represents a complex interplay between static anatomic structures and dynamic neurologic and physiologic processes. When an infant is born, the eyes are anatomically formed, but vision is truly a developmental sense. Events affecting the visual system during the first weeks, months, and years of life determine how fully vision potential will be realized, with earlier events playing the most important roles. Primary care providers, parents, and pediatric ophthalmologists are the guardians of this potential, and in many infants, without the intervention of all parties, the full potential for vision is lost.

Premature Infants

Babies born at approximately 24 weeks' gestation may have partially fused eyelids, remnants of a normal developmental stage. The lids should open spontaneously over the ensuing weeks. Preterm infants less than 28 to 30 weeks' gestation have a membrane over the pupil, vestiges of the tunica vasculosa lentis, an embryonic vascular network that covers the lens and is continuous with the border of the iris. This dulls the red reflex but resolves spontaneously by 36 to 40 weeks' gestational age. If it does not regress normally, persistent pupillary membranes and anterior polar cataracts may result (Fig. 12-2).

The dilator muscle of the pupil is not well developed for several months after term; therefore pupils may be small (miotic) and the anterior chamber shallow. The corneal diameter should be approximately 8 to 10 mm.

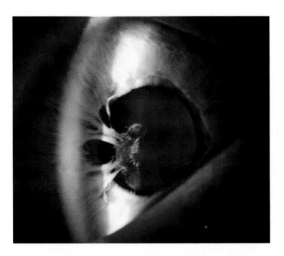

Fig. 12-2 Failure of completion of any of the normal prenatal steps of ocular development results in congenital eye anomalies. Here incomplete regression of tunica vasculosa lentis leaves a pupillary membrane and anterior lens plaque. Not all such anomalies are visually significant, but all should be referred to an ophthalmologist for evaluation.

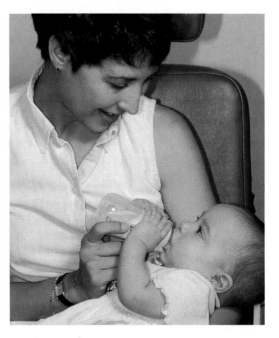

Fig. 12-3 The best stimulus for infant vision is a parent's face. By 6 weeks of age the infant should look at the parent's face and move eyes and head to follow as the parent changes position.

For premature infants before they reach term gestational age, the most important eye evaluation is an examination with the indirect ophthalmoscope by an ophthalmologist to detect retinopathy of prematurity (ROP). Primary care providers examining preterm infants can, however, look for reaction to light demonstrated by the infant squeezing the eyes shut and full spontaneous eye movements. An ophthalmologist should be involved in the care of these infants if they weigh 1500 g or less at birth, are 33 weeks' gestational age or younger, or have had oxygen therapy for more than 48 hours.

Term to 4-Month-Old Infants

A screening eye examination is generally part of all well-baby checkups, but because the eye and vision change so rapidly throughout infancy and childhood, the focus and assessment of each examination must also change.

Because the macula is not fully developed until 3 to 4 months of age, infants do not fixate well centrally, do not "lock onto" and follow objects, and may show variable crossing or drifting out of the eyes before this age.

To test children in this age range, the examiner should have the parent hold the infant in a feeding position with the baby looking at the parent's face (Fig. 12-3). The parent then moves the head from side to side. The baby should grossly follow this movement with eyes or head and should also blink when a light is directed into the eyes.

Next, a gross inspection is made of the eyes and face. The lids, brows, and globes should look symmetric. Any marked asymmetry is a warning signal, since the brain processes images from only one eye if the eyes are significantly different in any way.

Finally, the lights should be dimmed and the baby given a bottle, pacifier, or parent's finger to suck on. This usually elicits opening of the eyes. Normal infants may even have lid retraction and reveal visible sclera above and below the cornea. While the infant's eyes are open, the examiner uses a direct ophthalmoscope to look at the quality and symmetry of the red reflex. In blond or lightly pigmented infants this reflex is truly orange red. In more darkly pigmented infants the reflex looks dull orange or whitish orange. This should not be confused with leukokoria, which is a whitish appearance of the pupil on penlight or room light examination, usually differs between the two eyes, and generally prevents any reflex from being visible when the direct ophthalmoscope is used to check the red reflex. The key to judging responses as normal is symmetry and uniformity across the entire reflex (Fig. 12-4).

Sundowning, a tonic or intermittent downward deviation of the eyes (Fig. 12-5), may be benign in babies born prematurely if it is intermittent and persists for only a few weeks. Rarely, young term infants may show this sign intermittently for a few weeks. If the sundowning is constant; associated with poor feeding, nausea, vomiting, lethargy, bulging fontanelle, or abnormal head circumferences on a growth chart; or develops suddenly in an infant who never exhibited it before, it is a sign of increased intracranial pressure and mandates *immediate* referral to an ophthalmologist to prevent permanent brain and optic nerve damage or even death.

If the child is growing well, the fontanelle is flat, and the sundowning is persistent, it is often a sign of periventricular leukomalacia or other pathologic brain conditions. The risk of cerebral palsy is high in these children, and referral to a pediatric ophthalmologist is indicated.

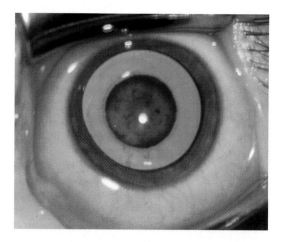

Fig. 12-4 Blocking of the red reflex by a cataract as viewed with the direct ophthalmoscope. Note the uniform orange glow around the edges of the cataract. The opacity blocks the red reflex in the center of the pupil.

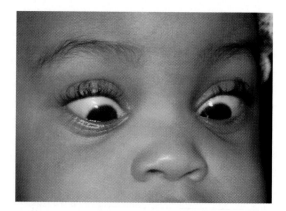

Fig. 12-5 Sundowning. Intermittent downward deviation of the eyes when lights are dimmed.

4-Month-Old Infants to Verbally Developed Children

The initial examination is the same as already outlined; however, central, steady fixation and following of a toy should be elicited. Using one thumb to cover one eye while the hand steadies the head, the examiner should check for central fixation and following with each eye (Fig. 12-6). Each eye should independently lock onto the toy and follow it smoothly and fully. If the child will cooperate, a stick-on occlusive patch may be used. If attention is poor, the lights can be dimmed and a toy illuminated. Next, the lights are dimmed and a light source is held a few inches from the child's eyes in the midline. The examiner is looking at the pupillary light reflex; it should be centered in each pupil (Fig. 12-7). If it is not, strabismus is present (Figs. 12-8 to 12-10). This method may miss an in-turning

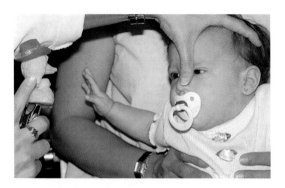

Fig. 12-6 Checking fixation in infants aged 4 months to verbal development. Often, dimming the lights and making noises are necessary to get young children's attention on a toy. For young children the thumb can be used to cover each eye in turn to watch fixation with the uncovered eye. Then the thumb is moved from one eye to the other (cover testing) to detect strabismus.

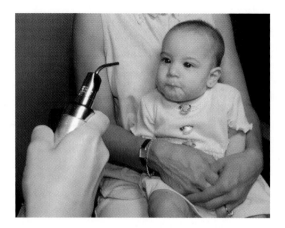

Fig. 12-7 Checking for symmetric pupillary light reflexes. Here a Fenhoff illuminator is used as a light source.

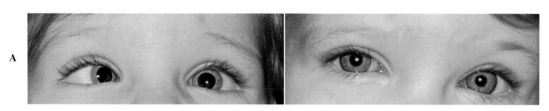

A   B

Fig. 12-8 A, In this example of esotropia the light reflex is off the center of the pupil in a temporal direction in the right eye. This child has congenital esotropia; both eyes are affected, but the fixating eye appears straight. **B,** Shortly after eye muscle surgery the corneal light reflexes are centered on both pupils.

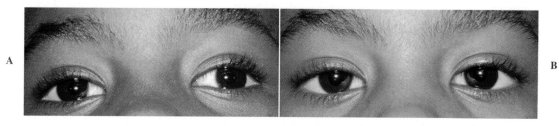

Fig. 12-9 Intermittent exotropia. **A,** The light reflex is off the center of the pupil in a nasal direction in the left eye when this child fixates in the distance. **B,** At near distance, control is better in exotropia, eyes are straight, and corneal light reflexes are centered.

Fig. 12-10 Pseudoesotropia. The eyes appear crossed because of large epicanthal skin folds *(1)* covering the sclera *(2).* This is normal before the nasal bridge develops fully. The corneal light reflexes are centered, proving the eyes are actually straight.

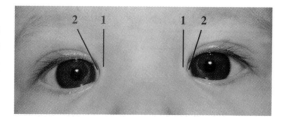

of the eyes (esotropia) as a result of accommodation, since a detailed target is needed to bring it out. If possible, the light is tapped on a toy to be sure the child is focusing at near distance. This method can also miss intermittent exotropia, a drifting outward that occurs more with distance viewing. A toy or other object is presented at the end of the room and the location of the pupillary light reflex examined while the child is fixating at a distance. The examination of the location of the pupillary light reflex to detect strabismus is the quickest and easiest method. Cover testing requires more practice and patience but is superior for detecting many types of strabismus (see Fig. 12-6). Fixation on a target is essential, and because children's attention spans are short, many toys for distance and near testing are needed. This is a standard setup in the pediatric ophthalmology office, but it may not be available for most primary care practitioners. Although children view these toys as simply being entertaining, accurate testing is impossible without them.

For cover testing, the child sits in the parent's lap. The clinician shows a toy at near distance and asks the child to touch or describe it to be sure fixation is occurring. One eye is rapidly covered; if the eyes are straight, no movement of the fellow eye should occur. The test is repeated for the other eye, thereby demonstrating constant deviations. If the child is older than 6 months of age, the test is repeated for distance. (Children younger than 6 months of age will not attend to distant targets.) Then the examiner again holds the target at near distance and slowly covers first one eye and then the other. If the eyes have no latent deviation, the uncovered eye should not move. If latent deviation (termed *phoria*) is present, the eyes shift back and forth as the cover is changed. The test is repeated for distance. Any child with a suspected deviation, latent or constant, should be referred to an ophthalmologist.

Verbal Children

Once children develop verbal abilities, the eye examination is much easier, but a few key points are worth noting. Corneal light reflex and cover testing should still be done as described. The major change is that objective measures of visual function, such as fixation and following, give way to subjective measures. As soon as children can speak well (usually by age 3 years), parents should be given a photocopy of the standard Allen or other calibrated pictures to practice at home with the child (Fig. 12-11). The first vision test in the office may not be accurate because of the child's unfamiliarity with the test.

The best way to test children before they know letters and numbers is to start with an Allen near card and put an occlusive patch over one eye. The examiner points to pictures on the card, starting at the largest and moving to the smallest, and has the child name them. The patch is changed to the other eye and the test repeated. Once the child is familiar with the symbols, keeping one eye patched, the examiner starts showing the cards in a flash card fashion while slowly walking backward to a distance of 20 feet. This pattern is repeated with the other eye. Children 3 to 5 years old may only read the cards at 15 feet instead of 20, but the distance should be the same for each eye and should improve on subsequent visits. The distance from the child and the figure size of the cards (20/30 for Allen cards) should be recorded. As an example, if the child sees the distance (20/30) Allen card at 20 feet, the vision is 20/30, normal for age. If the child only sees it to 10 feet, the vision is 10/30. This can be multiplied by 2 to obtain standard notation, in this case 20/60. Vision should be at least 20/40 or 20/50 at a distance for children younger than 5 years, but 20/20 to 20/30 for all ages at near distance. A vision measurement less than this or any difference in values between the eyes suggests a need for referral. In children older than 5 years, distance vision should be 20/20. For Allen cards, cards should be identified all the way to 20 feet; most Allen cards only test to 20/30, since children young enough to be illiterate generally read only 20/30, not 20/20 at distance.

Once children know numbers, a standard number chart can be used. Letters give the greatest accuracy, and once a child is old enough to read letters, attention is usually sufficient to cooperate with testing using a chart at the end of the room. Sometimes having a parent point to each letter helps with attention and accuracy.

The importance of using an occlusive patch rather than an occluder or covering of one eye cannot be overemphasized. If one eye sees poorly, children will peek to use the other eye to give the right answers (Figs. 12-12 and 12-13). Only an occlusive patch prevents this.

  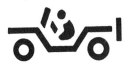

Fig. 12-11 Allen figures. Several such standard figures are available. This is the 20/30 size, which means a normal child should be able to identify it at 20 feet. These figures are reproduced at actual size, so if a sharp photocopy that is well lit and placed at 20 feet is interpreted correctly, visual acuity is at least 20/30.

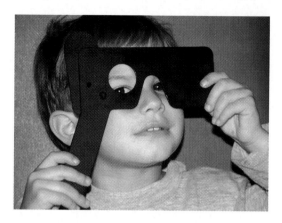

Fig. 12-12 Vision testing. Children often peek around standard occluders, especially if their better eye is covered.

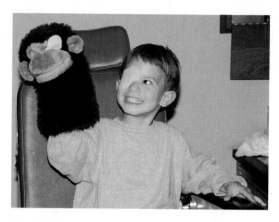

Fig. 12-13 An adhesive patch prevents peeking during vision testing.

Photoscreening is a new technology available to primary care offices. Flash pictures are taken of children's eyes to detect opacities, refractive errors, and strabismus. Although extremely useful in many cases, especially refractive amblyopia, photoscreening should be used as a well-child screening test, not an examination technique for children in whom a problem is suspected because certain disorders can be missed. All children with suspected ocular disorders should be referred to a pediatric ophthalmologist.

Red Reflex or Bruchner Test

Ideally, every child should have an examination of the red reflex at every well-child checkup. In the hands of an experienced examiner, this test can detect almost all major ocular problems of childhood. At a minimum it should be done at discharge from the hospital; once again before 3 months of age (to detect cataracts, which must be treated before 3 months to prevent blindness, and retinoblastoma, which if treated early, need not result in loss of the eye or life); again at 6 months; and then again at all well-child visits.

The lights are dimmed, the infant is given something to suck on, and while standing at arm's length, the examiner uses the direct ophthalmoscope to look at both pupils at once and then one at a time. For most examiners the ophthalmoscope should be set at 0, with the largest aperture open. If the pupils are small (miotic) or a good red reflex is not obtained, dilation of the pupils is recommended. For preterm infants up to 3 months of age, cyclopentolate hydrochloride/phenylephrine hydrochloride (Cyclomydril) should be used, one drop in each eye, which is repeated in 5 minutes. Then the examiner waits 20 minutes for dilation. More darkly pigmented irides take longer to dilate and may require another set of drops. The examiner must not exceed 4 drops in an hour. For term infants, cyclopentolate 0.5% and Neosynephrine 2.5% eyedrops are used, one drop in each eye and repeated in 5 minutes. After 6 months of age, cyclopentolate 1% and neosynephrine 2.5% are used, one drop in each eye and repeated in 5 minutes. Again, light irides dilate in about 20 minutes; dark irides take longer and may require another set of drops.

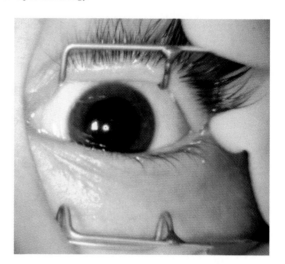

Fig. 12-14 Use of a lid speculum. An assistant holds the child snugly, especially the child's arms. Keeping gentle pressure on both sides of the speculum with one hand to compress it, the clinician uses the other hand to elevate the upper lid and slide one lip under. Without allowing the speculum to spring open, the lower lid is pulled down and the other lip slid under this lid. Next, pressure is removed from the speculum so that it will open the lids. A drop of proparacaine or tetracaine may be used in each eye before insertion. The procedure is not painful, but it is frightening to parents and child and reassurance is necessary.

The risk with these doses of eye medications are few. Tachycardia and facial flushing may result, but these are usually self-limited. These drops should be used with caution in children with cardiac disease or hypertension, and doses should be decreased for very lightly pigmented children. If all measures fail to get an infant to open the eyes, a lid speculum may be used (Fig. 12-14).

OCULAR DISORDERS OF INFANCY

CONJUNCTIVITIS

Symptoms

■ Usually no symptoms occur, but in severe cases, irritability may be present.

Signs

■ The disorder is usually bilateral but may be asymmetric.
■ Mild conjunctival injection is possible.
■ A watery, mucoid or mucopurulent discharge occurs.
■ Eyelids may adhere when the child awakens.
■ Eyelids may be erythematous or excoriated.
■ Preauricular lymph node may be present.

Differential Diagnosis

■ In infants younger than 1 week old, differential diagnoses include the following:
  • Toxic conjunctivitis from perinatal prophylaxis: The infant is usually initially seen with red lids and watery discharge.
  • Infectious disorders (usually acquired in the birth canal): Most often staphylococci, *Chlamydia,* herpes, and gonorrhea organisms are the infectious agents. The infant is initially seen with quiet lids and mucopurulent discharge, but symptoms can appear

identical to those of toxic conjunctivitis. If discharge is purulent and excessive (so-called hyperacute), gonorrhea is possible. Emergency referral to an ophthalmologist is required because blindness can result within 24 to 48 hours if the infection is not treated (Fig. 12-15).

■ In infants older than 1 week or those with community exposure, differential diagnoses include the following:

- Viral causes, specifically adenovirus or respiratory syncytial virus: Massive lid swelling may be present in infants, simulating cellulitis. A preauricular node or upper respiratory infection is often present.
- If the disorder is chronic and in particular unilateral, nasolacrimal duct obstruction should be considered.
- If the disorder manifests as photophobia, an enlarged cornea, and in particular watery and chronic discharge, congenital glaucoma must be ruled out or confirmed. Congenital glaucoma necessitates immediate ophthalmic referral and treatment.

Treatment

■ In infants younger than 1 week old with red lids and a watery discharge, toxic etiology is likely. All eye medications are ceased and the infant is observed for 24 to 48 hours. If no improvement is seen after 48 hours or discharge is mucopurulent, antibiotic drops (e.g., polymyxin B/trimethoprim [Polytrim], 1 drop 3 to 4 times a day or erythromycin ointment 4 times a day) are administered. If one of these agents was used for prophylaxis, it should not be readministered, since it may have been a causative factor. If the infant's condition does not improve in 48 hours, an ophthalmologist is consulted for cultures and further workup.

■ If the discharge is hyperacute, Gram stain and culture (chocolate agar) study is performed to look for gonorrhea; the infant is treated presumptively for gonorrhea with intravenous or intramuscular cefotaxime (Claforan) 25 mg/kg every 8 to 12 hours for 7 days. Hospital admission and an ophthalmologic consultation should be done immediately. Gonorrhea can penetrate an intact cornea rapidly. The mother is also tested.

■ If cultures or stains reveal *Chlamydia* organisms, the infant is treated systemically because of the risk of pneumonia. The mother should also be tested.

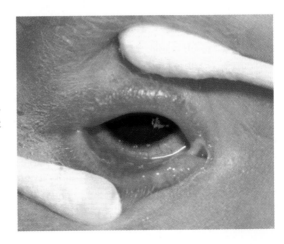

Fig. 12-15 Hyperacute gonorrheal conjunctivitis. Immediate topical and systemic antibiotics are needed to prevent blindness.

■ If *Haemophilus influenzae* is recovered from the infant, systemic treatment is performed. This infection often proves refractory to topical treatment and has a high risk of causing cellulitis and meningitis.

NASOLACRIMAL DUCT OBSTRUCTION

Symptoms

■ Usually no symptoms occur, but patients may have irritation of the eyelids and conjunctiva if the obstruction is longstanding or bacterial superinfection is present (Fig. 12-16).

Signs

■ The obstruction is usually bilateral but asymmetric.
■ The tear lake usually is elevated, and the lashes look wet.
■ With bacterial superinfection, a chronic mucopurulent discharge occurs, and the eyelids adhere in the morning. Later the periorbital skin becomes thickened and excoriated and the conjunctiva becomes injected.

Etiology

■ Most cases result from failure of the valve of Hasner to open; however, absence of the puncta or other anomalies of the system are rare causes (Fig. 12-17).
■ The origin is usually idiopathic and the disorder is very common.

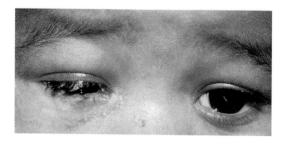

Fig. 12-16 Chronic nasolacrimal duct obstruction with bacterial superinfection. This child has been treated with topical and systemic antibiotics without resolution. If nasolacrimal duct obstruction is present, infection will not clear without probing. Note skin changes. All signs resolved 24 hours after probing.

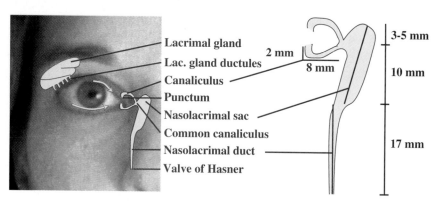

Fig. 12-17 Anatomy of the nasolacrimal system.

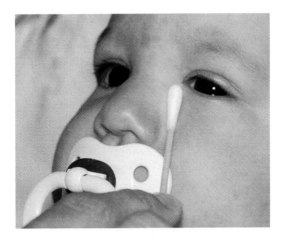

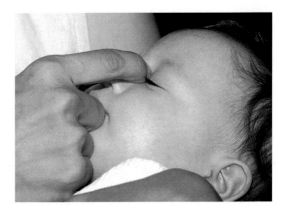

Fig. 12-18 Differentiating nasolacrimal duct obstruction from conjunctivitis in the office. The examiner presses firmly on the nasolacrimal sac with a cotton-tipped applicator while the parent immobilizes the child; the presence of reflux of mucopurulent material from the puncta is determined. If reflux is present, the diagnosis is nasolacrimal duct obstruction.

Fig. 12-19 Home massage over the nasolacrimal sac to open obstruction. This should be done 3 to 4 times a day, followed by an antibiotic drop such as polymyxin B/trimethoprim (Polytrim). If the obstruction does not resolve after 2 or 3 weeks and discharge is still present, referral for probing is indicated.

Associated Factors and Diseases

■ Infants with syndromes involving midface hypoplasia, clefting, and mass lesions such as dermoids of the canthal area are at increased risk.

Workup

■ To differentiate between conjunctivitis and nasolacrimal duct obstruction, the examiner presses a cotton-tipped swab firmly over the lacrimal sac and watches the puncta (Fig. 12-18). If a reflux of mucopurulent material is seen, the diagnosis is nasolacrimal duct obstruction, not solely conjunctivitis.

■ To differentiate between nasolacrimal duct obstruction and congenital glaucoma, the clinician measures intraocular pressure and examines the corneas and optic nerves. If tearing does not respond to treatment within a few weeks and no reflux from the sac occurs with pressure or the patient keeps the eyes closed when exposed to light and/or has large hazy corneas, referral to a pediatric ophthalmologist is necessary.

Treatment

■ About 75% of infants spontaneously open the obstruction within the first 6 months of life as long as bacterial infection is not present. Thus if the discharge is watery only, observation and daily massage over the lacrimal sac (rapid, downward pushing to pop open the valve of Hasner [Fig. 12-19]) are appropriate measures.

■ After 6 months of age, obstructions are far less likely to resolve and the child should be referred to an ophthalmologist.

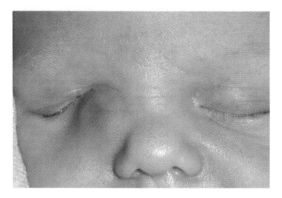

Fig. 12-20 Dacryocele. These are usually congenital and must be treated immediately by an ophthalmologist.

- With mucopurulent discharge, topical antibiotics (e.g., polymyxin B/trimethoprim [Polytrim] 1 drop 3 to 4 times a day) are administered for 1 to 3 weeks with massage and frequent cleansing of secretions. If the bacterial infection resolves, the system may open spontaneously.
- With a mass such as dacryocele, immediate referral to an ophthalmologist is necessary (Fig. 12-20).
- If antibiotic drops do not clear the mucopurulent discharge in 1 to 2 weeks, the patient should be referred to an ophthalmologist, regardless of age. These children have severe obstructions with bacterial colonization, and the condition will only worsen until probing is done.
- Nasolacrimal duct probing is 95% effective in opening obstructions if performed before 1 year of age. If undergone before the child is 2 years old, probing is approximately 85% successful. Because spontaneous opening is unlikely after 6 months of age or in the presence of infection and this procedure has a high rate of success only if done early, the treatment plan must be adjusted accordingly. Probing can be performed in the ophthalmologist's office without anesthesia if the child is younger than 3 or 4 months old. After this age, anesthesia is necessary.
- Silastic tubing can be placed to keep the system open in older children and those who fail probing.
- A balloon catheter procedure opens the system in recurrent cases.
- Creating a surgical passage among the tear lake, nasolacrimal sac, and nasal mucosa (dacryocystorhinostomy, or Jones' tube placement) is reserved for older children or those who fail probing and tubes. These are much more invasive surgeries and can often be avoided if early treatment is instituted.

RETINOPATHY OF PREMATURITY

Symptoms

- No symptoms occur.

Signs

■ The disorder is almost always bilateral but often asymmetric.

■ Pupils are small and immobile in the late stages, and iridic blood vessels are enlarged.

■ Most signs are only seen with the indirect ophthalmoscope. A ridge of abnormal vascular tissue grows from the retina into the vitreous. Blood vessels may become dilated and tortuous.

■ If advanced stages are not treated, retinal detachment is likely, causing blindness.

■ As children get older, strabismus (either esotropia or exotropia) can be seen as a late sequela.

■ Microphthalmia (a small eye) and phthisis (a shrunken eye) can result after retinal detachment.

Associated Factors and Diseases

■ Low birth weight, low gestational age, sepsis, and perinatal oxygen administration are risk factors for the disorder.

■ All babies born at 33 weeks' gestation or younger, weighing 1500 g or less, or having oxygen administered for more than 48 hours should be screened 6 weeks after birth by an ophthalmologist familiar with retinopathy of prematurity. If no retinopathy of prematurity is present, or the disorder resolves, these children still require follow-up with an ophthalmologist at approximately 3 months after discharge and throughout the first few years of life because of their increased risks of strabismus, high refractive error (i.e., need for glasses), amblyopia, optic atrophy, and retinal abnormalities.

Treatment

■ Once the treatment threshold is reached, cryotherapy or laser therapy of the retina must be performed, usually within 48 hours. An ophthalmologist trained in retinopathy of prematurity makes the determination of threshold disease based on strict criteria. Almost 95% of threshold infants who are treated retain vision, whereas in the past the majority developed blindness as a result of retinal detachment or scarring.

■ Throughout life, glasses, patching, surgery, and other modalities may be needed to treat the sequelae of retinopathy of prematurity.

CONGENITAL ANOMALIES

INTRAUTERINE INFECTIONS

Infections that cross the placenta, such as toxoplasmosis, rubella, cytomegalovirus, herpes virus, varicella virus, and human immunodeficiency (HIV) virus, often cause characteristic eye conditions. If an intrauterine infection is suspected, an ophthalmology consultation may help confirm the diagnosis. Vision is often affected, so early referral is essential.

CONGENITAL CATARACTS

Symptoms

■ Vision is mildly to severely decreased.

■ In severe cases in which essentially no vision is present, the infant may keep the eyes closed.

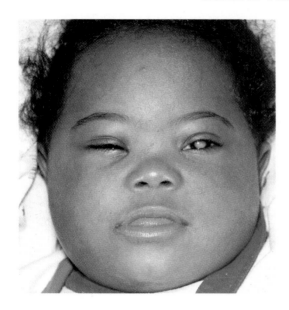

Fig. 12-21 Leukocoria. This child has a unilateral cataract. Leukocoria is seen as a white pupil when viewed with a penlight or in room light.

■ When the condition results in a partial cataract, the infant may squint, especially in bright sunlight, to decrease the resultant glare.

Signs

■ Leukocoria (white pupil) is present if the cataract is dense (Fig. 12-21).
■ The red reflex is abnormal.

Differential Diagnosis

■ Differential diagnoses include the following:
  • Cataract
  • Retinoblastoma
  • Coats' disease (an exudative retinal detachment caused by vascular anomalies)
  • Retinopathy of prematurity
  • Chorioretinal coloboma (white sclera where retina should be)
  • Corneal scar (Peters' anomaly)
  • Retinal detachment

Treatment

■ Congenital cataract is an emergency. The brain learns to see with the macula (the center of the retina where 20/20 vision is possible) most rapidly during the first 3 to 4 months of life. If vision is severely limited during this critical period of visual development, it cannot be restored completely. Thus congenital cataracts must be surgically removed, and optical rehabilitation with contact lenses or glasses must be in place *before* 3 to 4 months of age. Many patients can have near normal vision if treated promptly. If infants are treated after this age, some vision may be restored but the result is often in the 20/200 or legally blind range.

- An ophthalmologist determines the adequacy of an infant's visual stimulation in cases of partial cataracts.
- Persistent hyperplastic primary vitreous is a type of congenital cataract that may cause a small eye and painful glaucoma.
- All infants are screened for a red reflex before discharge from the nursery and at each well-baby checkup. If a cataract or other disruption of the red reflex is suspected, referral to an ophthalmologist is needed before the infant is 3 months of age.

CONGENITAL PTOSIS

The lid is primarily elevated by the levator muscle, which inserts onto the tarsal plate of the eyelid, and by the orbicularis oculi muscle, which encircles the eye. The levator is innervated by the third cranial nerve. The lid is also partially elevated by Müller's muscle, which is innervated by sympathetic fibers. These fibers travel from the brain out through the spine, around the neck, over the lung, then up around the carotid artery to innervate the pupil and muscle of the eyelid.

Symptoms

- If the ptosis is severe, vision is greatly decreased.
- If the condition is bilateral, the infant never opens the eyes or never focuses.

Signs, Etiology, and Differential Diagnosis

- An absent or a faint lid crease may signal a lack or an abnormal insertion of the levator aponeurosis. Lack of a lid crease is normal in Asian patients.
- One or both brows are often markedly elevated.

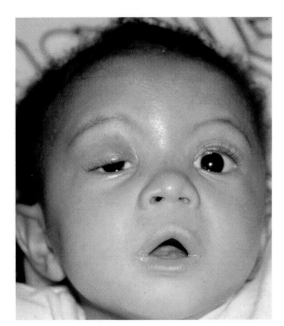

Fig. 12-22 Congenital ptosis. Baby keeps the chin up to see. Note elevated brows and lack of right lid crease.

■ The infant may keep a chin-up position (Fig. 12-22).

■ Mild ptosis with a lid crease, a small pupil (miosis), a difference in iris color (heterochromia), and an inability to sweat (anhidrosis) on one side of the face are signs of Horner's syndrome caused by sympathetic nerve interruption. In congenital cases a history of brachial plexus injury or difficult delivery may help determine the etiologic process.

■ If the lid is thickened or red, a hemangioma may be present.

Treatment

■ Surgical correction is necessary.

■ If untreated, amblyopia and loss of vision result in many cases. Ophthalmologic referral as soon after birth as possible is indicated.

■ If the condition is severe, surgical correction using a tarsal sling must be performed before the infant is 3 months of age.

■ Often ptosis induces refractive error (e.g., myopia, astigmatism), which must be treated with glasses.

■ Amblyopia may be dense and requires treatment with patching; if ptosis is asymmetric, amblyopia must be treated before the infant is 3 months of age.

CONGENITAL GLAUCOMA

Symptoms

■ Vision is decreased.

■ Photophobia occurs.

Signs

■ Excess tearing occurs, especially during daylight or in bright light.

■ The corneas are enlarged.

■ Hazy or cloudy corneas cause a diminished corneal reflex.

Differential Diagnosis

■ Nasolacrimal duct obstruction: Congenital glaucoma is often associated with blindness, whereas nasolacrimal obstruction is generally benign. Nasolacrimal duct obstruction often develops mucopurulent discharge and excess tearing over time. Even if no mucopurulent discharge is present on external examination, if gentle pressure is exerted on the nasolacrimal sac with a cotton-tipped swab, discharge can often be expressed. If this sign is not present and excess tearing continues for more than a few weeks, congenital glaucoma may be present. Simple nasolacrimal duct obstruction is not associated with photophobia; that is, in normal lighting the infant should have the eyes open and be looking around the room. If the infant is reluctant to do this and keeps the eyes closed much of the time even at age 2 or 3 months, either severe nasolacrimal duct obstruction with bacterial superinfection and irritation or congenital glaucoma may be present. Simple nasolacrimal duct obstruction should not be associated with any cloudiness or abnormal appearance of the eyes. Congenital glaucoma may be associated with other congenital anomalies, especially Turner's syndrome, Down syndrome, Rubinstein-Taybi syndrome, and Lowe syndrome.

Treatment

- Patients should be referred to an ophthalmologist.
- Medications, usually systemic or topical carbonic anhydrase inhibitors and topical β blockers, may be used for short-term management to relieve pressure; however, they are rarely sufficient to preserve vision.
- Surgery is almost always needed. Procedures quite different from adult glaucoma surgery are used and have an excellent success rate.

Follow-Up

- Most children need more than one operation, and concomitant problems such as amblyopia, high myopia, and strabismus are almost always present. Thus families need to be counseled that the condition is a lifelong ocular disorder requiring frequent follow-up. With close follow-up and despite a diagnosis of congenital glaucoma, many children today are not blind.

HEMANGIOMA

Symptoms

- Vision is decreased.
- In rare cases, respiratory or swallowing difficulties occur if the hemangioma is extensive.

Signs

- Ptosis or an irregular lid with or without an elevated, reddish mass occurs (Fig. 12-23).
- Hemangiomas are most visually significant when they are located on the upper lid; however, they may occur on the upper and lower lids and below the eyes and can involve the scalp or, rarely, the airway.
- Capillary hemangiomas are often present at birth but may be very small. They generally begin to grow within the first months of life and continue to grow throughout the first 1 to 2 years, then undergo slow regression.

Treatment

- Referral to a pediatric ophthalmologist is necessary, even for small hemangiomas of the upper lid or periorbital area before the infant is 3 months of age because of the known association of this condition with severe amblyogenic factors in the affected eye.

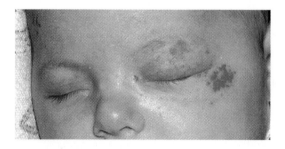

Fig. 12-23 Capillary hemangioma of the eyelid.

■ Referral to an ophthalmologist is necessary at any age if the hemangioma enlarges, causes ptosis, or occludes the pupil.

■ If vision is equal and little or no induced astigmatism or myopia is present, observation is usually sufficient.

■ In most cases the induced refractive error differs between the eyes. Glasses are prescribed and patching may be warranted to treat the amblyopia.

■ If the hemangioma is on the upper lid or another area that severely interferes with vision and it is enlarging, it is an ophthalmologic emergency. A course of systemic corticosteroids at 2 mg/kg/day for up to 1 or 2 weeks with a very slow taper thereafter often achieves excellent results. Intralesional injection of corticosteroids has also been advocated but may have severe complications.

Follow-Up

■ Patients must be monitored by a pediatric ophthalmologist and pediatrician.

■ Long-term follow-up care is required until the capillary hemangioma regresses.

PORT-WINE STAIN

Symptoms

■ No symptoms exist.

Signs

■ A large, flat, purplish lesion is found on the skin of the face or scalp. It may also be present on other parts of the body.

■ Glaucoma is likely to occur on the affected side, especially if the upper lid is involved.

■ Seizures and developmental delay are often also present. When intracranial involvement of the hemangioma occurs with these signs, Sturge-Weber syndrome is diagnosed.

Treatment

■ Because ipsilateral glaucoma occurs in approximately 50% of cases of port-wine stain (nevus flammeus) when it affects the upper eyelid, all children with the disorder should be referred for pediatric ophthalmic consultation as soon as the lesion is detected. Magnetic resonance imaging (MRI) scan, computed tomography (CT) scan of the brain, and an electroencephalogram may also be indicated.

■ Laser eradication of some cases is now possible, but this treatment's effect on the incidence of glaucoma is not known. Generally, the laser treatment must be performed within the first 2 years of life to be successful; therefore early referral is essential.

CONGENITAL ESOTROPIA AND EXOTROPIA

Variable, intermittent ocular misalignment is normal for the first 3 months of life; however, misalignment after 3 to 4 months of age is not normal. In addition, a constant misalignment of either or both eyes is always abnormal. Children who have a constant deviation of one or both eyes should be referred to an ophthalmologist immediately. This may be a sign of a developmental anomaly or tumor in the eye. Congenital esotropia occurs in children who have essentially normal eye movements for the first 3 to 4 months of life but whose eyes cross before 6 months of age. Congenital exotropia is a condition in which one or both eyes deviate outward toward the ear.

Symptoms

■ Early in the disease, double vision may occur.

■ Decreased stereopsis (depth perception) is present throughout life.

Signs

■ Strabismus, with one or both eyes pointing in toward the nose (esotropia) or outward toward the ears (exotropia), occurs.

■ Most patients with congenital esotropia are unable to abduct the eyes (look laterally) fully.

■ Nystagmus occurs in a small subset of patients with congenital esotropia.

■ A decreased ability to make eye contact and bond with parents occurs in some cases, which improves after treatment.

Differential Diagnosis

■ Early onset sixth nerve palsy or paresis may mimic congenital esotropia. This is often caused by increased intracranial pressure and is associated with nausea, vomiting, lethargy, and increased head circumference.

■ In premature infants the development of esotropia is related to neurologic causes: the disorder is often associated with periventricular leukomalacia and cerebral palsy. This type of esotropia may occur at the same age as congenital esotropia, but the ocular mis-alignment varies throughout the examination.

■ Congenital third nerve palsy is a possible cause.

■ For patients in whom no other symptoms are present and the perinatal or birth history is normal, the condition is an isolated finding in an otherwise healthy, normal infant.

Associated Factors and Diseases

■ Because of the relatively increased risk of intracranial pathologic disorders such as midline or other brain defects or megalocephaly, neuroimaging and ophthalmologic referral are needed.

■ Some children with severe esotropia may have motor delays because they can never look straight ahead when they are holding their heads straight. Their eyes are always pulled into the esotropic position. These children may turn their heads to the side to attempt to crawl or walk and often gain developmental motor milestones rapidly after surgery.

Treatment

■ Any patient with constant deviation or deviation that develops after the initial 3 to 4 months of life should be referred for ophthalmologic evaluation immediately.

■ For patients with amblyopia, treatment immediately after diagnosis is most effective and usually involves patching and/or glasses.

■ Stereopsis, the type of depth perception that results from the use of both eyes, can best be achieved in children with congenital esotropia or exotropia if surgery is performed before the age of 2 years. Approximately 65% of children need one surgery to straighten their vision; 35% will require a second surgery. Ideally, the eyes should be straightened, regardless of the number of surgical interventions needed, before the patient is 2 years old to increase the chance of stereopsis. The desire for stereopsis is twofold: (1) It achieves the normal visual experience for the child, and (2) if stereopsis is achieved, the brain may work to keep the eyes straight throughout life. In children who do not have stereopsis, even if the eyes are cosmetically straightened, they will probably drift again.

■ Immediate referral of patients for ophthalmologic and neurologic evaluation is needed if acute crossing is associated with nausea, vomiting, lethargy, increased head circumference, and sunsetting of the eyes. These are signs of increased intracranial pressure.

■ Parents need to be educated about the long-term nature of their child's treatment. Children with congenital strabismus often experience lifelong vision and stereopsis problems.

NYSTAGMUS

Nystagmus may be a sign of a life-threatening neurologic disorder or blindness. Thus any child who has nystagmus in the primary position should be referred to a pediatric ophthalmologist.

Symptoms

■ Vision is decreased.
■ Vision in the dark is decreased.

Signs

■ A constant, jiggling movement of the eyes may be horizontal, vertical, rotary, or a combination of these.
■ The disorder may be bilateral, unilateral, or asymmetric.
■ Compensatory head shaking or nodding is possible.
■ Weight loss may occur.
■ Failure to thrive may be present.

Differential Diagnosis

■ Differential diagnoses related to neurologic causes include the following:
  • Hydrocephalus
  • Diencephalic tumors
  • Toxicity from a number of medications, including phenytoin (Dilantin)
  • Arnold-Chiari malformation
  • Other brain tumors and anomalies
  • In rare cases, immaturity of the central nervous system (spasmus nutans), a benign condition possibly associated with head nodding and torticollis that is a diagnosis of exclusion necessitating diagnosis by an ophthalmologist or a neurologist
  • Middle ear abnormalities (rare in infants)
■ Differential diagnoses related to ocular abnormalities include the following:
  • Leber's congenital amaurosis (a congenital form of retinitis pigmentosa associated with severe blindness)

- Congenital stationary night blindness (a disorder in which glasses are needed and vision is extremely poor in dim illumination but that may be compatible with almost normal vision if glasses are worn and lighting is appropriate)
- Achromatopsia (a congenital abnormality of the retina associated with legal blindness and photophobia)
- Congenital motor nystagmus (a primary motor problem associated with decreased vision secondary to the nystagmus and that may be helped with eye muscle surgery)
- Albinism (partial and complete)
- Optic nerve hypoplasia

Associated Factors and Diseases

- Sometimes the etiology of the nystagmus points to other associated congenital anomalies to investigate. For example, optic nerve hypoplasia may be associated with deficiency of growth or thyroid hormone. Albinism is associated with a high risk of skin cancer, and sunscreen must be worn at all times. In partial forms of albinism, children appear to have normal pigment, but they are lighter than family members.

Workup

- The focus of the complete eye examination is to search for refractive errors, retinal abnormalities, and other clues to an ocular diagnosis.
- An electroretinogram and visual-evoked potential testing may be necessary.
- The head circumference is measured.
- If the findings of the electroretinogram are normal and no ocular clues exist, an MRI scan is performed.

Treatment

- Treatment depends on the underlying etiology.
- In patients with visual deprivation, treatment focuses on reversing the cause of the deprivation to lessen or eradicate the nystagmus. Ideally, treatment should be instituted within the first 3 months of life, but once nystagmus has begun, the condition has probably already persisted longer than 3 months. These conditions include very high refractive errors, untreated cataracts, and congenital cornea anomalies.
- Inherited retinal conditions often have an associated refractive error. Glasses may optimize vision but will not completely correct it or eliminate the nystagmus. These children benefit from early intervention programs to help them meet their developmental milestones, so early diagnosis is critical.
- Although some neurologic conditions are obviously treatable (e.g., hydrocephalus, diencephalic tumors) and some are not, the underlying etiologic process must be known.
- Some children with congenital motor nystagmus and in rare cases children with other types of nystagmus have a "null point," where they can turn their heads to dampen the nystagmus. Children who develop null points should keep their heads turned in this position to maintain the best vision. If the position is consistent, strabismus surgery can move the eye muscles into the most desirable position and achieve better vision with a normal head position.

COLOBOMA

Coloboma represents failure of closure of the fetal fissure during the development of the eye in utero. Normally the optic cup collapses on itself and the multilayered hemisphere grows closed around a central open space with the inferonasal aspect being the last to close. Failure of complete closure results in only a partial circle of pigment for the iris and a defect in the optic nerve or inferonasal retina and choroid. White, bare sclera is visible inside the eye when a chorioretinal coloboma is present.

Symptoms

- No symptoms occur.
- Vision may be decreased.

Signs

- A keyhole or teardrop pupil is possible, with the open area located inferiorly or inferonasally.
- Leukokoria is possible if a large chorioretinal coloboma is present.
- In *forme fruste* presentations the retinal coloboma looks like a small chorioretinal scar and the pupil, instead of having a large keyhole or notch appearance, may simply be mildly larger or oval compared with the other pupil (Fig. 12-24).
- Nystagmus is possible if the defect is severe, but the condition is usually not apparent until the patient is 3 months of age.
- A small, malformed eye (microphthalmia) is possible.
- In some children the CHARGE association—which consists of coloboma, heart abnormalities, choanal atresia, retardation, genitourinary anomalies, and ear malformations—is evident.

Etiology

- Up to 22% of colobomas may be inherited in an autosomal dominant pattern with extremely variable expressivity.

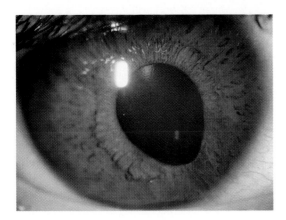

Fig. 12-24 Very mild iris coloboma causing teardrop pupil. All such children must have a complete eye examination to rule out associated chorioretinal coloboma, which may severely affect vision. This child also has a small retinal coloboma, but with glasses and amblyopia therapy, visual acuity improved from 20/200 to 20/30.

Treatment

- For patients with high refractive errors, glasses are needed. These children often develop amblyopia because of the asymmetry of the colobomas and their eyes must be patched. Immediate treatment is needed for the increased risk of cataract and glaucoma development.
- Referral for pediatric ophthalmologic evaluation is indicated as soon as the coloboma is detected or suspected.
- For inherited colobomas, examination of the parents is necessary to identify any mild manifestations; the risk of recurrence is 50% for subsequent children.

CORNEAL LEUKOMA

Symptoms

- Vision is decreased.

Signs

- The cornea appears white or gray.
- The disorder is unilateral or bilateral.
- The opacity is central or peripheral.
- The disorder may be associated with a small, malformed globe (microphthalmia).
- The lesion may be elevated (corneal dermoid).

Differential Diagnosis

- Differential diagnoses include the following:
  - A hazy cornea resulting from congenital glaucoma with increased intraocular pressure causing cornea edema
  - Peters' anomaly, a developmental abnormality of the cornea that results in corneal clouding

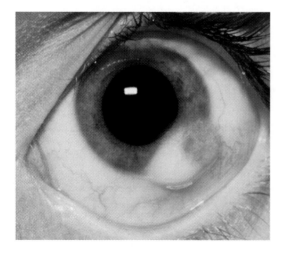

Fig. 12-25 Corneal dermoid.

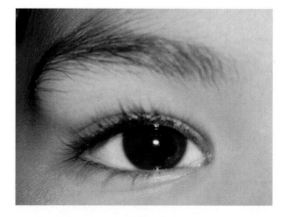

Fig. 12-26 Temporal brow dermoid.

- Forceps injury, causing damage to the cornea and acute corneal edema with haziness
- Dermoid, a white elevated lesion on the cornea (Fig. 12-25) that can also occur under the skin in the brow area (Fig. 12-26), causing intense inflammation if traumatic rupture occurs
- Corneal ulcer in cases of congenital or neonatal herpes
- Sclerocornea, a rare developmental anomaly in which the cornea does not form and the entire front of the eye is white

Treatment

■ Corneal leukomas are always an emergency, and immediate consultation with a pediatric ophthalmologist is essential.

■ Exact treatment depends on the type and cause but ranges from dilation of the eye with drops and patching of the other eye to corticosteroid and antibiotic treatment to corneal transplantation. Because corneal opacities produce dense, irreversible amblyopia if not treated within the first few months of the patient's life, referral is critical.

RETINOBLASTOMA

Symptoms

■ Usually, no symptoms occur.

■ Vision may be decreased.

Signs

■ A white pupil (leukokoria) is present in patients with advanced retinoblastoma.

■ Different color of each iris (heterochromia) occurs in advanced retinoblastoma.

■ Proptosis results if the tumor has spread into the orbit.

■ The cornea is enlarged if glaucoma has developed.

■ The patient is lethargic and experiences failure to thrive if a pineal tumor (trilateral retinoblastoma) or metastatic retinoblastoma is present.

■ Multiple other abnormalities, including developmental delay, occur if the retinoblastoma is precipitated by a large deletion of chromosome 13.

■ Multiple other tumors occur in other family members or the affected child during life.

Differential Diagnosis

■ Differential diagnoses are the same as those for leukokoria.

■ Retinoblastoma needs to be confirmed or ruled out in any child who does not have a good red reflex or has any other signs of retinoblastoma. Referral for ophthalmologic consultation is essential. Because some tumors hug the wall of the eye and are not present in the visual axis, accurate diagnosis by a primary care physician using a direct ophthalmoscope, especially if dilating drops are not used, can be difficult or impossible. A parental history of intermittent white reflex, or "cat eye," or of the eyes always looking different on flash photographs should be enough to prompt a referral. NOTE: Photoscreening can miss retinoblastoma when the tumor is in certain locations.

Treatment

■ If retinoblastoma is caught and treated early, the sight and life of the child may be saved.

- For small tumors, laser treatment, cryotherapy, and radioactive plaque treatment, combined with chemotherapy in some cases, may restore vision or save the eye.
- For orbital extension, radiation therapy and chemotherapy are often very successful.
- For distant metastases, the prognosis is worse but chemotherapy and radiation therapy have a significant success rate.
- For very advanced ocular tumors, removal of the eye (enucleation) is performed.
- Children with the hereditary form of retinoblastoma, that is, a positive family history, bilateral tumors, positive blood test, or an early age of onset should be monitored closely throughout life for new malignancies, especially sarcomas. The risk of all malignancies is increased.

HETEROCHROMIA

Symptoms

- No symptoms occur.

Signs

- Irides have different colors.
- Pupil on the side of the lighter iris is possibly smaller than normal, so pupillary size must be examined carefully.

Differential Diagnosis

- Heterochromia may represent a benign entity or be the harbinger of a life-threatening disorder.
- Nevus of the darker iris is possible if the pupils are of equal size.
- Waardenburg's syndrome is possible if a white forelock of hair is present on the side of the lighter iris. Deafness is often an associated condition.
- Horner's syndrome is possible if one pupil is miotic, especially if that side also has ptosis. (The two most common causes of Horner's syndrome are birth trauma and neuroblastoma.)
- Heterochromia can also occur with ocular inflammation or trauma, retained intra-ocular foreign body, and retinoblastoma.

Treatment

- Treatment depends on the etiologic process.
- All children with heterochromia should be referred for an ophthalmologic examination to determine whether the disorder is benign.

OCULAR DISORDERS OF CHILDHOOD

CONJUNCTIVITIS

Symptoms

- Itching occurs.
- Pain is present.
- Rarely, vision is blurred.

Signs

- The disorder is usually bilateral but may be asymmetric.
- Conjunctival injection occurs.
- A watery mucoid or mucopurulent discharge is evident.
- Eyelids may adhere on the patient's awakening.
- A preauricular lymph node may be present.
- Nodules or vesicles are present on the conjunctiva.

Differential Diagnosis

- *Viral conjunctivitis*—In young children a diffuse conjunctivitis often accompanies upper respiratory infections and many viral illnesses. Chickenpox and measles may have an associated conjunctivitis. Chickenpox lesions can occur on the conjunctiva and be seen as small vesicles on the white part of the eye. At times, these may become erythematous. A very red, painful eye in a patient with chickenpox may be a symptom of a more severe superinfection and should be examined by an ophthalmologist immediately.

  The most common type of viral conjunctivitis is adenoviral conjunctivitis (see Figs. 4-3 to 4-6). This generally presents with red, profusely watery eyes and a palpable preauricular lymph node. It is often contracted at day care facilities or from family members. Adenoviral conjunctivitis generally runs a 2-week course with worsening symptoms during the first week and then slow improvement during the second week. It is contagious throughout the entire course. In some severe cases a thick, white pseudomembrane forms on the inside of the lower and upper eyelids. Bleeding of the conjunctiva may occur. Some strains cause infiltrates of the cornea beginning 10 to 14 days after the acute infection. This may severely decrease vision and leave some permanent scarring.

- *Herpes simplex conjunctivitis with corneal involvement*—All age groups can contract herpes simplex conjunctivitis. A dendrite (see Fig. 5-7) may be seen on the cornea. Vesicular lid lesions also are common.

- *Bacterial conjunctivitis*—In children, bacterial conjunctivitis is much less common than viral conjunctivitis (see Figs. 4-7 and 4-8). If it does occur, nasolacrimal duct obstruction should be confirmed or ruled out.

- *Chronic conjunctivitis*—The chronic form of conjunctivitis should never occur in children. Persistence of symptoms for longer than a few weeks may signal toxic exposure, underlying iritis, or another disorder. Watery discharge and photophobia point to possible developmental glaucoma. Referral to an ophthalmologist is indicated in all cases.

- *Vernal conjunctivitis*—Found only in children and adolescents, vernal conjunctivitis is a type of allergic conjunctivitis and may be associated with other atopic disorders. The primary symptom is intense itching. The lids may be droopy and discolored from chronic eye rubbing. It generally is cyclic, occurring only at certain times of the year (e.g., spring). Children are usually first seen with thickened conjunctiva around the limbus of the eyes that can be excruciatingly uncomfortable. Prolonged treatment may be necessary. Children should be referred to an ophthalmologist at once if severe pain and discomfort are associated with conjunctivitis.

Associated Factors and Diseases

■ As children age, the risk of iritis increases. This can be seen with viral illnesses such as coxsackievirus, chickenpox, and other acute viral conditions and with juvenile rheumatoid arthritis and other inflammatory conditions. The conjunctiva appears diffusely pink, but no discharge usually occurs. The pupil may be small (miotic), and photophobia is often present. Because untreated iritis can cause cataract, glaucoma, and permanent scarring in the front of the eye, children with this constellation of signs should be referred to an ophthalmologist immediately.

Treatment

■ No treatment modifies the course of viral conjunctivitis. Artificial tears, which may be obtained over the counter, are generally soothing to the eye in the early stages. Topical antibiotic drops are not administered unless there are signs of a bacterial superinfection (a thick, mucopurulent discharge and crusting and adherence of the eyelids). Use of antibiotics for viral ocular infections only increases resistant strains, causes increased irritation from the toxicity of the antibiotics to the cornea, and does not hasten the patient's recovery from the illness.

■ For bacterial superinfection, antibiotic drops (e.g., polymyxin B/trimethoprim [Polytrim] ophthalmic drops 1 drop 4 times a day in each eye) are administered for 7 days. If the infection worsens on this regimen or recurs after the drops are stopped, the child should be referred to an ophthalmologist for appropriate culturing of the conjunctiva.

■ With no discharge, a small (miotic) pupil, and/or photophobia, iritis is a possible cause. Treatment involves the use of corticosteroids and cycloplegic dilating drops, so iritis should only be diagnosed with a slit lamp and treated by an ophthalmologist.

■ Herpes conjunctivitis and keratoconjunctivitis can have the same symptoms and signs as iritis, but if the patient is treated with corticosteroids, loss of the eye can result. These diagnoses are more appropriately made by an ophthalmologist.

OCULAR TRAUMA

Symptoms

■ Symptoms vary and include pain, photophobia, decreased vision, and tearing.

Signs

■ Lid swelling and ecchymosis occur.
■ Conjunctival injection is evident.
■ Subconjunctival hemorrhage can occur.
■ Blood in the eye (hyphema) may be observed.
■ The pupil may be irregular or peaked.
■ A large or small, poorly reactive pupil may be present.
■ A poor red reflex may be noted.

Differential Diagnosis

■ On rare occasions, children try to conceal the actual events of an injury to avoid possible punishment. If unexplained pain, photophobia, or decreased vision occur, trauma should always be suspected.

■ Children often have severe pain, nausea, vomiting, somnolence, and lethargy after intra-ocular bleeding. Layered red blood cells may be seen filling the anterior chamber (hyphema) just behind the cornea (see Fig. 15-16). Glaucoma may result and, if untreated, can cause permanent damage to the optic nerve. In children who have sickle cell disease or sickle trait, a hyphema is more likely to cause severe glaucoma.

■ Any child who has suffered blunt trauma has an increased risk of developing glaucoma throughout life even if glaucoma does not develop at the time of the initial trauma.

■ Nonaccidental trauma, or the shaken baby syndrome, must be suspected in young children with trauma for which the history does not match clinical findings. Retinal hemorrhages may be diagnostic. The presence of retinal hemorrhages in an infant with lethargy, vomiting, and old fractures is pathognomonic and requires notification of authorities. Because retinal hemorrhages may not always be visible with the direct ophthalmoscope, immediate referral to a pediatric ophthalmologist is necessary for examination using indirect ophthalmoscopy (Fig. 12-27).

Treatment

■ For severe blunt or penetrating trauma, the clinician places a protective shield over the eye, using a metal Fox shield or paper or Styrofoam cup that has been cut so that the bottom can be taped over the eye. Excessive manipulation of lids by personnel unaccustomed to examining eyes can result in pressure on the eye and further damage. An immediate ophthalmologic evaluation is critical. Nonsteroidal antiinflammatory agents decrease clotting and are contraindicated. The child is kept quiet until ophthalmologic evaluation is obtained. Antiemetics are administered if the child experiences nausea because vomiting worsens intraocular bleeding or may cause extrusion of ocular contents in the case of a penetrating injury.

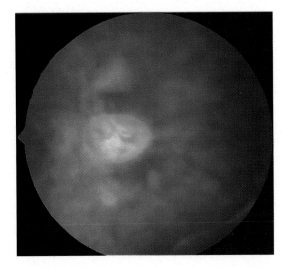

Fig. 12-27 Retinal hemorrhage in the shaken baby syndrome. Visualization with the direct ophthalmoscope is not always possible. This child died of his injuries.

■ For penetrating trauma a tetanus shot is administered if the child's tetanus vaccine is not up to date. Treatment with a broad-spectrum intravenous antibiotic (e.g., cefazolin 25 to 50 mg/kg/day divided into three doses) is initiated. Because of the possibility of surgical intervention, the child is allowed nothing by mouth that would delay an operation. If the trauma involves chemicals in the eye and no rupture, the clinician irrigates the eye with sterile saline solution, usually using 1 to 2 L. This procedure is better tolerated if tetracaine or another topical ocular anesthetic is used initially. Determining the amount of the substance to which the eye was subjected is the first step; often only a small amount of toxic material entered the eye and excessive irrigation may cause more abrasion than the original injury.

Follow-Up

■ Prevention is the best treatment, so children should be advised to wear polycarbonate safety goggles for sports and other high-risk activities. BB guns are a major cause of severe eye injuries in children.

PRESEPTAL AND ORBITAL CELLULITIS

Symptoms

■ For patients with preseptal cellulitis, erythema, warmth, and swelling of the eyelids occur.

■ For patients with orbital cellulitis, irritability, lethargy, decreased vision, high fever, and a more toxic appearance are present.

Signs

■ Preseptal cellulitis is marked by the following:
  • The skin of the eyelids is red and swollen and sharply circumscribed or diffuse.
  • Conjunctival injection may be present.
  • Mucopurulent discharge from the nasolacrimal system may occur if this is the source of infection.
■ Orbital cellulitis is marked by the above signs in addition to the following:
  • Small or diffuse areas of infection that may cause marked motility disturbance
  • Proptosis (a pushing of the eyeball forward because of a mass of infection behind the globe) depending on the location of the infection
  • A large focus of pus near the optic nerve causing the optic nerve to begin to lose function, a decrease in vision, a sluggishly reactive pupil, and a possible afferent pupillary defect

Etiology

■ Cellulitis can result from the following:
  • Ethmoid sinus disease
  • Lacerating trauma around the eye
  • Bacterial infection with nasolacrimal duct obstruction
  • Buccal mucosa infection
  • Stye or chalazion

■ Because the orbital septum in children is extremely thin and does not provide a good barrier against infection from the anterior skin surface, preseptal cellulitis may move rapidly posterior into the orbit, often into the subperiosteal space, causing an abscess. From this location, it may move back to the brain and cause a brain abscess and meningitis. The younger the child, the more rapidly this progression can take place.

Differential Diagnosis

■ Differential diagnoses include the following:
  - Retinoblastoma
  - Ruptured dermoid tumor
  - Orbital pseudotumor
  - Leukemic infiltrate of the orbit

Treatment

■ For children younger than 2 years of age even if the cellulitis is preseptal, hospital admission for intravenous antibiotic administration and observation is needed because of the rapidity with which the infection can move posteriorly. If the child is younger than 3 years of age, appears in a toxic state, or has an elevated white cell count and fever, a full septic workup, including lumbar puncture, is indicated. Broad-spectrum antibiotics are administered, particularly agents targeting gram-positive organisms.

■ For children 2 years of age and older in whom the disease is clinically preseptal, oral antibiotics are administered; these patients are not admitted to the hospital but are carefully followed. If a patient does not respond within 48 hours or worsens at any point, the child is admitted and intravenous antibiotics are administered.

■ In children with signs of orbital involvement, an immediate CT scan of the orbits is needed to detect an abscess or a nidus of infection. If a small subperiosteal abscess is noted, intravenous antibiotics are initially administered for up to 48 hours. In younger children, intravenous antibiotic regimens often resolve an orbital cellulitis even when an abscess is present. If the patient's condition does not improve or worsens in 48 hours, surgical drainage of the abscess is needed.

■ A lumbar puncture is indicated in all these patients before antibiotic administration begins. However, if a lumbar puncture cannot be immediately performed, antibiotics are administered first, particularly in an acutely ill child.

■ If a patient's mental status changes, a CT scan of the brain with contrast is indicated to confirm or rule out a brain abscess.

■ Any immunosuppressed child with erythema around the eyelids should be immediately referred for ophthalmologic evaluation. Mucormycosis is a possible diagnosis, particularly in children with malignancies. In general, mucormycosis is treated with debridement; this disorder does not respond well to the administration of intravenous amphotericin alone.

HEADACHE

Parents and physicians often assume headaches are related to eye disease or eyestrain. This is rare in children, but uncorrected refractive error should always be addressed.

Symptoms

- Headaches occur.
- Vision may be blurred or decreased.

Signs

- Usually, no signs are present.

Differential Diagnosis

- *Migraine*—Severe unilateral or bilateral headache, especially if associated with nausea or vomiting and relieved only by sleep, is often a migraine. The onset in most cases is in early childhood. The classic scintillating scotoma or wavy lines across the field of vision occur in only a minority of patients. However, a history of this phenomenon is almost diagnostic for migraine. Often a family history of migraine headaches is reported. Before the age of puberty, boys and girls experience migraines with equal frequency. After puberty, the incidence of migraines decreases in boys but increases in girls. Thus a hormonal etiology is suspected.
- *Tension or stress headaches*—Often present in children, tension or stress headaches are generally not as prolonged as a migraine. They often occur toward the end of the day at school and are relieved by acetaminophen or aspirin. Children may associate them with reading, but often only a certain class such as mathematics precipitates the headache.

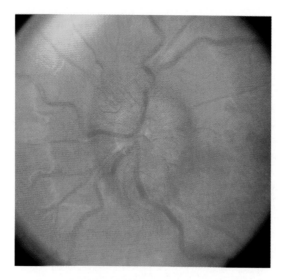

Fig. 12-28 Elevated optic nerve head (papilledema) in a child with headache for 1 week, otitis media, and transverse sinus thrombosis from mastoiditis. Symptoms and signs resolved with serial lumbar puncture, antibiotic administration, and heparin therapy.

- *Increased intracranial pressure*—If a headache is chronic and unremitting, does not improve with sleep or any medication, and is worse in the morning or associated with decreased vision, nausea, vomiting, double vision, or crossing of the eyes, increased intracranial pressure must be suspected. If the child is young enough, head circumference plots should be reviewed. In older children a careful history is needed and physical examination performed for precocious puberty, ataxia, weight loss, and altered mental status, signs of craniopharyngioma and posterior fossa tumors. A fundoscopic examination to detect papilledema (an elevation of the optic nerve, often with hemorrhage on the nerve [Fig. 12-28]) should be performed. If these signs or symptoms are present, the case should be referred to an ophthalmologist as an emergency.

Treatment

- In cases of apparent migraine, triggers should be identified. These often include certain foods such as chocolate, uncorrected refractive error, skipping of meals, lack of sleep, and menses. If the headaches still persist once all triggers have been addressed, many appropriate medications are available. They must be used with care in children, and consultation with a pediatric neurologist is recommended.
- In cases of milder, possibly tension-related headaches, stress-reducing activities are emphasized. Parents and children often perceive that the child's eyes are the source of the problem in tension headaches. The only ocular problems that cause headaches are high uncorrected astigmatism, high hyperopia in older children, and convergence insufficiency. If vision seems decreased in these cases, examination by a pediatric ophthalmologist is needed.

STYES AND CHALAZIA

Symptoms

- Usually no symptoms occur, but mild pain or discomfort may be present.
- In rare cases, vision is blurred as a result of induced astigmatism.

Signs

- An elevated, slightly tender, bright red nodule is present on the outer lid surface or a very erythematous circumscribed area of the conjunctival lining of the eyelid is evident in the early stages (see Fig. 3-16).
- In later stages, the lesion becomes nontender but remains round and very firm, loses its reddish color, but does not disappear (see Fig. 3-17).

Differential Diagnosis

- In children, lesions of this type are almost always hordeola (styes), which is the acute phase, or chalazia, which is the chronic phase.
- In rare cases, basal cell or other types of cancer are present.
- In children with neurofibromatosis a neuroma of the eyelid can occur.
- The lesions of molluscum contagiosum are usually much smaller than styes and have an umbilicated center.
- The lesions of tuberous sclerosis are not usually confined to the lids and can thus be differentiated.

Treatment

- For styes (hordeola), rapid institution of very warm compresses used for 15 to 20 minutes several times a day with or without topical erythromycin ointment in the eye often brings about resolution. Children who are predisposed to styes and chalazia get them repeatedly unless lid hygiene is practiced. This involves using commercially available eye scrub pads or baby shampoo on a warm, wet washcloth to scrub along the base of the eyelashes daily. The meibomian glands, which open near the base of the eyelashes, become plugged in individuals who have thick secretions, causing the stye. In older children and adolescents in whom tetracycline may be used safely without damaging the teeth, a regimen of oral tetracycline is needed if recurrent hordeola are resistant to daily lid scrubs.
- For chalazia, warm soaks, antibiotics, and scrubs are not effective. These must be removed by an ophthalmologist. In older, cooperative children, this procedure can be performed in the office setting with local anesthesia. For very young children, removal requires anesthesia in the operating room. Large chalazia can cause refractive errors, specifically astigmatism. Thus in young children, these should be treated aggressively, and if vision is decreased, an opthalmologic consultation is needed.

STRABISMUS

The peak occurrences of benign esotropia are before 6 months of age (congenital) and between 2 and 4 years (accommodative). Congenital exotropia is rare; intermittent exotropia is quite common. It is often seen fleetingly in the first year of life; one third of these children develop a more frequent occurrence during early childhood and adolescence.

Symptoms

- Double vision and loss of depth perception occur initially. Blindness (amblyopia) slowly results if strabismus is not treated. Very young children are usually not aware of either symptom.

Signs

- The pupils of the eye are misaligned.
- In esotropia, one or both eyes are deviated inward.
- In exotropia, one or both eyes are deviated outward.
- In hypertropia, one eye is deviated upward. In some syndromes, one or both eyes cannot move fully in one or more directions.

Differential Diagnosis

- For acute acquired esotropia, differential diagnoses include the following:
  - Increased intracranial pressure causing sixth nerve palsy or paresis
  - Acute viral sixth nerve palsy
  - Accommodative esotropia
  - Undetected congenital esotropia
- For acute acquired exotropia, differential diagnoses include the following:
  - Acute third nerve palsy
  - Intermittent exotropia with a breakdown of fusion
  - Undetected congenital exotropia

■ In cases of vertical misalignment of the eyes, differential diagnoses include the following:
- Acute fourth nerve palsy
- Decompensated congenital fourth nerve palsy
- Partial third nerve palsy
- Dissociated vertical deviation in a child who had a congenital horizontal misalignment
- Other congenital eye muscle syndromes

Treatment

■ All patients with strabismus should be immediately referred to an ophthalmologist.
■ In children with esotropia, treatment involves the following:
- If the cause is sixth nerve paresis from increased intracranial pressure, normalization of intracranial pressure, usually via neurosurgery, generally results in resolution of the sixth nerve palsy within 6 months. Amblyopia therapy is needed during this time. Any sixth nerve palsy that does not resolve within 6 months after the insult requires eye muscle surgery.
- Viral sixth nerve palsies usually disappear spontaneously once the underlying illness resolves; however, amblyopia therapy during and after the paresis is often necessary in young children.
- Accommodative esotropia is the most common cause of eye crossing in children 2 to 4 years of age and is usually caused by uncorrected hyperopia (Fig. 12-29). These

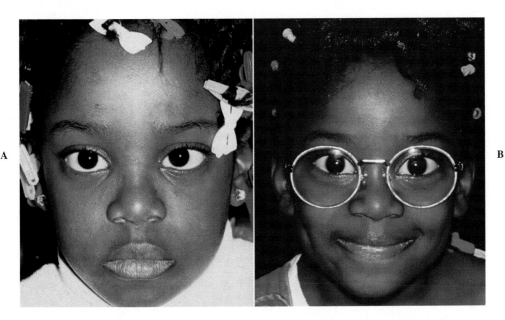

A   B

Fig. 12-29 A, Accommodative esotropia. In this child, fixation with the right eye is preferred; the pupillary light reflex is temporal to the center of the pupil in the left eye because it is crossing in. Vision was not normal even in the right eye because of high hyperopia. **B,** After wearing of full hyperopic correction in spectacles, the eyes are straight (i.e., pupillary light reflexes are centered), vision is 20/20 in each eye, and stereopsis (depth perception) returned to normal. This is only possible if glasses are quickly prescribed once crossing begins.

children require cycloplegic refraction by a pediatric ophthalmologist and must wear their spectacles all the time. As the eye grows, the hyperopia often decreases. Some children can have their prescription strength decreased over serial examinations and may not need glasses and have straight eyes by approximately 9 years of age. If the glasses are not worn, permanent esotropia requiring surgical correction and amblyopia causing blindness of one eye usually result. Some children also require a bifocal to correct crossing at near distance.

- In children with exotropia, treatment involves the following:
  - Intermittent exotropia is more difficult to treat, with options including eye exercises, glasses, and surgical correction.
  - Third nerve palsy exotropia is extremely difficult to treat. Surgery can often help cosmetic alignment, and intensive patching therapy for amblyopia is required, but normal stereopsis usually cannot be achieved.
- In children with hypertropia, treatment involves the following:
  - Acute fourth nerve palsy may be a viral entity or a disorder secondary to an intracranial pathologic disease. Prompt referral to an ophthalmologist is recommended.
  - Decompensated congenital fourth nerve palsy should be treated if a significant head tilt occurs. The treatment of choice is surgery. Exercises do not help this condition, although concomitant exercises for the foreshortened neck muscles may be necessary. Rarely, even surgical correction of the torticollis is necessary if the neck does not straighten after the eye muscle surgery has been performed. In other vertical muscle palsies and abnormalities, correction is more complex and beyond the scope of this chapter.

AMBLYOPIA

Symptoms

- Vision is decreased in one eye, typically to the range of legal blindness (20/200).
- The amblyopia is bilateral in some cases.
- When the disorder is unilateral, children rarely complain or notice the visual deficit.

Signs

- In some cases, no signs occur. The eyes appear normal. Visual acuity is decreased on standardized testing provided the fellow eye is completely occluded to prevent peeking.
- Strabismus is possible, with the poorly seeing eye turning inward in very young children and outward in older children. Decreased stereopsis can be detected on standard stereopsis testing.
- In rare cases an afferent pupillary defect is present in the affected eye.

Differential Diagnosis

- For children with severely decreased vision in one eye, differential diagnoses include the following:
  - Amblyopia
  - Refractive error
  - Congenital abnormality of the retina or optic nerve
  - Cataract
  - Malingering

- In children with bilateral decreased vision, visual acuity is reduced in both eyes to the 20/200 range; nystagmus is present if the deficit occurred within the first 3 months of life and absent if the deficit occurred later. Differential diagnoses include the following:
  - Bilateral refractive errors
  - Bilateral amblyopia
  - Bilateral congenital optic nerve or retinal dysfunction

Treatment

- The mainstay of treatment is early correction of the underlying cause, followed by patching of the better eye under a strictly prescribed regimen that is based on the child's age.
- Deprivation amblyopia is seen in patients with congenital cataracts, hemangiomas of the eyelid, severe congenital ptosis, and corneal leukomas. If this condition is present at birth, it must be completely corrected, including optical correction, before 3 to 4 months of age for the child to have any potential for normal vision. This type of amblyogenic factor generally must be picked up by the pediatrician on the baby's nursery exit examination or a well-baby checkup.
- Amblyopia resulting from uncorrected refractive error is a very common type of amblyopia that is often undiagnosed until the child is too old for the most appropriate treatment. This condition is missed because the refractive error occurs in only one eye or because one eye has a much greater refractive error than the other. The brain favors the better-seeing eye unless spectacles or contact lenses are prescribed. Usually the eyes stay straight and appear normal. Only careful testing for a difference in brightness on the red reflex test with photoscreening or reading of an eye chart in verbal children with complete occlusion of the better eye can detect this type of amblyopia. Spectacle or contact lens correction is sufficient if the condition is detected early. If the amblyopia is detected later, patching of the fellow eye must also be instituted. If both eyes have equal, high refractive errors and glasses are not worn before the age of 8 or 9 years, vision will never be perfect because of bilateral refractive amblyopia.
- Strabismic amblyopia is caused by the underlying esotropia, exotropia, or vertical deviation. Because the brain cannot process two images at once, it ignores one image and one eye loses the ability to see. Again, timing of diagnosis and treatment is critical. If strabismus is present from birth and amblyopia begins very early, complete correction is not possible unless treatment is started within the first months or years of life. If the strabismus begins between 2 and 4 years of age and is rapidly corrected, no amblyopia may result. The longer the amblyopia is untreated, the denser and harder to reverse it is. Generally, refractive and strabismic amblyopia can be effectively treated up to the age of 9 years, whereas deprivation amblyopia does not have a good outcome after a child is 4 months to a year old in most cases. Strabismus must be treated before children reach 2 years of age for them to have the best chance of regaining stereopsis.
- Organic amblyopia results from an anatomic abnormality of the eye such as dragging of the retina in retinopathy of prematurity, coloboma, and optic nerve hypoplasia. The potential for vision in the eye is not 20/20; however, amblyopia therapy must be instituted shortly after birth for the patient to attain the greatest possible vision.

REFRACTIVE ERRORS

Symptoms

- Vision is decreased.
- Eye strain occurs.
- Diplopia is sometimes present.

Signs

- Squinting is observed.
- Blinking of the eyes is excessive.
- The child rubs the eyes.
- The child performs poorly on distant tasks at school.
- The child has poor tolerance for extended periods of reading.

Differential Diagnosis

- Although refractive errors are the cause of decreased vision in the majority of cases, other differential diagnoses include the following:
  - Midline brain tumors that compress the optic chiasm
  - Tumors of the optic nerves
  - Optic neuritis
  - Iritis
  - Inherited retinal degenerations
  - Corneal dystrophies
  - Developmental cataracts

Workup

- Any child who fails a vision screening test or whose parents have noted decreased vision should be referred to a pediatric ophthalmologist for a complete ophthalmologic examination and cycloplegic refraction. This test objectively measures refractive errors and does not rely on a child's answers to a vision test. It also allows for close examination of the optic nerve and retina. Because many progressive disorders result in few signs initially, all children who have decreased vision that is not immediately improved to normal with spectacles should be monitored closely for the development of neurologic and other signs.
- An ophthalmologist should determine the need for glasses in infants using the retinoscope and dilation with cyloplegic drops.

Treatment

- Not all refractive errors in children need to be treated. Unless associated with esotropia, small amounts of hyperopia do not mandate treatment. Minimal myopic correction or correction for small amounts of astigmatism need not be instituted until children begin school.
- High refractive errors are associated with bilateral amblyopia and developmental delays, particularly delayed walking. In these children, spectacle correction should be immediate.

- Because the natural developmental desire is to see clearly, glasses are readily accepted and worn by infants if the refractive error significantly interferes with vision. Even small infants keep them on and search for them if the glasses markedly improve vision. Often an infant who has been wearing glasses appropriately will become less tolerant of wear, which usually indicates that the prescription has changed and should precipitate another referral to the pediatric ophthalmologist. The eye grows very rapidly during infancy, and lenses may need to be changed every 3 to 6 months for the first 2 years of life. Slightly less frequent changes in lenses are needed over the next couple of years. After a child is 4 years of age, yearly examinations are usually acceptable.
- Refractive errors have a genetic basis, although they do not follow simple mendelian inheritance patterns. Thus if parents have high refractive errors, children should be seen at an early age to rule out or confirm refractive errors. All children who wear glasses should be questioned about sports participation and should have a separate pair of prescription wrap-around safety goggles for sports.

INHERITED RETINAL AND CORNEAL DEGENERATIONS

Many retinal degenerations such as retinitis pigmentosa are hereditary. Decreased night vision is often an early symptom. Photophobia can occur during childhood in cases of inherited corneal dystrophies. Any child with a family member who has significant early onset vision problems should have a baseline examination early in life and again if symptoms occur. DNA blood tests are now available for some inherited eye disorders.

SYNDROMES

Approximately 25% of the U.S. population is nearsighted (myopic), and although myopia begins in childhood, it is usually of low to moderate degree and increases slowly throughout adolescence. If high myopia or rapidly progressive myopia is present before 6 years of age, an underlying syndrome should be sought. Homocystinuria and Marfan syndrome have associated less subluxation that causes high myopia. These disorders can be life threatening. Stickler syndrome is an autosomal dominant disorder that includes cleft palate, early arthritis, partial deafness, and high myopia. High hyperopia and astigmatism are associated with albinism. Any child with a very high refractive error, especially myopia, should have a complete workup by a pediatric ophthalmologist.

Orbital Disease

Ted H. Wojno

ANATOMY

The bony orbit is a four-sided pyramid with the apex pointed posteriorly (Fig. 13-1). The medial orbital wall is composed mainly of the ethmoid bone. The lateral wall is composed of the zygomatic bone anteriorly and the greater wing of the sphenoid bone posteriorly. The superior wall is composed of the frontal bone, whereas the inferior wall is formed by the maxillary and zygomatic bones. The optic foramen transmits the optic nerve and ophthalmic artery. The superior orbital fissure transmits the third, fourth, opthalmic division of fifth, and sixth cranial nerves.

The four rectus muscles are involved in horizontal and vertical movements of the globe (Fig. 13-2). The superior and inferior oblique muscles are involved in the globe's torsional movements, and the orbital fat cushions and supports the globe. The pink lacrimal gland is located just under the superolateral orbital rim. The clinician can easily visualize this structure, which is responsible for reflex tearing, by retracting the upper lid superolaterally and having the patient look inferonasally (Fig. 13-3). The lacrimal drainage system begins with the puncta and canaliculi, which join to enter the lacrimal sac (Fig. 13-4). The sac empties into the nasolacrimal duct, which passes through the medial wall of the maxillary sinus and empties into the nose under the inferior turbinate.

PRESEPTAL CELLULITIS

For preseptal cellulitis in children, see Chapter 12.

Symptoms

- Warm, erythematous, tender swelling of the lids may extend over the nasal bridge to the opposite side.

Signs

- Usually a low-grade fever and elevated white blood cell count are found.
- Vision, pupillary reflexes, and extraocular movements are normal.
- Blood cultures are negative unless the organism is *Haemophilus influenzae* or *Streptococcus pneumoniae*.

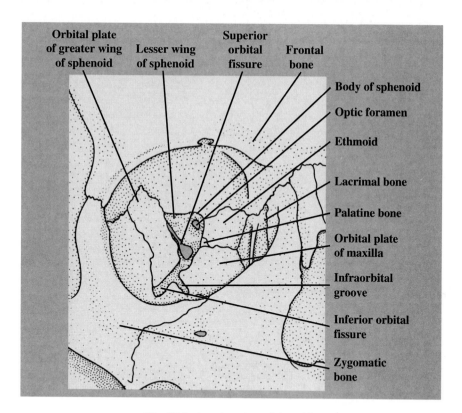

Fig. 13-1 Anterior view of the orbit.

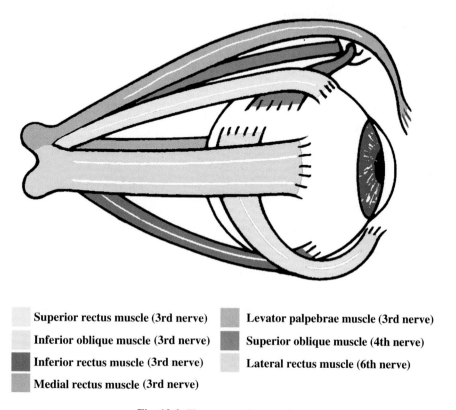

Superior rectus muscle (3rd nerve)	Levator palpebrae muscle (3rd nerve)
Inferior oblique muscle (3rd nerve)	Superior oblique muscle (4th nerve)
Inferior rectus muscle (3rd nerve)	Lateral rectus muscle (6th nerve)
Medial rectus muscle (3rd nerve)	

Fig. 13-2 The extraocular muscles.

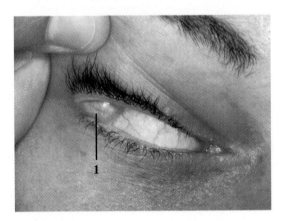

Fig. 13-3 The normal lacrimal gland *(1)*.

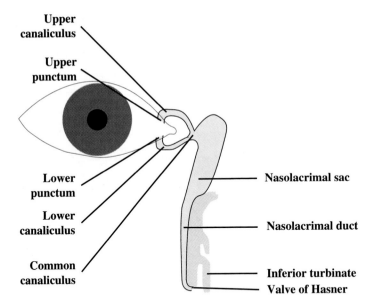

Fig. 13-4 The nasolacrimal excretory system.

Etiology

- An upper respiratory tract infection or sinusitis can result in the disorder. The most common causative organisms in adults are *Streptococcus* species, *Staphylococcus aureus,* and mixed flora.
- Lid trauma (blunt or perforating) can lead to preseptal cellulitis. The most common causative organisms are *Streptococcus pyogenes, S. aureus,* and fungus (if organic material was involved).
- The disorder can result from superficial lid infections such as a stye (hordeolum) or impetigo.
- Conjunctivitis can cause the disorder.
- Dacryocystitis can lead to the disorder.
- In rare cases, septicemia results in the disorder.

Differential Diagnosis

- Differential diagnoses include the following:
  - Orbital cellulitis
  - Orbital pseudotumor
  - Carotid-cavernous fistula

Workup

- A CBC is performed.
- Culture of an open wound, purulent nasal drainage, conjunctival discharge, or any weeping vesicles is performed.
- Computed tomography (CT) scan of orbits and sinuses is performed if indicated.
- Blood cultures are performed if *H. influenzae* or *S. pneumoniae* is suspected.

Treatment

- In cases of mild to moderate preseptal cellulitis without localized abscess, an oral, broad-spectrum antibiotic (e.g., amoxicillin/clavulanate [Augmentin] 250 to 500 mg 3 times a day) is administered. If the patient is allergic to penicillin, oral erythromycin (250 to 500 mg 4 times a day) is given.
- In cases of severe preseptal cellulitis, an intravenous, broad-spectrum antibiotic (e.g., cefuroxime [Zinacef] 750 mg to 1.5 g 3 times a day) is administered. If the patient is allergic to penicillin, intravenous clindamycin (300 mg 4 times a day) and intravenous gentamicin (1 mg/kg 3 times a day) are administered.
  NOTE: Antibiotic dosages should be adjusted in the presence of renal impairment. Peak and trough levels of gentamicin are used to adjust dosage. Blood urea nitrogen (BUN) and creatinine levels are followed closely.
- In cases of localized abscess formation, an oral or intravenous, broad-spectrum antibiotic is administered depending on the severity of the abscess. Incision and drainage with or without a drain may be performed depending on the severity of the abscess.
- For lesions with extensive crusting, after incision and drainage, or in cases of penetrating injury, a topical broad-spectrum ophthalmic ointment such as polymyxin B/bacitracin (Polysporin) is used.

Follow-Up

- The focus of follow-up is to ensure that orbital cellulitis does not develop.

ORBITAL CELLULITIS AND ABSCESS

For orbital cellulitis in children, see Chapter 12.

Symptoms

- The symptoms are the same as those for preseptal cellulitis. Orbital involvement can lead to vision loss and double vision.

Signs

- Usually a low grade fever and elevated white blood cell count are found.
- Proptosis, restricted motility, sluggish pupillary reflex, and decreased vision occur (Fig. 13-5).

Workup

- Workup is the same as that for cases of preseptal cellulitis.
- A fundoscopic examination may reveal retinal hemorrhages, venous congestion, and disc edema.
- A CT scan displays diffuse infiltration of orbital fat that may progress to abscess formation (Fig. 13-6).
- Blood cultures are usually negative.

Etiology

- Underlying causes are the same as those for preseptal cellulitis.
- Surgical procedures that violate the orbital septum such as strabismus, retinal detachment repair, and orbital surgery can lead to the disorder.

Differential Diagnosis

- Differential diagnoses are the same as those for preseptal cellulitis.

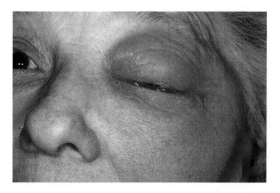

Fig. 13-5 Orbital cellulitis resulting from ethmoid sinusitis.

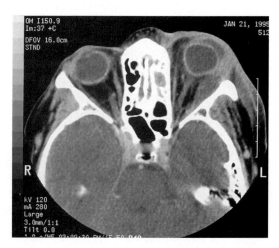

Fig. 13-6 An axial CT scan of the patient in Fig. 13-5 shows diffuse infiltration of the left orbital structures.

Treatment

- An intravenous, broad-spectrum antibiotic (e.g., cefuroxime [Zinacef] 750 mg to 1.5 g 3 times a day) is used. If the patient is allergic to penicillin, intravenous clindamycin (300 mg 4 times a day) and intravenous gentamicin (1 mg/kg 3 times a day) are used.
    NOTE: Antibiotic dosages should be adjusted in the presence of renal impairment. Peak and trough levels of gentamicin are used to adjust dosage. BUN and creatinine levels are followed closely.
- Surgical drainage is needed for a large abscess or small abscess that does not resolve on an intravenous antibiotic regimen in 2 or 3 days.
- Sinus drainage is performed if appropriate.

Follow-Up

- The focus of follow-up is to ensure that cavernous sinus thrombosis does not develop.

NASOLACRIMAL DUCT OBSTRUCTION
Symptoms and Signs

- Tearing occurs.

Etiology and Associated Factors and Diseases

- Previous nasal or sinus disease, surgery, or trauma can lead to stenosis of the naso-lacrimal duct.
- The disorder can have an idiopathic origin.
- In rare cases, a tumor may also be present.

Differential Diagnosis

- Tearing secondary to ocular irritation should be ruled out or confirmed.

Workup

- Probing and irrigation of the nasolacrimal system is performed to confirm the presence of an obstruction.

Treatment

- If the patient and physician feel the symptoms warrant intervention, a surgical fistula is created by connecting the lacrimal sac to the nasal mucosa, thus bypassing the obstructed nasolacrimal duct (dacryocystorhinostomy).

DACRYOCYSTITIS
Symptoms

- Tearing, pain, and mucopurulent drainage occur in dacryocystitis (infection of the lacrimal sac).

Signs

- Tearing, swollen lacrimal sac, and mucopurulent drainage are evident (Fig. 13-7).
- In rare cases, preseptal cellulitis occurs.

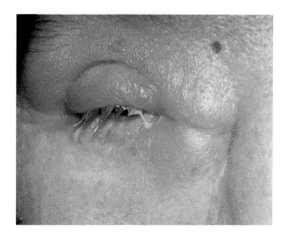

Fig. 13-7 Acute dacryocystitis. This acute infection involves erythema and enlargement lateral to the nasal bridge. Mucopurulent conjunctivitis is also present.

Etiology

■ Nasolacrimal duct obstruction can lead to infection of the lacrimal sac.

Differential Diagnosis

■ An ethmoid mucocele should be ruled out or confirmed.

Workup

■ Digital pressure over the lacrimal sac may cause reflux of the mucopurulent material.

Treatment

■ In cases of acute dacryocystitis an oral, broad-spectrum antibiotic (e.g., amoxicillin/clavulanate [Augmentin] 250 to 500 mg 3 times a day) is administered. If the patient is allergic to penicillin, oral erythromycin (250 to 500 mg 4 times a day) is used.
■ Incision and drainage are appropriate interventions if a large abscess has formed.
■ Dacryocystorhinostomy or dacryocystectomy is performed when the infection is quiescent.
■ In cases of chronic dacryocystitis, dacryocystorhinostomy or dacryocystectomy is performed.

DACRYOADENITIS

Symptoms

■ Lateral lid swelling, pain, and tearing occur in dacryoadenitis (inflammation of the lacrimal gland).

Signs

■ The lacrimal gland is swollen, tender, and erythematous (Fig. 13-8).
■ Inferonasal globe displacement occurs.

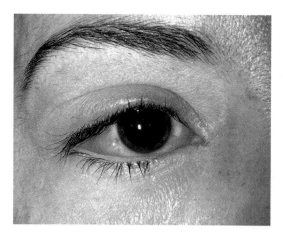

Fig. 13-8 Acute viral dacryoadenitis. The superior temporal lid is erythematous, and the lid margin is S shaped as a result of the underlying enlargement of the lacrimal gland.

Etiology

- Commonly the inflammation is idiopathic.
- Less common inflammations include sarcoidosis, vasculitis, and Sjögren's syndrome.
- Uncommonly, infectious bacterial and viral agents (e.g., mononucleosis, mumps, herpes zoster) can lead to the disorder.

Differential Diagnosis

- Tumor of lacrimal gland should be ruled out or confirmed.

Workup

- Signs of bacterial or viral infection are sought.
- Signs of other inflammatory disorders are sought.
- A CT scan or an MRI of the orbits is performed.
- A biopsy of the lacrimal gland is undertaken if indicated.

Treatment

- In cases of idiopathic inflammation, oral corticosteroids are administered.
- In cases of a specific inflammation the underlying disorder is treated.
- In cases of infectious agents the following apply:
  - Oral, broad-spectrum antibiotics (e.g., amoxicillin/clavulanate [Augmentin] 250 to 500 mg 3 times a day) is used for bacterial infection. If the patient is allergic to penicillin, oral erythromycin (250 to 500 mg 4 times a day) is administered.
  - In cases of viral infection, the underlying disorder is treated.

Follow-Up

- A biopsy of the lacrimal gland is performed if the condition fails to resolve with appropriate therapy.

CANALICULITIS

Symptoms

■ Tearing, pain, and mucopurulent discharge occur.

Signs

■ Swelling and erythema are noted over the involved canaliculus (Fig. 13-9).
■ Mucopurulent discharge results when digital pressure is applied over the involved canaliculus.

Etiology

■ Infectious organisms that can lead to the disorder include *Actinomyces* species (most common) and *Streptomyces* species, which are often associated with stones in the canaliculus (dacryolith).

Differential Diagnosis

■ Differential diagnoses include the following:
  • Dacryocystitis
  • Tumor

Treatment

■ Curettage of the canaliculus is performed by an ophthalmologist to remove the stones.
■ Surgical incision of the canaliculus (canaliculotomy) is performed to remove the stones.
■ Nasolacrimal duct probing and irrigation confirm patency of the distal system.

Follow-Up

■ The focus of follow-up is to monitor for recurrences, which are uncommon if the canaliculus was incised.

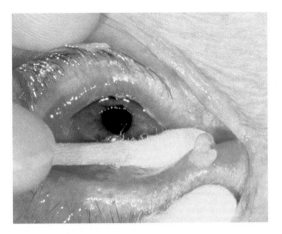

Fig. 13-9 Canaliculitis includes conjunctivitis, inflamed and pouting punctum, and expressible discharge from the canaliculus.

THYROID EYE DISEASE

Symptoms

- In mild cases, irritation, burning, foreign body sensation, and tearing occur.
- In moderate cases, double vision, aching discomfort, and blurred vision occur.
- In severe cases, visual loss and pain from corneal ulceration occur.

Signs

- The onset is gradual.
- Lid retraction occurs, with superior or inferior scleral show (Fig. 13-10).
- The patient is unable to close the eyes (lagophthalmos).
- The disorder is usually bilateral, although often asymmetric.
- Ocular motility is restricted (Fig. 13-11).
- Exophthalmos is evident (Figs. 13-10 and 13-12).
- Conjunctival blood vessels are dilated, especially over medial and lateral rectus muscles.
- Swelling of the conjunctiva, lids, and brows is noted.
- A loss of visual acuity, visual field, and color vision occurs.

Etiology

- A thyroid abnormality can lead to the disease.
- Patient may be hyperthyroid, hypothyroid, or euthyroid when the orbital disease occurs.
- Some patients have autoimmune thyroiditis (Hashimoto's disease).
- Ophthalmic disease may precede or follow glandular disease by many years.
- Most commonly, ophthalmic disease develops shortly after the patient undergoes treatment for hyperthyroidism.

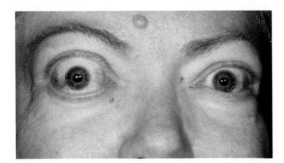

Fig. 13-10 A patient with thyroid eye disease showing both exophthalmos and lid retraction. Note the dilated conjunctival blood vessels over the medial and lateral rectus muscles.

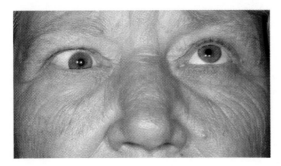

Fig. 13-11 A patient with severe ocular motility disturbance resulting from thyroid eye disease. The patient is attempting to look up.

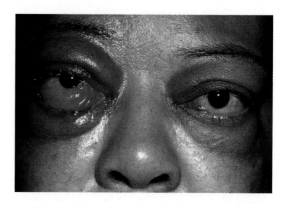

Fig. 13-12 A patient with severe exophthalmos and orbital congestion resulting from thyroid eye disease.

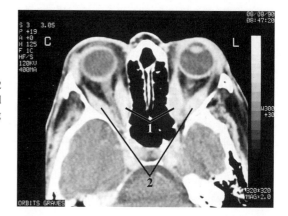

Fig. 13-13 An axial CT scan of the patient in Fig. 13-12 shows fusiform enlargement of the medial *(1)* and lateral *(2)* rectus muscles in both eyes producing compressive optic neuropathy at the orbital apex.

Differential Diagnosis

■ Differential diagnoses include the following:
   • Conjunctivitis
   • Orbital pseudotumor
   • Myasthenia gravis
   • Orbital tumor

Associated Factors and Diseases

■ Ophthalmopathy remains active for an average of 2 years and much longer in some patients.

Workup

■ A complete battery of thyroid tests is needed.
■ Careful monitoring of the patient's thyroid status is performed if the thyroid tests have normal findings.
■ A CT scan or an MRI is needed if the ophthalmic diagnosis is not completely confirmed (Fig. 13-13).

- A thorough ophthalmologic examination and computerized visual field testing are performed to diagnose early visual loss and other sight-threatening conditions. Visual loss is caused by enlarged extraocular muscles compressing the apical portion of the optic nerve (compressive optic neuropathy).

Treatment
- In mild cases, artificial tears are used for lubrication.
- In moderate to severe cases the following apply:
  - The head of the bed is elevated to reduce congestion.
  - Oral prednisone (20 to 100 mg/day) is used to treat congestion, inflammation, and compressive optic neuropathy. Unfortunately, when the dosage is reduced, the ophthalmopathy flares again quickly. Oral prednisone is usually a temporizing therapy.
  - Orbital radiation is performed for congestion, inflammation, and compressive optic neuropathy. This may shorten the overall course of the disease or decrease the severity. This therapy begins working in 1 month, and it may cause radiation retinopathy.
  - Orbital decompression is performed for congestion, compressive optic neuropathy, and exophthalmos. Beneficial effects may be noted within days. Ocular motility disturbances may worsen. Long-term side effects include sinusitis and facial paresthesias.
  - Eye muscle surgery (strabismus surgery) is performed after the disease is quiescent to correct double vision.
  - Repair of lid retraction is performed after the disease is quiescent or during the active phase if severe exposure is present.

Follow-Up
- Ophthalmologic examination is needed every 3 to 6 months during the active phase and yearly thereafter to monitor for ophthalmopathy, which may recur.
- Visual field testing is performed as needed to exclude the possibility of compressive optic neuropathy.

ORBITAL PSEUDOTUMOR
Symptoms
- The acute variety, in which the onset is hours to a few days, is the common form and involves severe pain, proptosis, visual loss, restricted ocular motility, malaise, and fatigue.
- The subacute to chronic variety, in which the onset is weeks to months, is the uncommon form.
- Symptoms experienced depend on the location and rapidity of onset. In general, the more acute the onset, the more dramatic the symptoms.

Signs
- The disorder is usually unilateral.
- See Box 13-1 for classification.

Etiology
- The origin of the disorder is idiopathic.

Text continued on page 224

Box 13-1
Classification of orbital pseudotumor

Diffuse
- Generalized orbital involvement occurs (Figs. 13-14 and 13-15).

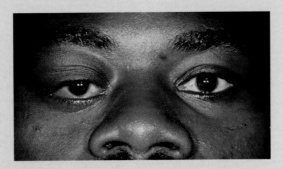

Fig. 13-14 Diffuse orbital pseudotumor. This 30-year-old man had a 2-day history of pain, proptosis, motility restriction, and visual loss involving the right eye.

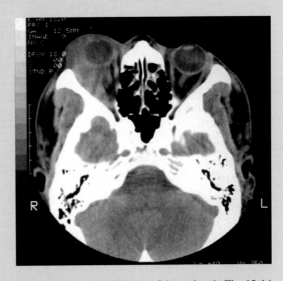

Fig. 13-15 An axial CT scan of the patient in Fig. 13-14 showing diffuse orbital inflammation on the right side.

Box 13-1
Classification of orbital pseudotumor—cont'd

Posterior tenonitis
- The inflammation is restricted to the posterior half of the connective tissue surrounding the globe (Tenon's capsule) (Figs. 13-16 and 13-17).

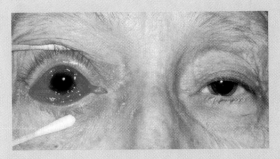

Fig. 13-16 Orbital pseudotumor, posterior tenonitis. This 86-year-old woman had a 3-day history of pain, lid and conjunctival swelling, and visual loss of the right eye.

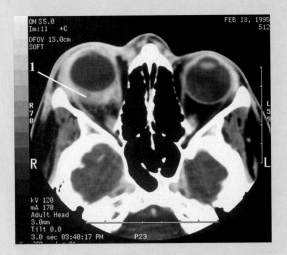

Fig. 13-17 An axial CT scan of the patient in Fig. 13-16 shows that the inflammation is restricted to posterior Tenon's capsule (1) of the right eye.

Continued

Box 13-1

Classification of orbital pseudotumor—cont'd

Orbital myositis
■ The inflammation is restricted to one or a few extraocular muscles (Figs. 13-18 and 13-19).

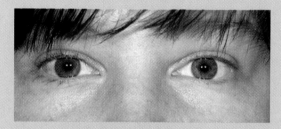

Fig. 13-18 Orbital pseudotumor, myositis. This 30-year-old woman had a 1-week history of double vision and pain in the left eye.

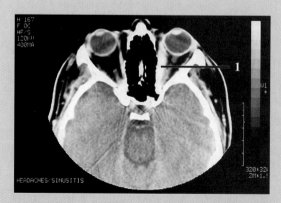

Fig. 13-19 An axial CT scan of the patient in Fig. 13-18 shows orbital myositis involving the left medial rectus muscle *(1)*.

Box 13-1
Classification of orbital pseudotumor—cont'd

Dacryoadenitis
■ The inflammation is restricted to the lacrimal gland (Figs. 13-20 and 13-21).

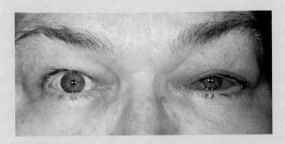

Fig. 13-20 Orbital pseudotumor, dacryoadenitis. This 64-year-old woman had a 1-month history of pain, swelling, and erythema of the left eye nonresponsive to oral antibiotics and topical corticosteroid drops.

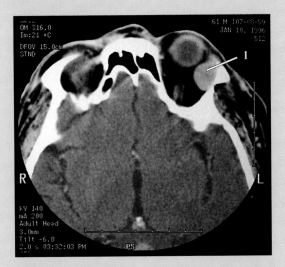

Fig. 13-21 An axial CT scan of the patient in Fig. 13-20 shows enlargement of the left lacrimal gland *(1)*.

Differential Diagnosis

- Differential diagnoses include the following:
  - Thyroid eye disease
  - Specific orbital inflammation (e.g., sarcoidosis, vasculitis)
  - Orbital cellulitis
  - Orbital tumor

Workup

- A biopsy is often necessary because orbital pseudotumor is a diagnosis of exclusion. Polymorphous inflammatory cell infiltrate with variable degrees of fibrosis is noted.
- A CT scan or an MRI is indicated.
- The diagnosis of orbital pseudotumor is made when there is a low index of suspicion for other causes of these symptoms.

Treatment

- Prednisone (80 to 120 mg/day) is administered and tapered over 4 to 8 weeks. This usually gives rapid (1 to 3 days) and permanent resolution of symptoms.
- Low-dose orbital radiation (20 to 30 Gy) is an acceptable alternative if the patient relapses after corticosteroids are tapered (uncommonly) or if the patient cannot take corticosteroids.
- Immunosuppression may be needed with Cytoxan, Imuran, or cyclosporine if the patient fails to respond to corticosteroids and radiation therapy, which is a rare occurrence.

Follow-Up

- The disorder rarely recurs.

Systemic Disease and Therapies

Emmett F. Carpel

SYSTEMIC DISEASES

ANKYLOSING SPONDYLITIS

Ankylosing spondylitis is an immune-mediated disease with arthritis as its major manifestation. The rheumatic changes involve the sacroiliac and vertebral joints. The incidence of the disorder is higher in males than in females. The ocular manifestation is anterior uveitis.

Symptoms
- Vision is decreased.
- Pain occurs.
- A burning sensation is reported.
- Brow ache occurs.
- Light sensitivity is noted.

Signs
- Perilimbal injection is evident.
- Cells and flare are usually seen on slit lamp examination.
- Pupils may be small.

Treatment
- Patients should be referred to an ophthalmologist.
- Cycloplegia and topical corticosteroids are used for anterior uveitis.
- The ocular prognosis is generally very good.

BEHÇET'S DISEASE

Behçet's disease is a systemic vasculitis of small blood vessels with major mucocutaneous and ophthalmic manifestations. The clinical diagnosis is based on a triad of uveitis and oral and genital ulcers, which are the clinically most consistent sign. Skin lesions (erythema nodosum), arthritis, and neurologic involvement also occur.

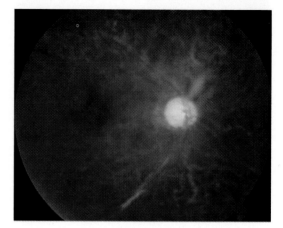

Fig. 14-1 End-stage retinal disease in Behçet's disease as a result of recurrent retinal vascular occlusive episodes. Note markedly attenuated retinal vessels, fibrosis, and optic atrophy.

Symptoms

■ Pain, redness, and light sensitivity occur if anterior uveitis is present.

■ Vision is decreased if the retina or optic nerve is involved.

Signs

■ In cases of anterior uveitis, conjunctival injection, anterior chamber cells and flare, corneal cellular precipitate, and an accumulation of white cells in the anterior chamber (hypopyon) are found.

■ Retinal vasculitis occurs.

■ Optic nerve atrophy can occur (Fig. 14-1).

Treatment

■ Patients should be referred to an ophthalmologist.

■ Cycloplegia and topical corticosteroids are administered.

■ Systemic immunosuppression may be necessary for retinal or systemic vasculitis.

■ Systemic corticosteroids, cyclosporin A, azathioprine, and a combination of azathioprine and cyclophosphamide have been used for treatment.

■ The prognosis is poor even with aggressive treatment. Severe vasculitis may lead to a loss of vision.

DERMATOMYOSITIS

Dermatomyositis is a collagen vascular disease that primarily involves the skin and muscle. It is an immune complex–mediated vasculopathic disorder and may occur with other collagen diseases such as rheumatoid arthritis, systemic lupus erythematosis, scleroderma, and polyarteritis nodosa. Muscle weakness, especially of the proximal limb muscles, may occur over weeks or with an acute onset. Muscle pain may be present.

Symptoms

■ Usually no symptoms occur.

■ Pain, redness, and light sensitivity are noted if anterior uveitis is present.

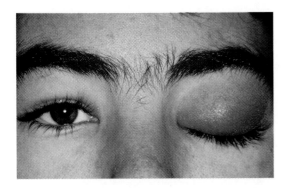

Fig. 14-2 A heliotrope rash on the upper lid has a violaceous discoloration.

- A heliotrope discoloration of upper eyelids often occurs in patients with telangiectasia (Fig. 14-2).
- Periorbital and conjunctival edema are reported.
- Anterior uveitis is rarely found.
- Retinopathy may manifest as cotton-wool spots.
- Hemorrhages, variable pigmentation of the fundus, and optic atrophy caused by occlusive vasculitis occur rarely.

Treatment
- No specific ocular therapy is necessary unless anterior uveitis is present.
- The ocular prognosis is generally good.

DIABETES

Diabetes is a metabolic vasculopathy in which the major cause of permanent visual loss results from retinal vascular disease. (For a more detailed description of diabetic retinopathy, see Chapter 9.)

Symptoms
- Patients display no symptoms.
- A sudden change in visual acuity occurs; most often the patient becomes nearsighted.
- A sudden, painless visual loss is associated with vitreous hemorrhage.
- A gradual visual loss is often caused by cataracts.
- A sudden, painful visual loss is associated with neovascular glaucoma.

Signs
- A change in the refractive error occurs (i.e., glasses need to be stronger or weaker).
- Small, poorly reactive pupils (pseudo–Argyll Robertson pupils) are found.
- Cortical spokes (Fig. 14-3) or snowflake-type cataracts are evident.
- Retinal hemorrhages, exudates, microaneurysms, neovascularization, and vitreous hemorrhage occur (see Chapter 9).

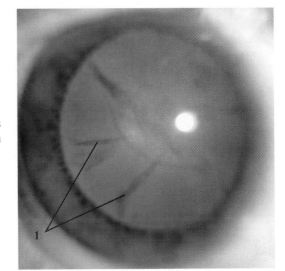

Fig. 14-3 Spokelike clefts in the lens cortex *(1)*. Cataracts may occur at an earlier age in patients with diabetes than in the general population.

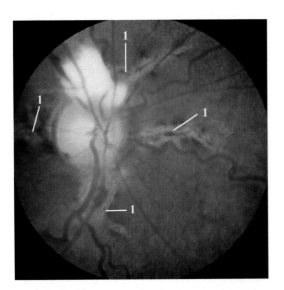

Fig. 14-4 Ehlers-Danlos syndrome—Angioid streaks *(1)*. These irregular, hypopigmented lines are a result of degeneration and breaks in Bruch's membrane. Angioid streaks are also seen in pseudoxanthema exasticum, sickle cell disease, and Paget's disease (osteitis deformans).

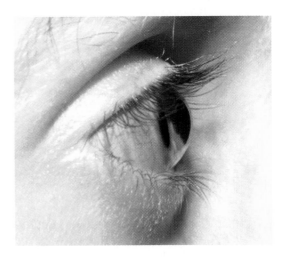

Fig. 14-5 Ehlers-Danlos syndrome is characterized by poor cross-linking of collagen. This results in joint hypermobility, skin hyperextensibility, easy bruising, and a propensity toward tissue rupture. A blue sclera (as seen here) results from thinning of the sclera.

EHLERS-DANLOS SYNDROME

Symptoms

- No symptoms occur.
- Vision loss may result as a complication of angioid streaks.

Signs

- Angiod streaks are found in the retina adjacent to the optic disc (Fig. 14-4). Retinal bleeding may occur as a result of these streaks. Other causes of angioid streaks include sickle cell disease, Paget's disease of the bone, lead poisoning, and other collagen disorders such as Weill-Marchesani syndrome and pseudoxanthoma elasticum.
- Extreme thinning of the cornea (keratoglobus) can occur with Ehlers-Danlos syndrome type VI (Fig. 14-5).

Treatment

No specific ocular treatment exists. However, with sudden visual loss resulting from subretinal neovascular membrane associated with angioid streaks, laser photocoagulation may be indicated. Patients with extremely thin corneas (keratoglobus) must wear safety glasses at all times because minor trauma can result in globe rupture and blindness.

HIV INFECTION

The human immunodeficiency virus (HIV) is a retrovirus that destroys the cells of the body's immune system, resulting in a host of systemic and ophthalmic problems.

Molluscum Contagiosum

Molluscum contagiosum is a nodular, umbilicated lesion often up to 2 to 3 mm in size (see Fig. 3-18). These lesions occur more often in HIV-infected patients and are seen on the eyelids in many patients. They can cause a chronic conjunctivitis. Treatment usually focuses on evacuating the contents of the crater, but simple excision is probably a more definitive treatment.

Herpes Zoster Ophthalmicus

Herpes zoster ophthalmicus is seen with increased frequency in young adults with HIV infection, and it may be the initial sign of HIV infection. It typically begins with a rash or vesicles in the distribution of the fifth cranial nerve (see Fig. 5-9). Ocular involvement includes corneal inflammation, glaucoma, and uveitis. The eye findings may progress as the skin lesions resolve. (For treatment, see Chapter 5.)

Kaposi's Sarcoma

Kaposi's sarcoma is a bluish-purple vascular tumor frequently seen on the eyelid or conjunctiva in HIV-infected patients. These lesions are usually painless and discrete and may appear as flat patches, elevated papules, or raised nodules. When the lesions occur on the conjunctiva, the disorder may initially manifest as a hemorrhagic conjunctivitis, most commonly inferiorly (Fig. 14-6). Treatment options include surgical excision, cryotherapy, radiotherapy, and chemotherapy, or no treatment may be implemented.

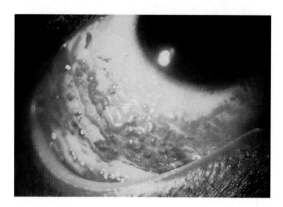

Fig. 14-6 Kaposi's sarcoma mimics subconjunctival hemorrhage or hemangioma, but the nodularity and thickness of the vessels are distinctive.

Cotton-Wool Spots

Cotton-wool spots are the most common ocular finding in early HIV-related retinopathy. They represent a nerve fiber layer infarct caused by a microvasculopathy. They appear identical to cotton-wool spots seen in patients with diabetes (see Fig. 9-10) or hypertension. Distinguishing between cotton-wool spots and very early cytomegalovirus retinitis may be difficult; observation leads to the correct diagnosis. No specific treatment of cotton-wool spots is indicated.

CMV Retinitis

See Chapter 9.

HYPERLIPIDEMIA

Symptoms

■ Usually no symptoms occur.

Signs

■ The following signs may be associated with hyperlipidemia but not invariably so:
   • Heavy arcus of the cornea (especially in patients under age 50) (Fig. 14-7)
   • Xanthelasma (especially in those under age 50), although most xanthelasma is not associated with increased lipids (see Fig. 3-11)
   • Lipid deposition in the retina (lipemia retinalis), a rare finding that may be seen when serum triglyceride levels exceed 2500 mg/ml

Treatment

■ Systemic treatment of hyperlipidemia is undergone if indicated.
■ Xanthelasma may be excised for cosmetic purposes.
■ Lipid deposition in the retina usually resolves when the triglyceride levels are normalized.

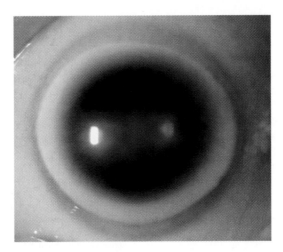

Fig. 14-7 Arcus senilis. A heavy deposition of lipid in the peripheral cornea at a young age (i.e., younger than 50 years) may be associated with hyperlipidemia. Arcus usually occurs as a normal aging change.

HYPERTENSION

Symptoms

- Usually no symptoms occur.
- With malignant hypertension, blurred vision, blind spots, and visual loss may be present.

Signs

- Ocular:
  - Externally, no signs are noted.
  - Retinal findings include focal narrowing of retinal arterioles or general narrowing, vessel light reflex changes, nerve fiber layer hemorrhages, and cotton-wool spots (see Chapter 9).
- Additional signs with malignant hypertension:
  - Papilledema is evident.
  - Lipid exudates are found in a star configuration (Fig. 14-8).
  - Macular edema occurs.

Treatment

- The elevated blood pressure is treated.

INFLAMMATORY BOWEL DISEASE

Inflammatory bowel disease, most notably Crohn's disease, and ulcerative colitis may have associated ocular findings in the anterior segment of the eye.

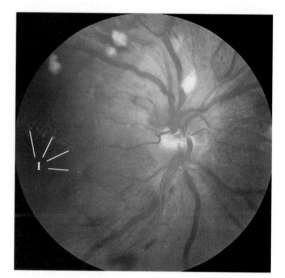

Fig. 14-8 Advanced hypertensive retinopathy. Lipid deposits in the macula *(1)*, cotton-wool spots, small flame hemorrhages, vascular light reflex changes, venous tortuosity, and early disc edema are present.

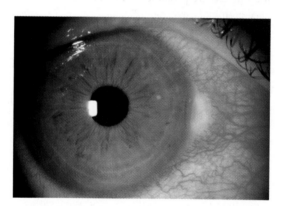

Fig. 14-9 Crohn's disease with sclerokeratitis.

Symptoms

- Pain and redness occur if episcleritis or scleritis is present.
- Pain, light sensitivity, and redness are noted if anterior uveitis is present.

Signs

- In cases of episcleritis and scleritis, local or diffuse scleral injection occurs.
- In cases of anterior uveitis, perilimbal injection, anterior chamber cell and flare, and corneal cellular precipitates are findings.
- Limbal corneal infiltrates may not stain with fluorescein and usually occur adjacent to an area of scleritis (Fig. 14-9).

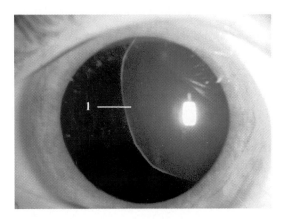

Fig. 14-10 Marfan syndrome—Luxation of crystalline lens *(1).*

- Cataracts are possible if the patient has been taking systemic corticosteroids for long periods.
- Dry eye and night blindness are possible findings in severe cases and are secondary to vitamin A deficiency with malabsorptive states.

Treatment

- Patients should be referred to an ophthalmologist.
- Topical corticosteroids and cycloplegics help control inflammation of the cornea or in the anterior chamber.
- Scleritis and associated limbal corneal infiltrates may respond to topical corticosteroids, but in some cases, systemic immunosuppression (e.g., oral corticosteroids) is needed.

MARFAN SYNDROME

Marfan syndrome is an autosomal dominant disorder of connective tissue that has ocular, skeletal, and cardiovascular findings. The basic defect is in collagen (fibrillin deficiency).

Symptoms

- Monocular diplopia occurs.
- A painless decrease in vision is noted.
- Fluctuating vision occurs.

Signs

- A subluxation or luxation of the lens, usually upward, occurs and is best seen with a dilated examination (to allow visualization of the edge of the lens with a slit lamp) or occasionally with gross examination (Fig. 14-10). A tremulousness of the iris known as *iridodonesis* may indicate a lack of normal lens support.
- Glaucoma may be an associated finding.
- The axial length of the eye increases, resulting in myopia.

Treatment

■ Contact lenses are prescribed if the luxated lens is out of the visual axis.

■ Lens extraction is performed if the luxated lens obstructs the visual axis.

MUCOPOLYSACCHARIDOSES

The mucopolysaccharidoses are a group of lysosomal storage diseases caused by a deficiency of the enzymes that degrade glycosaminoglycans. Subtypes are categorized by enzyme deficit, inheritance pattern, and clinical features.

Symptoms

■ Central vision is poor.

■ Night vision is poor.

Signs

■ Corneal clouding is manifest by diffuse, fine punctate opacities in the stroma that are homogenous and bilateral (Fig. 14-11).

■ Depending on the type of storage disease, a pigmentary retinopathy may be manifest by a salt-and-pepper appearance of the retina.

■ Papilledema and optic atrophy are possible.

■ Glaucoma is often an associated disease.

Treatment

■ No specific treatment for the eyes is prescribed.

■ With extreme corneal clouding, a corneal transplant may be performed.

■ Prognosis is related to which subtype the patient has.

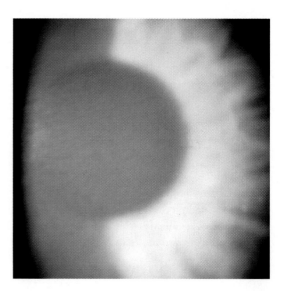

Fig. 14-11 Diffuse corneal clouding in Morquio syndrome, an autosomal recessive disorder of mucopolysaccharide metabolism.

MYOTONIC DYSTROPHY

Myotonic dystrophy is an inherited autosomal dominant disorder that involves body musculature with significant associated ophthalmic findings.

Symptoms

- Foreign body sensation, tearing, and a burning sensation occur if corneal drying and exposure are present.
- Double vision with extraocular muscle involvement occurs.
- Vision is decreased if cataracts are present.

Signs

- Ptosis and weakness of the orbicularis muscles is found.
- Pupils are sluggishly reactive.
- The cornea may have fine punctate fluorescein staining caused by poor blinking, exposure, or decreased lacrimal secretions (Fig. 14-12).
- Iridescent flecks or metachromatic granules are found in the lens. Cortical cataracts also may be seen.
- Defective eye movements, even ophthalmoplegia, occur.
- Intraocular pressure is low.
- The macula and retinal periphery display fine pigmentary granules.

Treatment

- Ocular treatment includes lubrication with preservative-free tears and ophthalmic lubricating ointments at bedtime.
- Surgery is performed for ptosis and cataracts when indicated.
- NOTE: These patients are at increased risk for complications from general anesthesia when muscle relaxants are used, and the anesthesia team should be made aware of the diagnosis.
- The prognosis for retention of vision is good.

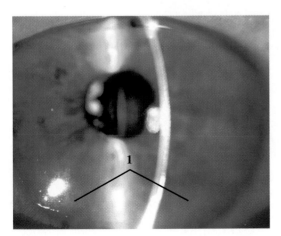

Fig. 14-12 Myotonic dystrophy—exposure keratopathy *(1)*.

NEUROFIBROMATOSIS (RECKLINGHAUSEN'S DISEASE)

Neurofibromatosis is an autosomal dominant disorder that may have significant ophthalmic involvement.

Symptoms

- No symptoms occur.
- Excessive tearing secondary to lid abnormalities may occur.
- A painless loss of vision is secondary to glaucoma or optic nerve glioma.

Signs

- Neuromas of the lid, often a plexiform neuroma, are found.
- Regional gigantism includes enlargement of the globe (buphthalmos) and may also be associated with congenital glaucoma.
- The iris may display an increased number of nevi or Lisch nodules, which are smooth, round, and translucent (Fig. 14-13).
- Optic atrophy may be caused by glaucoma or optic nerve glioma.

Treatment

- When the diagnosis of systemic disease is made, patients should have a baseline ophthalmic examination even if they currently have no symptoms.
- Elevated intraocular pressure is addressed if present.
- Plastic surgery may be indicated for disfiguring cosmetic problems.

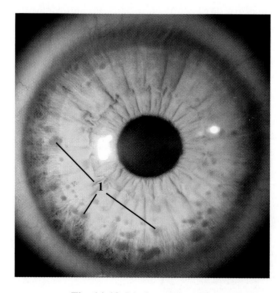

Fig. 14-13 Lisch nodules *(1)*.

- The ocular prognosis is generally good. Vision loss secondary to optic nerve glioma or glaucoma may occur.
- Neuroimaging should be obtained for progressive optic atrophy to rule out optic nerve glioma.
- Excision of the tumor (and optic nerve) is indicated when the tumor enlarges in a blind eye without chiasmal involvement. When the tumor involves the chiasm, radiotherapy is used.

OSTEOGENESIS IMPERFECTA

Osteogenesis imperfecta is a heritable disorder of connective tissue with skeletal, ear, and eye manifestations. The several subtypes are classified by degree of involvement.

Symptoms
- No symptoms occur.

Signs
- The major ocular sign is a blue sclera (Fig. 14-14). The color may be slate to dark blue depending on the thickness of the sclera.
- Corneal thinning (keratoglobus) may occur.
- Congenital glaucoma may occur.
- Optic atrophy may be found secondary to skull fractures with nerve compression.

Treatment
- No specific ocular therapy is indicated.
- The ocular prognosis is generally very good.

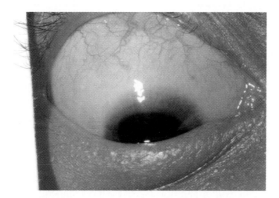

Fig. 14-14 Osteogenesis imperfecta is an inherited disorder characterized by bone fractures, deafness, and blue sclera.

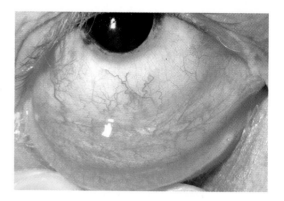

Fig. 14-15 Polycythemia vera. Engorged blood vessels of conjunctiva give rise to patient reports of redness of the eyes.

POLYCYTHEMIA VERA

Polycythemia vera is a blood disorder in which blood volume, blood viscosity, and an absolute number of red blood cells (RBCs) are increased with resultant decreased blood flow.

Symptoms

- No symptoms may occur.
- Redness results from vascular congestion in the conjunctiva.
- Episodic blurring of vision is caused by retinal hemorrhages.
- A painless loss of vision may result from optic nerve involvement or central retinal vein occlusion.

Signs

- Vascular congestion may be found, and prominent conjunctival vessels may mimic chronic conjunctivitis (Fig. 14-15).
- Hyperemia of the disc and a dark-purplish hue of the fundus may occur.
- Scattered deep retinal hemorrhages and papilledema may occur.
- In rare cases, the disorder is associated with central retinal vein occlusion.

Workup

- Retinal examination shows darkening, dilation, and tortuosity of the retinal veins; retinal arteries may appear normal.

Treatment

- Treatment is systemic without any specific ocular therapy.

REITER'S SYNDROME

Reiter's syndrome is defined by three associated problems: arthritis, urethritis, and eye inflammation (conjunctivitis and/or anterior uveitis). Mucocutaneous lesions frequently occur.

Symptoms

- Nonspecific irritation and a burning sensation occur.
- Pain, redness, and light sensitivity occur if anterior uveitis is present.
- Pain and redness are noted if episcleritis or scleritis is present.

Signs

- With conjunctivitis a nonspecific conjunctival infection without a significant follicular or papillary response is found. A watery, mucoid discharge may also occur.
- With uveitis, perilimbal injection is noted, and cells and flare may be seen on slit lamp examination.
- With episcleritis or scleritis, which are extremely rare, sectoral or diffuse scleral injection is noted.

Treatment

- For conjunctivitis, no specific therapy is indicated. Artificial tears may be used for comfort.
- For iritis, cycloplegic agents and topical corticosteroids are administered.
- The ocular prognosis is generally excellent.

RHEUMATOID ARTHRITIS

Rheumatoid arthritis is a systemic, multisystem collagen vascular disease associated with inflammatory joint pain. It may also cause infiltration and scarring of the salivary and lacrimal glands. The arthritis is polyarticular and usually symmetric and involves adults in middle age, with a higher incidence in females than in males.

Symptoms

- A foreign body and burning sensation occur if dry eye is present.
- Vision loss may occur.

Signs

- A dry eye with punctate staining of the corneal epithelium is noted (see Fig. 5-4).
- If present, scleral thinning is slow and painless without inflammation (scleromalacia perforans; see Fig. 6-6) or with active inflammation and pain (necrotizing scleritis; Fig. 14-16).
- Corneal thinning may be found adjacent to the scleral inflammation (Fig. 14-17). These ulcers may progress to perforation.

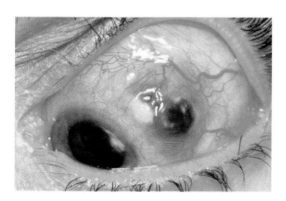

Fig. 14-16 Necrotizing scleritis in rheumatoid arthritis. Active scleral inflammation surrounds an area of the tissue loss. Uveal tissue can be seen in the areas of scleral loss.

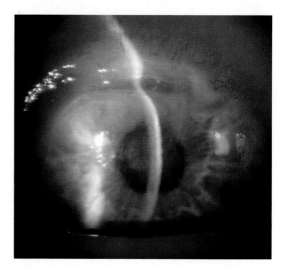

Fig. 14-17 Peripheral corneal ulcer in rheumatoid arthritis. The cornea is markedly thinned, with corneal vascularization.

Treatment

- Lubricants, especially preservative-free artificial tears, are used.
- Punctal occlusion is performed by an ophthalmologist.
- Topical corticosteroids should not be prescribed because of the possibility of necrosis and perforation of the cornea.
- For corneal and scleral thinning, systemic immunosuppression is usually effective.
- Ocular perforation requires surgical repair.

SARCOIDOSIS

Sarcoidosis is a chronic granulomatous disease that is multisystemic and may directly or indirectly affect any part of the eye.

Symptoms

- Pain, redness, and light sensitivity occur if iritis is present.
- A foreign body sensation, dryness, and irritation are reported if dry eye is present.
- If the optic nerve is involved, if a vitreous hemorrhage is present (rare), or if a cataract is present, vision is decreased.
- Pain may occur around the area of the lacrimal gland.

Signs

- A nodule (granuloma) may be present in the lids. Orbital inflammation may be manifest by lacrimal gland tenderness.
- Conjunctiva may display injection or nodules (Fig. 14-18).
- Cornea may show drying and fine punctate staining with fluorescein.
- Uveitis may manifest as cells on the endothelium or clumps of cells described as "mutton-fat" keratic precipitates (Fig. 14-19) and anterior chamber cell and flare. The iris may be adherent to the lens (posterior synechiae).

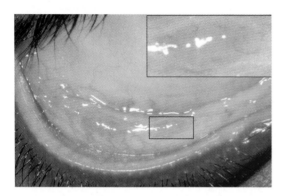

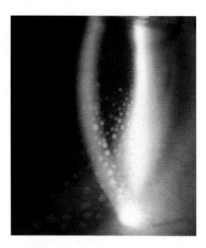

Fig. 14-18 Multiple sarcoid nodules in the inferior fornix. The solid raised lesions may resemble follicles *(inset)*.

Fig. 14-19 Granulomatous uveitis. Mutton-fat large keratic precipitates are on the corneal endothelium.

- Nodular lesions are possible on the iris.
- The lens may have a cataract.
- The fundus may show inflammatory changes of the disc noted by hyperemia or swelling.
- Candle wax–type drippings may be seen on the retinal surface in a linear pattern along the retinal veins.
- Retinal vasculitis with secondary retinal neovascularization may occur.

Treatment

- This chronic disease requires an ophthalmologist to monitor care.
- For uveitis, cycloplegia and topical and systemic corticosteroids are administered.
- The prognosis is good with mild to moderate inflammation. However, with severe or chronic involvement, band keratopathy, cataract, and glaucoma may lead to visual loss.
- Permanent visual loss is usually caused by glaucoma or optic neuropathy.

SJÖGREN'S SYNDROME

Sjögren's syndrome is often associated with rheumatoid arthritis and is the result of direct infiltration of inflammatory cells into the lacrimal and salivary glands. Dry eye (xerophthalmia) and dry mouth (xerostomia) are the dominant sequelae. This is most often seen with increasing age in women.

Symptoms

- Dry eye occurs.
- A foreign body sensation is reported.
- A burning sensation occurs.

Signs

- Mild conjunctival injection is noted.
- Keratoconjunctivitis sicca results in punctate fluorescein staining of the corneal epithelium (see Fig. 5-4).
- Mucus debris is found in the tear film.

Treatment

- Artificial tears, especially preservative free (e.g., Bion Tears, Hypotears Preservative Free, Refresh Plus) because they must be administered frequently, are used.
- Punctal occlusion is performed by an ophthalmologist.
- The eyelids are taped at night if a history of nocturnal lagophthalmos is reported. (NOTE: Sleeping with the eyes open is a relatively common phenomenon.)
- The ocular prognosis is generally good, but severe visual loss may occur with corneal necrosis. The patient's quality of life is significantly affected by the dryness, and continued attempts to maintain a moist environment are indicated (e.g., use of moisture chamber glasses or goggles).

STEVENS-JOHNSON SYNDROME

Stevens-Johnson syndrome (erythema multiforme) is an immunologically mediated syndrome that may occur in response to a microbial (e.g., herpes simplex) or pharmacologic (e.g., sulfonamide) agent. It is an immune complex vasculitis with inflammatory signs. When mucous membrane involvement dominates, Stevens-Johnson syndrome is the diagnosis.

Symptoms

- Pain occurs.
- Visual loss is noted.

Signs

- Conjunctival hyperemia and eventually scarring are found.
- Eyelid closure is incomplete.
- The amount of tears decreases.
- Corneal epithelial defects stain readily with fluorescein and may progress to ulceration.
- Depending on the disease severity, the cornea may become dry and exposed because of conjunctival scarring and poor eyelid closure (Fig. 14-20).

Treatment

- Treatment includes eradication or cessation of the offending microbial or pharmacologic agent.
- In the acute stages, extremely frequent (i.e., every half to 1 hour) use of preservative-free tears (e.g., such as Bion Tears, Hypotears Preservative Free, Refresh Plus) is indicated. Even more effective and protective are lubricating, preservative-free ointments (e.g., Hypotears, Refresh PM).
- The use of topical and systemic corticosteroids is controversial.
- The disease usually resolves in 2 to 3 weeks.
- The visual prognosis is good unless severe corneal drying and ulceration have occurred.

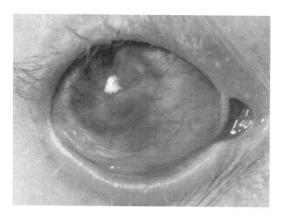

Fig. 14-20 Stevens-Johnson syndrome. Conjunctival and corneal scarring are seen.

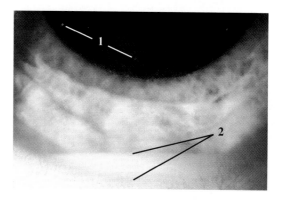

Fig. 14-21 Syphilitic uveitis. Small cellular precipitates *(1)* on the posterior cornea and a layered hypopyon *(2)* are seen.

SYPHILIS

The spirochete *Treponema pallidum,* which causes syphilis, leads to various systemic and ocular problems.

Symptoms

- Pain, light sensitivity, and redness occur if iritis is present.
- Pain and redness are reported if episcleritis or scleritis is present.
- Vision is decreased or there are visual field changes if the retina or optic nerve is involved.

Signs

- Iritis manifests as perilimbal injection, anterior chamber cells and flare, corneal cellular precipitates (Fig. 14-21), and a possibly engorged iris vasculature.
- Sectoral or diffuse scleral injection occurs with episcleritis and scleritis.
- Vasculitis may be seen in the retina with inflammatory changes adjacent to vessels.
- Swelling of the optic disc may ultimately lead to optic atrophy.
- An associated edema is found adjacent to the disc extending to the macula in cases of neuroretinitis.
- Classic Argyll Robertson pupils are noted. The pupils are poorly reactive or nonreactive to light but briskly reactive when the patient fixates on a near target.

Workup

- RPR and VDRL tests have positive findings early in the disease.
- The fluorescent treponemal antibody absorption (FTA-ABS) test is essential to detect active tertiary disease or previous infection. (NOTE: Most laboratories perform only the VDRL or RPR test unless the clinician insists on an FTA-ABS test.) If the finding is positive and the patient has signs of tertiary disease, a neurologic evaluation with consideration of lumbar puncture is indicated. The HIV status should be checked in any patient with signs and symptoms of syphilis because syphilis is a frequent associated finding.

Treatment

- Systemic penicillin (or alternatives depending on patient allergy) is prescribed.
- Local ophthalmic treatment includes cycloplegia and topical corticosteroids for iritis, topical corticosteroids or oral nonsteroidal antiinflammatory agents for episcleritis, and oral corticosteroids for scleritis.
- The ocular prognosis is excellent with early treatment.

SYSTEMIC LUPUS ERYTHEMATOSIS

Systemic lupus erythematosis (SLE) is a collagen vascular disease that usually involves the skin, kidney, and eye but may affect any organ. Its manifestations result from immune-mediated vasculitis and necrosis of the small vessels and capillaries. Fibrin, immuno-globulins, and complement deposition take place in these structures.

Symptoms

- No symptoms occur.
- Pain over the brow and redness are noted if scleritis is present.
- Foreign body sensation, burning, and dryness occur if dry eye is present.

Signs

- Sectoral or diffuse injection and tenderness of the sclera occur with scleritis (Fig. 14-22).
- Dry eye displays fine punctate staining of the corneal epithelium with fluorescein dye.
- Usually no peripheral ulceration occurs in SLE as is seen with rheumatoid arthritis.
- Retinopathy manifests as cotton-wool spots.
- Blotchy retinal hemorrhages are found in the posterior pole.
- Roth spots, a retinal hemorrhage with a whitish center, are noted (see Fig. 9-26).

Treatment

- For surface ocular problems, artificial tears are used.
- For episcleritis, systemic nonsteroidal antiinflammatory agents are administered. If no response occurs, topical corticosteroids may be used under the care of an ophthalmologist.
- For scleritis, systemic immunosuppression (primarily corticosteroids) is used.

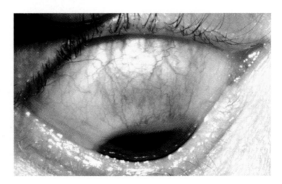

Fig. 14-22 Focal episcleritis or scleritis in a patient with systemic lupus erythematosus.

THYROID DISEASE

For a discussion of thyroid-related eye disease, see Chapter 13.

WEGENER'S GRANULOMATOSIS

Wegener's granulomatosis is a necrotizing granulomatous vasculitis with multiorgan system involvement, especially the eye, respiratory tract, and kidneys.

Symptoms

- Pain, light sensitivity, and redness occur if iritis is present.
- Pain and redness are reported if scleritis or keratitis is present.

Signs

- In cases of iritis, perilimbal injection, anterior chamber cell and flare, and corneal cellular precipitates are found.
- In cases of scleritis, local or diffuse scleral injection or necrosis is present (Fig. 14-23). Keratitis and progressive marginal corneal inflammation and ulceration are additional findings (Fig. 14-24).

Treatment

- Ocular treatment involves administration of cycloplegic agents and topical corticosteroids for associated iritis or episcleritis. Systemic nonsteroidal antiinflammatory agents may be beneficial for scleritis. The mainstay of treatment involves administration of systemic corticosteroids and/or cytotoxic agents such as cyclophosphamide.
- This disorder is best handled by a team of physicians.
- The ocular prognosis is guarded because severe necrosis and vision loss may occur. However, eye involvement is often controlled with aggressive systemic immunosuppressive therapy.

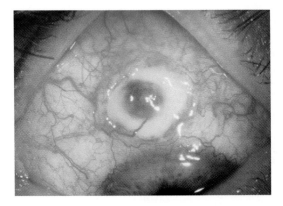

Fig. 14-23 Wegener's granulomatosis, necrotizing scleritis. A ring of avascular necrotic sclera surrounds an area of protruding uvea.

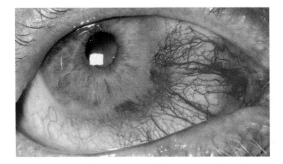

Fig. 14-24 Wegener's granulomatosis, peripheral sclerokeratitis.

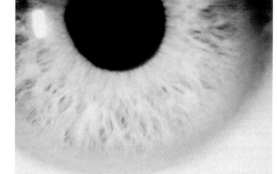

Fig. 14-25 Wilson's disease. A Kayser-Fleischer ring, which is a gold-yellow ring, extends to the limbus without a clear interval.

WILSON'S DISEASE

Hepatolenticular degeneration results from a defect in copper metabolism that causes copper to be deposited in the liver and basal ganglia. A deficiency of ceruloplasmin in the blood leads to defective excretion of copper by the liver lysosomes.

Symptoms

- Normally, no eye complaints are reported.
- Blurred vision is possible in cases of advanced cataracts.

Signs

- The most notable ocular sign is a Kayser-Fleischer ring that is a gold-brown or blue-green peripheral corneal opacification resulting from the deposition of copper in Descemet's membrane (Fig. 14-25). Usually the superior and inferior cornea are involved first. This finding may be seen in the absence of hepatic or neurologic disease and may require gonioscopy to identify early copper deposition.
- Copper deposition in the lens capsule causes a spokelike cataract ("sunflower cataract"). Usually no symptoms occur, and the cataract is best identified with a dilated slit lamp examination.

Treatment

- Systemic penicillamine is often used. Ocular myasthenia may be seen as a side effect of this treatment.
- With treatment, the ocular prognosis is excellent, and if the disease is diagnosed early, the systemic prognosis is vastly improved.
- The cataracts and Kayser-Fleischer ring may resolve with treatment.

SYSTEMIC THERAPIES

AMIODARONE USE

This medication is used in cardiac arrhythmias.

Symptoms

- No symptoms occur in the vast majority of patients.
- Vision loss or blurring may be noted if corneal changes are present.
- Rarely, sudden vision loss may occur with optic neuropathy.

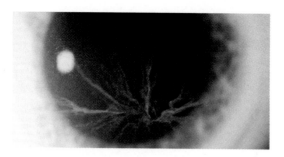

Fig. 14-26 Amiodarone deposits in a typical serpiginous, whorl configuration in the corneal epithelium (cornea verticillata).

Signs

- Verticillate or stellate white-brown lines are found in the interpalpebral area of the corneal epithelium (Fig. 14-26).
- Rarely, disc edema with vision loss occurs.

Differential Diagnosis

- Clinicians need to rule out any condition or medication that produces a similar corneal epithelial line such as Fabry's disease and chloroquine, hydroxychloroquine, indomethacin, and other nonsteroidal antiinflammatory drugs.
- See Chapter 11 for other causes of optic neuropathy.

Treatment

- With visual loss a prompt ophthalmologic examination is recommended; the risk-benefit ratio may favor discontinuing the drug.
- The corneal changes are reversible, but some cases of optic neuritis may progress to permanent vision loss. The optic neuropathy may represent an ischemic optic neuropathy rather than a true toxic effect. Regular ophthalmologic examinations are recommended during amiodarone therapy.

CHLOROQUINE USE

Chloroquine hydrochloride is an antimalarial, amebicidal agent. In the past it was used for the treatment of collagen vascular diseases but presently is seldom used because of the availability of hydroxychloroquine, which has much less ocular toxicity.

Symptoms

- No symptoms occur.
- Vision is blurred.
- Focusing is difficult.
- Night blindness occurs.
- Blind spots (scotomata) are present in the visual field.
- Reading is difficult because words "disappear."

Signs

- Punctate or linear, whorl-shaped lesions are found in the corneal epithelium on slit lamp examination. These deposits may be seen early after treatment initiation. They are usually not visually significant.

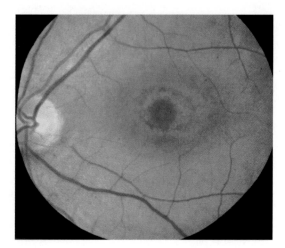

Fig. 14-27 Chloroquine maculopathy, advanced. A well-defined bull's-eye pattern is evident.

- The retina displays mild pigment stippling of the macula, a decrease or loss of the normal foveal reflex, and if the disorder is progressive, a bull's-eye pattern maculopathy (Fig. 14-27). In extreme cases, optic atrophy with narrowing of the retinal arterioles and pigmentary changes in the retinal periphery may be seen.

Workup

- A baseline ophthalmic examination, including visual acuity, slit lamp examination, fundus examination, and examination of the central visual field, is needed.

Treatment

- The drug is immediately discontinued for any visual symptoms that are not explained by problems with accommodation.
- Chloroquine is thought to be safe at a dosage of 4.0 mg/kg/day or less.

Follow-Up

- An ophthalmologic evaluation is repeated every 3 months.

CORTICOSTEROID USE
Symptoms

- No symptoms occur.
- Blurred vision can be relatively acute with refractive changes or gradual with cataractous changes.
- Headache and transient vision loss occur with pseudotumor cerebri.

Signs

- A refractive error change toward myopia results from corticosteroid-induced blood glucose changes (systemic corticosteroids).
- Pseudotumor cerebri manifests as papilledema from increased intracranial pressure (systemic corticosteroids).

- Intraocular pressure is increased (systemic and topical corticosteroids).
- A posterior subcapsular cataract is found (systemic and topical corticosteroids) (see Fig. 7-5).
- The drug use may potentiate herpes simplex infection of the cornea or eyelids (systemic and topical corticosteroids).

Treatment

- A careful analysis of the risk-to-benefit ratio of topical and oral corticosteroids is needed.
- The intraocular pressure increase is usually reversible after discontinuation of corticosteroids. However, cases of permanent increases in intraocular pressure have been reported.
- The cataractous changes are irreversible, and cataract surgery may be necessary.

CYTOSINE ARABINOSIDE USE

Cytosine arabinoside (Cytarabine) is an inhibitor of DNA synthesis and, when used systemically, may have eye findings.

Symptoms

- Vision is blurred.
- A foreign body sensation occurs.
- Light sensitivity is noted.

Signs

- Corneal epithelial cysts are found (Fig. 14-28).
- Hemorrhagic conjunctivitis is present.

Treatment

- Corneal lesions are reversible by cessation of medication.
- Administration of topical corticosteroid drops may prevent the hemorrhagic conjunctivitis and epithelial cysts, but their use should be regulated by an ophthalmologist.

DIGOXIN USE

Digoxin is a cardiac glycoside that causes ocular symptoms when blood levels of the drug are in the toxic range.

Symptoms

- Vision is blurred.
- Yellow-orange vision (xanthopsia) occurs.

Signs

- No signs are present.

Treatment

- The dosage is decreased to achieve proper therapeutic levels.

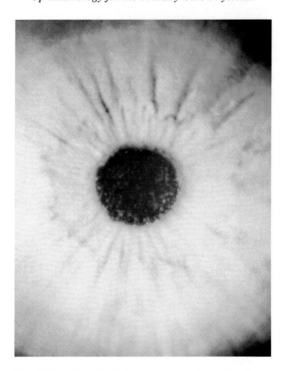

Fig. 14-28 Magnified slit lamp view of multiple intra-epithelial cysts associated with the use of the anti-metabolite cytosine arabinoside (cytarabine).

ETHAMBUTOL USE

Ethambutol is an antituberculous medication that may have reversible or irreversible ocular toxicity.

Symptoms
■ No symptoms occur.
■ Visual acuity or visual field loss is noted.
■ Color vision loss occurs.
■ Paracentral blind spots (scotomata) are present.

Signs
■ The optic nerve may appear normal.
■ Optic atrophy occurs.

Workup
■ A baseline ophthalmic examination should be performed before treatment and every 6 months thereafter.

Treatment

- The effects seem dosage related, and ocular effects are almost never seen at dosages of 15/mg/kg/day and are rarely seen up to 25/mg/kg/day.
- The drug is immediately discontinued once changes in visual acuity, color vision, or visual field defects are documented. After discontinuation, the decrease in visual acuity may continue but often improves after several months. The effects may be synergistic with Isoniazid (INH).

ISONIAZID USE

Isoniazid (INH) is an antituberculous medication that may have reversible or irreversible ocular toxicity.

Symptoms

- No symptoms occur.
- Visual acuity or visual field loss is reported.
- Color vision loss occurs.
- Paracentral blind spots (scotomata) are present.
- Visual hallucinations (bright colors in bizarre patterns) or blurring of vision are early manifestations of overdosage.

Signs

- The optic nerve may appear normal.
- Optic atrophy occurs.

Workup

- A baseline ophthalmic examination is needed before treatment and every 6 months thereafter.

Treatment

- The effects seem dosage related, and ocular effects tend to occur when dosages exceed recommended levels (usually 300 mg/day).
- The drug is immediately discontinued once changes in visual acuity, color vision, or visual field defects are documented.

PHENOTHIAZINE USE

Virtually any phenothiazine can cause pigment deposition in the lens and cornea, although this is not visually significant. Thioridazine (Mellaril) is the most common phenothiazine associated with retinal findings, particularly at dosages greater than 700 mg/day.

Symptoms

- Usually no symptoms occur.
- Mild night visual dysfunction is possible.
- Vision is blurred.
- Color vision loss is reported.

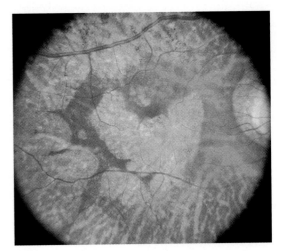

Fig. 14-29 Advanced pigmentary changes in the macula and retinal periphery resulting from thioridazine (Mellaril) toxicity.

Signs

■ A fine, brown pigment dusting of the cornea or lens may be seen. This is usually subtle and involves experienced slit lamp–examination technique.

■ Pigmentary retinopathy is found in the midperipheral retina. Advanced cases may involve the macula (Fig. 14-29).

Treatment

■ Pigment deposition in the cornea and lens is not visually significant and does not require a change in treatment.

■ Thioridazine (Mellaril) is discontinued if signs or symptoms of retinal toxicity occur. Early retinal changes may be reversible.

Follow-Up

■ An annual ophthalmology follow-up (every 6 months with Mellaril) is suggested.

PLAQUENIL USE

Hydroxychloroquine (Plaquenil) is used in the treatment of collagen vascular disease. A host of ocular side effects have been reported with this drug, but in general, the incidence of ocular toxicity with Plaquenil is less than that with chloroquine. The most observable effects are in the cornea, which are usually reversible, and the retina, which may be reversible or permanent.

Symptoms

■ No symptoms occur.

■ Vision is blurred.

■ Focusing is difficult.

■ Night blindness occurs.

■ Blind spots (scotomata) are present in the visual field.

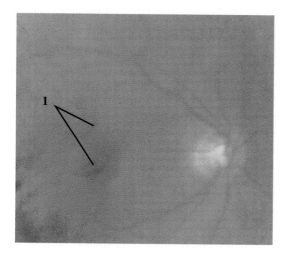

Fig. 14-30 Plaquenil toxicity. Although rarely seen, retinal toxicity may occur with Plaquenil use. This early case exhibits very subtle, nonspecific macular pigment changes *(1)*.

Signs

- Punctate to linear, whorl-shaped lesions in the corneal epithelium may be seen on slit lamp examination. These deposits may be seen early after the patient begins medication. These are usually not visually significant.
- The retina may show mild pigment stippling of the macula (Fig. 14-30) and a decrease or loss of the normal foveal reflex. If the effects are progressive, a bull's-eye pattern of maculopathy occurs in which pigment clumps are centrally surrounded by a ring of relative hypopigmentation encircled by a zone of relative hyperpigmentation. In extreme cases, optic atrophy, pallor of the disc with narrowing of the retinal arterioles, and pigmentary changes in the retinal periphery may be seen.

Workup

- A baseline ophthalmic examination, including visual acuity, slit lamp examination, dilated fundoscopic examination, and examination of the central visual field is indicated.

Treatment

- Ocular changes are virtually never seen with antimalarial prophylaxis but occur when the drug is used daily for systemic lupus erythematosus or rheumatoid arthritis. Recent evidence suggests the rate of dosage is important, with Plaquenil 6.5 mg/kg/day (of ideal body weight) or less a safe dosage in which retinopathy is virtually never seen.
- With early documented pigment changes on the retina or visual field changes, discontinuation of the drug may reverse any initial visual acuity or visual field effects. Rarely, visual field effects may progress after medication is discontinued. The frequency of retinal toxicity may increase in older age groups (60 years of age or older), but age-related macular degeneration changes are also more likely to occur with increasing age.
- All patients should be advised to use sunglasses (UV protection) and a hat with a brim in sunny climates because light may play a role.
- Immediate evaluation of any patient displaying symptoms is performed.

Follow-Up

■ The frequency of follow-up in these patients while on medication is controversial. The manufacturer still recommends every 3 months. However, many ophthalmologists feel that the incidence of retinal findings is so rare with Plaquenil that every 6 months or even annual follow-ups are sufficient. Because the retinal changes may be reversible if found early and irreversible if found too late, a follow-up every 6 months appears reasonable in the usual patient who is symptom free. Thus a recommendation for ophthalmic follow-up in a patient without symptoms is as follows:

- Patient on a low dosage (e.g., 200 mg/day)—Once a year
- Patient on a dosage approaching but not exceeding 6.5 mg/kg/day (ideal body weight)—Every 6 months
- Patient on a dosage of >6.5 mg/kg/day—Every 3 to 4 months in most cases
- With decreased renal function—Downward adjustment of the dosage and evaluation of ocular status every 3 to 4 months
- Patient with history of or concomitant gold or phenothiazine therapy—Adjustment of the dosage and monitoring of the ophthalmic status every 3 to 4 months because the threshold for retinal toxicity may be lower

TAMOXIFEN USE

Tamoxifen is a nonsteroidal antiestrogen that may have asymptomatic or symptomatic ocular effects.

Symptoms

■ No symptoms occur.
■ Vision is blurred.

Signs

■ Crystalline deposits are found in the retina (Fig. 14-31).
■ In rare cases, cystoid macular edema occurs.

Treatment

■ No treatment is indicated unless visual acuity changes are documented, in which case the drug is discontinued.

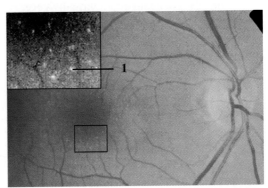

Fig. 14-31 Tamoxifen deposition. White-yellow crystalline deposits are seen in the retina *(1)*.

Ocular Trauma

Wayne A. Solley and Geoffrey Broocker

PERIORBITAL OR OCULAR CONTUSION

Symptoms

- The patient relates a history of trauma to the eye or periorbital region.
- Periorbital erythema or ecchymosis is found superiorly and/or inferiorly and may involve the contralateral eye (Fig. 15-1).
- The patient reports minimal pain.
- The degree of periorbital edema varies.
- Vision is minimally decreased or blurred.

Signs

- Periorbital ecchymosis and edema are present.
- Quiet eye with no anterior chamber reaction is found unless iritis is present.
- Subconjunctival hemorrhage is possible.
- The eye shows full motility, with slight pain on eye movement possible.

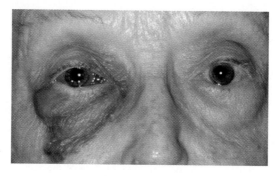

Fig. 15-1 Periorbital contusion.

Differential Diagnosis

■ Differential diagnoses include the following:
  • In children, child abuse
  • If contusions are bilateral in an infant, child abuse or neuroblastoma
  • Periorbital neoplasm, such as hemangioma or lymphangioma, that has hemorrhaged
  • When visual acuity is mildly decreased, traumatic iritis or corneal abrasion
  • When visual acuity is markedly decreased, hyphema (an often-missed diagnosis), vitreous hemorrhage, traumatic optic neuropathy, and lens subluxation (Fig. 15-2)

Workup

■ A general eye examination is performed on both eyes; dilated examination is mandatory. The red reflex is examined through the dilated pupil to evaluate lens position and clarity.
■ Plain x-ray films and/or computed tomography (CT) scanning of the orbit is needed if orbital fracture is suspected. Entrapment of orbital soft tissue in an orbital blow-out fracture is often seen clearly on CT.

Treatment

■ If no severe ocular or periocular injury is seen, cool compresses are applied and the patient is reassured. If the injury is sports related in a child, use of safety glasses or goggles should be encouraged.
■ Nonemergency ophthalmologic follow-up is needed, specifically a careful peripheral retinal examination. Trauma severe enough to cause substantial periorbital edema and ecchymosis can cause a tear in the retinal periphery that may not cause symptoms initially but may result in a retinal detachment if not identified.
■ Patients with evidence of hyphema should be immediately referred to an ophthalmologist.

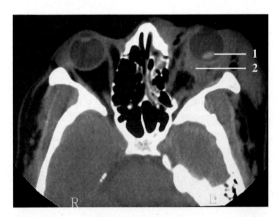

Fig. 15-2 Orbital CT scan showing sequelae of blunt orbital or ocular injury. This patient was struck with a can of soda, causing a dislocated lens *(1)*, retrobulbar hemorrhage *(2)*, and blow-out fracture of the medial orbital wall.

CORNEAL ABRASION

Symptoms

- A history of mild trauma to the eye, possibly caused by a fingernail, tree branch, contact lens, make-up brush, or foreign body, is reported.
- Photophobia, conjunctival injection, and involuntary lid closure (blepharospasm) occur.
- Pain and foreign body sensation may be quite severe.
- If the abrasion is in the central cornea, visual acuity is decreased (20/80 to 20/200).

Signs

- Conjunctival hyperemia, swollen eyelids, and tearing are noted.
- Slip lamp examination shows an epithelial defect but often a clear cornea. A surface irregularity may be identified with a penlight. Minimal cellular reaction is seen in the anterior chamber. If corneal haze or moderate to severe flare and cell is noted in the anterior segment, especially with an associated discharge, bacterial superinfection may be present.
- Fluorescein dye is absorbed by areas devoid of epithelium and outlines the defect (Fig. 15-3).
- Immediate relief occurs with topical anesthesia (e.g., proparacaine, tetracaine). Topical anesthetics are used only to confirm the diagnosis and are not prescribed for long-term relief.

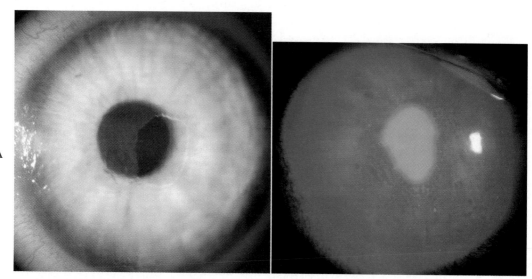

A   **B**

Fig. 15-3 Corneal epithelial abrasion. **A,** Epithelial defect without fluorescein highlighting the defect. An irregularity in the otherwise smooth corneal surface is the key to identifying the defect if no fluorescein is available. **B,** Classic fluorescein staining of an epithelial defect.

Differential Diagnosis

■ Differential diagnoses include the following:
  • Viral keratitis (herpes simplex or zoster), often with corneal dendrites (see Fig. 5-7)
  • Corneal or conjunctival foreign body, especially under the conjunctiva of the upper lid, which can cause "ice-skate track" abrasions as the foreign body is repeatedly swept linearly over the epithelium
  • Recurrent erosion, which is identical to primary epithelial defects but occurs long after the initial corneal trauma (see Fig. 5-18)
  • Ultraviolet corneal injury (welder's flash)

Workup

■ The size and extent of denuded epithelium are documented. Location is important because any complications (infections) in the central portion of the cornea may have lasting visual consequences.
■ The eyelids are everted to search for a foreign body, especially if the history suggests one may be present (e.g., glass from an automobile accident, vegetable matter from bark). Linear corneal abrasions should alert the examiner a foreign body is possible.

Treatment

■ For contact lens–associated corneal abrasions, see p. 260.
■ For non–contact lens–associated abrasions, the following apply:
  • Cycloplegia (e.g., homatropine 5% 3 times a day) is administered.
  • Antibiotic ointment appropriate for the injury is used. Polymyxin B/bacitracin (Polysporin) or erythromycin ophthalmic ointment 2 times a day and at bedtime is effective for most abrasions. Tobramycin ophthalmic ointment is used for abrasions caused by vegetable matter (for improved gram-negative coverage).
  • A firm pressure patch is applied for 24 hours if the abrasion is large (more than 5 to 10 mm) or the patient is in severe pain. (See Chapter 1 for proper patch application.) Although pressure patching promotes wound healing, the chance of infection is increased when a warm environment is created by the patching. In circumstances in which microbial contamination exists, a pressure patch is not used.
  • Analgesia is given for pain; sometimes a narcotic analgesic is needed (e.g., Tylenol with Codeine).
  • Under *no* circumstances should topical anesthetics be prescribed or given to the patient. Not only do anesthetics retard wound reepithelialization, but the loss of the cornea's normal pain response predisposes the patient to a much more severe injury.
  • Patients with a large central abrasion or high-risk abrasion should be referred to an ophthalmologist for management and follow-up care.

Follow-Up

■ All abrasions are monitored daily until they have completely resolved. If healing takes longer than 2 or 3 days, the patient should be referred to an ophthalmologist.
■ A pressure patch is never used for more than 24 hours. If patient compliance with follow-up is questionable, antibiotic ointment and cycloplegia are applied to heal the abrasion without the added risk of patching.
■ If visual acuity is markedly decreased (less than 20/400), more severe ocular injury needs to be ruled out, especially if the history suggests severe trauma.

CONTACT LENS INJURY

Symptoms

■ Pain, foreign body sensation, photophobia, tearing, and blepharospasm occur immediately after insertion or removal of a contact lens.

■ Blurred vision, conjunctival hyperemia, and pain occur during contact lens wear. The presence of these symptoms on awakening suggests hypoxic corneal injury.

Signs

■ Conjunctival hyperemia and ciliary flush, which is a manifestation of circumlimbal injection (redness around the corneoscleral junction), are noted.

■ An epithelial defect is present if an abrasion exists.

■ The contact lens is immobile and corneal edema is diffuse (in cases of tight lens syndrome/hypoxic corneal injury).

Etiology

■ Direct trauma to the corneal epithelium with insertion or removal of the lens can result in injury.

■ A foreign body between the lens and cornea can cause injury (Fig. 15-4).

■ Hypoxic injury to the cornea results from improper contact lens fit, improper lens material for the patient's needs, or overwear by the patient (e.g., sleeping in a daily wear lens). While the patient sleeps, the oxygen available to the cornea is markedly decreased, and with a low oxygen-permeable lens, the corneal epithelium becomes hypoxic and edematous.

■ Toxic product buildup in the contact lens can result in injury.

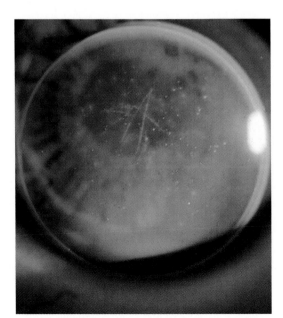

Fig. 15-4 Foreign body between hard contact lens and cornea. Note the vertical "dust trails" or ice skate tracks caused by the vertically moving foreign body.

Differential Diagnosis

■ Differential diagnoses include the following:
  • Early microbial keratitis (e.g., bacterial keratitis)
  • Corneal or conjunctival foreign body
  • Ultraviolet corneal injury

Workup

■ A complete eye examination of both eyes, including slit lamp, fluorescein staining, and eversion of the lids to search for hidden foreign bodies, is indicated. Fluorescein is not used in an eye with the soft contact lens in place because the lens will absorb the fluorescein and turn green permanently. Hard or gas-permeable contact lenses do not turn yellow on fluorescein instillation.

Treatment

■ The contact lens is removed; a suction cup can assist in removal of hard contact lenses. The patient is instructed not to wear the lens until the abrasion is completely healed (usually 10 to 14 days).

■ If an abrasion exists, a topical ophthalmic ointment that covers gram-negative organisms (e.g., gentamicin, tobramycin) is administered frequently (e.g., every 2 hours). Patients should be referred to an ophthalmologist for management because a significant risk exists for gram-negative bacterial corneal infection (especially *Pseudomonas* infection) in soft contact lens wearers. Patches are not used because any gram-negative infection can progress rapidly to corneal ulceration.

■ For overwear or tight lens syndrome, use of the contact lens is discontinued until the patient is assessed by an ophthalmologist; immediate referral is indicated. Lens fit, oxygen permeability, and the overall health of the cornea must be addressed. Chronic hypoxia can lead to corneal neovascularization and scarring.

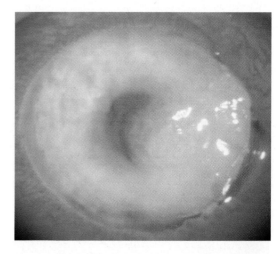

Fig. 15-5 Extensive *Pseudomonas* bacterial corneal ulcer associated with soft contact lens wear.

Follow-Up

■ For patients with abrasions, daily follow-up is mandatory.

■ As a rule, contact lens–associated abrasions heal completely in a short time, although they may take longer than non–contact lens–associated abrasions. Management is fairly easy, but an error (e.g., prolonged patching in a contact lens wearer, inadequate follow-up, neglect of antibiotic coverage) can cause severe corneal infection (ulceration) that threatens the ultimate visual outcome (Fig. 15-5).

ACUTE ULTRAVIOLET RADIATION INJURY

Symptoms

■ A history of welding or sunbathing (indoor sunlamp) without protective eyewear is reported.

■ Moderate to severe pain occurs.

■ Red eyes, tearing, blurred vision, photophobia, and blepharospasm occur.

■ Symptoms occur 6 to 12 hours after the activity; the patient sometimes awakens with these symptoms the day after the activity.

Signs

■ Dense punctate staining of the cornea occurs on fluorescein instillation; the central cornea is often more involved than the superior and inferior portions.

■ Injection or edema of the eyelids is noted.

■ Mild corneal edema or injected conjunctiva is evident.

■ Minimal to no anterior chamber cell and flare occurs.

Differential Diagnosis

■ Differential diagnoses include the following:
  • Toxic epitheliopathy from drugs or chemicals, for example, multidose artificial tear overuse, which causes a reaction to the tear preservative; corneal anesthesia caused by topical anesthesic abuse (e.g., proparacaine, tetracaine); and exposure to crack cocaine smoke
  • Exposure keratopathy (e.g., thyroid eye disease, seventh nerve palsy, any lid abnormality causing poor closure)
  • Severe dry eye syndrome (usually sparing the upper portion of the cornea)

Workup

■ A complete eye examination of both eyes, including fluorescein instillation and lid eversion, is indicated.

■ Questions should focus on recent welding or sunlamp use without eye protection.

■ If no history of ultraviolet exposure is reported, use of topical medications and drugs is addressed.

Treatment

■ Cycloplegic agents (e.g., homatropine 5% 3 times a day) are administered.

■ Antibiotic ointment (e.g., polymyxin B/bacitracin [Polysporin], erythromycin ointment 2 to 3 times a day) is applied.

■ For severe ultraviolet keratopathy, pressure patching is bilateral if the patient has assistance. If this is not possible, the more affected eye is patched and an antibiotic is used in the less involved eye.

■ Systemic analgesics are usually needed.

Follow-up

■ The patch is removed after 24 hours. If the condition is improved, antibiotic ointment use continues for an additional 2 to 3 days, and then symptoms should be resolved. If symptoms persist after 24 hours, the eye is repatched and reevaluated in 24 hours.

■ Referral to an ophthalmologist is not usually needed unless the condition does not improve after 1 or 2 days.

■ The prognosis is very good. The high absorption of ultraviolet rays in the corneal tissues usually protects the inner eye tissue from severe damage except with massive exposure. The lens is the next most susceptible tissue to injury but only becomes cataractous in cases of prolonged exposure to ultraviolet rays or markedly high levels of ultraviolet energy.

SUBCONJUNCTIVAL HEMORRHAGE

Symptoms and Signs

■ An acute, dense, "blood red" discoloration of the subconjunctival space is often noted on awakening (Fig. 15-6).

■ The conjunctival appearance ranges from a flat, red spot with no chemosis of the conjunctiva to massive hemorrhagic conjunctival suffusion, possibly extending over the lid margin.

■ The hemorrhage often appears after Valsalva's maneuver (e.g., coughing spells, constipation with straining, heavy lifting) is performed.

Etiology

■ Blunt trauma that may seem insignificant can lead to the disorder.

■ The disorder can result from rupture of small conjunctival vessels with Valsalva's maneuver.

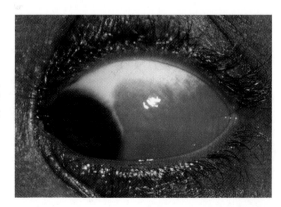

Fig. 15-6 Subconjunctival hemorrhage. This usually results from Valsalva's maneuvers and is benign. In the setting of severe trauma, however, it may obscure a more significant injury to the globe.

- Microbial conjunctivitis (e.g., viral hemorrhagic conjunctivitis, adenoviral or pneumo-coccal conjunctivitis) is possible, especially if the disorder is associated with discharge or ocular discomfort.
- Hypertension, usually accelerated, can result in the disorder.
- The disorder can occur with a bleeding disorder, including those in patients using oral anticoagulants.
- Trauma to the globe and orbital periosteal injury are etiologic processes. Significant subconjunctival hemorrhage and a suggestive history should prompt inspection for possible orbital fracture. Zygomatic arch fracture should be suspected with a lateral subconjunctival hemorrhage that extends far posteriorly.

Differential Diagnosis

- Ruptured globe is considered, especially with trauma involving missiles (metal on metal or grinding injury) or a large subconjunctival hemorrhage, which may obscure a scleral rupture beneath the hemorrhage. A complete subconjunctival hemorrhage is often a sign of retrobulbar blood that has progressed forward in the potential space between the conjunctiva and globe. The posterior extent of the hemorrhage is therefore hidden. Fractures of the periorbital region or ruptured globe must be ruled out in these cases.
- Bleeding diathesis is a possible diagnosis, especially if multiple episodes of hemor-rhage have occurred.
- Conjunctival neoplasm with associated hemorrhage is considered.
- Conjunctival Kaposi's sarcoma (reddish-purple subconjunctival mass) must be ruled out or confirmed.

Workup

- The history should include abnormal clotting, oral anticoagulant use, and any Valsalva's maneuvers (e.g., weightlifting, constipation, severe coughing or sneezing [especially with chronic obstructive pulmonary disease or asthma], scuba diving).
- If the history suggests the possibility of severe injury, a complete eye examination, including intraocular pressure evaluation (unless globe rupture is suspected), is needed.
- If the patient history details spontaneous, recurrent subconjunctival hemorrhage, clot-ting studies are indicated.
- Blood pressure is measured.
- If a retrobulbar hemorrhage is suspected in a patient (usually in cases of trauma), accurate assessment of intraocular pressure, which can be markedly elevated, must be performed.

Treatment

- Reassurance is paramount; artificial tears help alleviate any discomfort. The patient is informed that the blood may take up to 2 weeks to clear.
- If clotting studies are abnormal (with recurrent spontaneous hemorrhage), referral for hematologic evaluation is necessary.
- If the hemorrhage is associated with trauma and a ruptured globe is possible, imme-diate referral to an ophthalmologist is indicated.

Follow-Up

■ The prognosis is excellent for a primary spontaneous subconjunctival hemorrhage. The patient is reevaluated in 2 to 3 weeks if the hemorrhage does not clear or recurs.

CONJUNCTIVAL FOREIGN BODY

Symptoms

■ A foreign body sensation, tearing, red eye, and ocular irritation and pain occur.

■ A history of working underneath a car, boat, or machinery when a low-velocity foreign object entered the eye is reported. Conversely, high-speed missile injury (e.g., explosions, propelled foreign body from industrial equipment, lawn mowers, power tools) may also lodge a foreign body in the conjunctiva.

Signs

■ Conjunctival hyperemia, laceration, or obvious foreign body is found.

■ Conjunctival or subconjunctival hemorrhage obscures the foreign body.

■ Linear, vertical corneal abrasions (ice-skate track abrasions) indicate retained foreign bodies in the superior tarsal conjunctiva (Fig. 15-7).

Differential Diagnosis

■ Differential diagnoses include the following:
  • Ruptured globe and intraocular foreign body with ocular penetration, especially with high-speed missile injury
  • Corneal foreign body, corneal abrasion, and contact lens–associated injury
  • Other causes of ocular discomfort and redness (e.g., episcleritis, scleritis)

Workup

■ Depending on the patient history a complete examination of both eyes, including intraocular pressure and slit lamp evaluation to assess anterior chamber depth and inflammation, iris defects, and lens clarity, is necessary.

■ Lid eversion and dilated fundus examination are performed.

■ If the patient history relates a high-speed missile or metal-on-metal injury, a CT scan of the orbits, which must specify axial/coronal 2-mm cuts through the orbits, is needed to help detect an intraocular or intraorbital foreign body.

■ If visual acuity is markedly decreased, a more severe injury than superficial conjunctival foreign body should be explored.

Treatment

■ If globe penetration is suspected or undetermined, immediate referral to an ophthalmologist, shielding of the eye, and minimal manipulation of the globe are indicated.

■ With suspected superficial foreign body and no ruptured globe, the foreign body is removed under topical anesthesia (e.g., a drop of proparacaine or tetracaine). Irrigation with saline solution removes loosely adherent conjunctival foreign bodies. If the foreign material is slightly embedded in the conjunctiva and resistant to saline irrigation, it is removed at the slip lamp with a jeweler's forceps under topical anesthesia (a cotton-tipped applicator soaked in tetracaine or proparacaine and applied to the

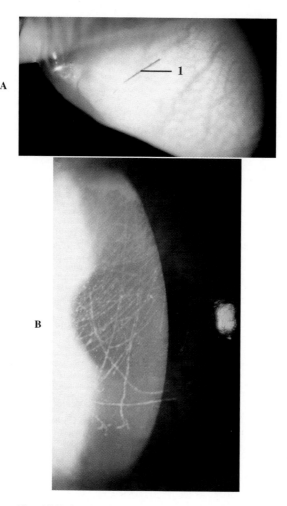

Fig. 15-7 A, A grasshopper leg *(1)* embedded in the superior tarsal conjunctiva. **B,** Dust trail corneal linear abrasions are found in the same patient.

region for 25 seconds). The foreign body must be completely seen (i.e., does not penetrate through the sclera and into the intraocular space) before removal. If it does extend further, immediate referral to an ophthalmologist and no manipulation of the globe are necessary steps.

- With multiple foreign bodies the clinician irrigates with saline solution, removes the readily accessible portion with forceps, and sweeps the fornices with cotton-tipped applicators soaked in a topical anesthetic.

- After removal, a topical antibiotic (e.g., polymyxin B/bacitracin [Polysporin] ophthalmic ointment) and artificial tears are used as needed. If a significant number of foreign bodies remain, immediate referral to an ophthalmologist is indicated.

Follow-Up

■ Follow-up is performed as needed if a single or a few foreign bodies were easily removed and no further discomfort was experienced.

CONJUNCTIVAL LACERATION

Symptoms

■ A history of trauma (especially with sharp objects) is reported.

■ A red eye, mild foreign body sensation (much less uncomfortable than that in a corneal abrasion), and mild pain occur.

Signs

■ The conjunctival defect is noted on slit lamp examination, often with fluorescein pooling in the defect.

■ Hemorrhage (conjunctival or subconjunctival) may obscure the injury (Fig. 15-8).

■ White sclera is often visible in the base of the laceration if it is overlying the globe.

Differential Diagnosis

■ Differential diagnoses include the following:
  • Serious injury to the globe (rupture) and orbital structures, including intraocular and intraorbital foreign bodies
  • Subconjunctival foreign bodies

Workup

■ As with all seemingly benign injuries of the periocular structures, a detailed history of the injury is imperative. The nature of the injury dictates the level of suspicion of severe ocular injury. For example, reports of a high-speed projectile or severe car accident with broken glass resulting in a conjunctival laceration raise suspicion of a more severe injury. A fingernail or other less severe mechanism of injury is less likely to cause serious ocular injury.

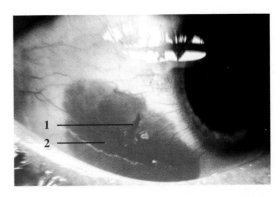

Fig. 15-8 Note the small laceration in the conjunctiva *(1)* with surrounding subconjunctival hemorrhage *(2)*. In this patient, no associated subconjunctival foreign body or scleral injury occurred.

- A complete eye examination in both eyes including fluorescein staining to outline the defect, is needed. The base of the laceration is evaluated carefully to rule out the presence of retained foreign bodies in the subconjunctival space and ensure that no scleral penetration or laceration has occurred. This area is explored with caution. If the globe is violated, even minimal pressure on the eye (even from the patient squeezing the lids together) can extrude intraocular contents and jeopardize the visual outcome. The clinician carefully examines the conjunctiva using topical anesthesia and a cotton-tipped applicator soaked in the anesthetic (e.g., tetracaine, proparacaine).
- The tetanus status of the patient is assessed.
- With suspicion of a ruptured globe or an intraocular or intraorbital foreign body, a CT scan with axial and coronal thin cuts through the orbits is indicated.

Treatment

- The patient is immediately referred to an ophthalmologist.
- For small lacerations (< 1.0 cm) in which a severe injury is not suspected, an antibiotic ointment (e.g., polymyxin B/bacitracin [Polysporin] 2 or 3 times a day) is administered for 1 week depending on the extent of the laceration.
- For large lacerations (> 1.0 cm) a suture may be needed for closure. An ophthalmologist performs this procedure with a microscope or loupes.

Follow-Up

- A patient with a small laceration is referred to an ophthalmologist if the laceration does not heal properly or the foreign body sensation persists.
- The prognosis is excellent.

CORNEAL FOREIGN BODY

Symptoms

- A history of acute foreign body sensation, red eye, tearing, and blurred vision is related. Often the patient can identify the moment the foreign body entered the eye.
- The pain is severe early and gradually becomes more tolerable. If the foreign body contains iron, rust will deposit in the cornea, causing pain.
- Blepharospasm (involuntary lid closure) is possible.

Signs

- Conjunctival injection, eyelid edema, and a mild anterior chamber reaction are seen.
- The foreign body is usually easily observed in the cornea with slit lamp or penlight examination (Fig. 15-9).
- A corneal stromal infiltrate is usually present if the foreign body has been present for more than 24 hours. The infiltrate may be noninfectious, but microbial keratitis must be suspected, especially if the foreign material is vegetable in origin (e.g., bark, thorn).
- Iron foreign bodies often form rust rings in the anterior corneal stroma and are seen as a reddish-orange haze around the foreign body on slit lamp examination.
- A dense cellular reaction in the anterior chamber or hypopyon suggests ulceration of the cornea or penetration of the globe by the foreign body and secondary endophthalmitis.

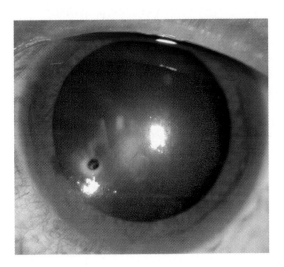

Fig. 15-9 A small, iron foreign body may be seen on external examination.

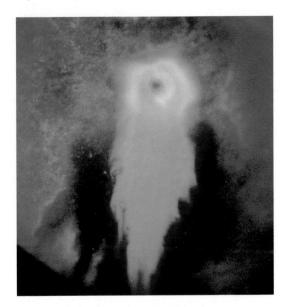

Fig. 15-10 Seidel-positive wound.

Differential Diagnosis

■ Differential diagnoses include the following:
  • Corneal abrasion or laceration
  • Conjunctival foreign body

Workup

■ NOTE: Use of topical anesthesia can greatly assist in determination of visual acuity and facilitates the patient's cooperation with the remainder of the examination.

■ A complete eye examination in both eyes is indicated, including careful slit lamp examination of the cornea to assess the depth of penetration of the foreign body. If the foreign body is seen protruding into the anterior chamber, the globe is penetrated and at high risk for infection. No further manipulation of the foreign body should be attempted under any circumstances to prevent dislodging it and decompressing the eye.

■ Lid eversion is essential to rule out a hidden foreign body under the superior tarsal conjunctiva. The inferior fornix is examined carefully.

■ With a suspected high-speed metal-on-metal or other projectile injury, a dilated fundus examination with indirect ophthalmoscopy by an ophthalmologist is essential. This will rule out globe rupture with intraocular foreign body. CT scanning or B-scan ultrasound may also be indicated.

■ For deep foreign bodies, Seidel's test is performed to determine whether fluid (aqueous) is leaking from the eye:
  • The examiner places a drop of anesthetic (e.g., proparacaine) in the eye to be tested and on a sterile fluorescein strip. Excess anesthetic drips off the strip, which is then used to "paint" the area on the eye where the leak is suspected.

- The examiner uses the cobalt-blue filter on the slit lamp to observe the area. An aqueous leak manifests as a bright green stream as the aqueous dilutes the dye (Fig. 15-10). This is deemed *Seidel positive;* a *Seidel-negative* wound does not eliminate the possibility of intermittent leakage.

Treatment

- For globe penetration, the eye is shielded and the patient is immediately referred to an ophthalmologist.
- For superficial foreign material, simple irrigation often removes the material. If this procedure is unsuccessful, a cotton-tipped applicator can be used. The clinician instills a drop of topical anesthesia (e.g., proparacaine) into the eye and wets a sterile cotton-tipped applicator with saline solution or topical anesthetic. Most foreign bodies can be easily removed with minimal manipulation. If this procedure is also unsuccessful, the back of a sterile blade can be used to gently scrape the foreign body off the cornea. A foreign body spud or sterile jeweler's forceps are also effective. Hypodermic needles should *not* be used for corneal foreign body removal to prevent further corneal injury.
- For deep foreign material, referral to an ophthalmologist is indicated. Overaggressive manipulation or "digging" for a foreign body can cause more scarring and corneal damage. Similarly, overuse of an ophthalmic burr to remove a deep rust ring may cause extensive scarring that can compromise visual acuity. Removal in the operating room may be needed for deep, large, central, or infectious foreign bodies (such as vegetable matter).
- Corneal rust rings may be removed with an ophthalmic burr, a procedure probably best performed by an ophthalmologist. Patients with central rust rings should be referred to an ophthalmologist for management within 24 hours of the initial diagnosis. The natural propensity of corneal rust rings is for them to migrate superficially and become a white scar.
- Patients with numerous foreign bodies (as with an explosive injury) should be immediately referred to an ophthalmologist. If an attempt is made to remove each small object, undue scarring may result.
- After the foreign body is removed, the patient is given topical antibiotics (e.g., polymyxin B/bacitracin [Polysporin] ophthalmic ointment) until the epithelial defect has healed.

Follow-Up

- The patient is seen daily until the epithelium heals; this ensures no infectious complications.
- The residual corneal defect (epithelial defect) is treated as a corneal abrasion. If the corneal defect is large and central and associated with a discharge or other signs of infection (e.g., severe pain, corneal clouding, marked anterior chamber reaction), the patient should be immediately referred to an ophthalmologist. Topical corticosteroids are not used.
- Multiple, deep, central, iron-containing foreign bodies confer the worst visual prognosis. Patients with injuries caused by small, single, peripheral foreign bodies generally have excellent visual outcomes.

CORNEAL LACERATION

A corneal laceration may be full or partial thickness. Patients with partial-thickness lacerations have excellent prognoses and can be treated with patching and antibiotics, much like patients with corneal abrasions. Patients with deep or full-thickness lacerations should be urgently referred for ophthalmologic evaluation.

Symptoms

- A history of trauma with a sharp object or projectile (high velocity) is reported.
- Pain, decreased vision (depending on the depth and location of the laceration), involuntary lid closure (blepharospasm), and a red eye are noted.
- The patient may have observed a brief flow of fluid (aqueous) from the eye immediately after the injury.

Signs

- A positive Seidel's test finding is indicative of full-thickness corneal laceration.
- A gaping corneal wound is seen.
- The iris prolapses out the corneal wound, or the iris and cornea touch where the iris has plugged the corneal defect. A corneal laceration of this type is nearly always associated with a "peaking" or "teardrop" shape to the pupil in the direction of the corneal defect (Fig. 15-11).
- Other signs of a penetrated globe include an asymmetric anterior chamber depth when compared with that of the uninvolved eye, a hyphema, conjunctival injection and chemosis, reduced (in most cases) or elevated (in few cases) intraocular pressure, lens injury, and pupillary asymmetry. Vision is markedly decreased.

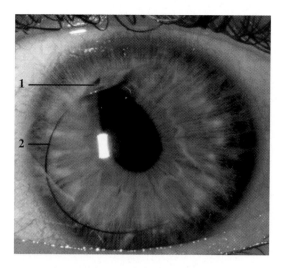

Fig. 15-11 Acute corneal laceration with prolapsed iris *(1)* and resultant peaked pupil. An eyelash *(2)* has entered the anterior chamber.

Workup

- A complete eye examination of both eyes, including Seidel's test, is indicated. If rupture of the globe becomes evident (or rupture is suspected), the examination ends, the eye is shielded, and the patient is referred to an ophthalmologist immediately. Excessive manipulation of the globe or exertion of pressure on the eyelids during an examination may result in extrusion of intraocular contents.
- A CT scan of the orbits is needed to evaluate possible intraocular or intraorbital foreign bodies.
- A slit lamp examination is performed to examine the extent and depth of the corneal injury. Distinguishing deep, nonpenetrating lacerations from penetrating, well-opposed wounds, is often difficult. For this reason, if the extent of the injury is questionable, the patient should be referred to an ophthalmologist immediately.

Treatment

- All patients are immediately referred to an ophthalmologist for evaluation because if a penetrating injury is not diagnosed, disastrous infectious complications may result. For protection a shield is placed over the eye without a patch.
- Antibiotic ointment is not used in any patient with a suspected ruptured globe because the medication may enter the eye.
- For a suspected or confirmed full-thickness laceration, operative intervention is usually necessary and broad-spectrum intravenous antibiotics are administered. For example, adults receive 1 g of cefazolin (Ancef) every 8 hours. Children receive 25 to 50 mg/kg/day of cefazolin (Ancef) in three divided doses.
- The patient's tetanus immune status is addressed.

SCLERAL LACERATION OR RUPTURE

Symptoms

- A history of trauma, often with a high-velocity projectile or sharp object, is reported.
- Conjunctival swelling, red eye, pain, decreased vision, and possible inadvertent lid closure (blepharospasm) occur.

Signs

- A defect is noted in the conjunctiva or sclera, with or without subconjunctival hemorrhage (Fig. 15-12). Marked hemorrhagic chemosis (swelling) may obscure the underlying scleral injury.
- Uveal or vitreous prolapse occurs through the scleral wound. The prolapse may appear as a brownish discoloration beneath the conjunctiva, sometimes mistaken for blood. The pupil may be abnormally shaped (e.g., peaked).
- The intraocular pressure is low in most cases. Less commonly, the intraocular pressure is normal or elevated.

Etiology

- Usually, sharp objects or missiles (e.g., metal-on-metal projectile injury, broken glass, knife wound, bullet) cause the injury.
- Severe blunt trauma (e.g., from a fist, bottle, or club) is a common cause.

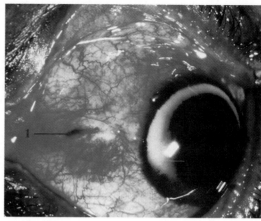

Fig. 15-12 Scleral laceration. This lesion *(1)* was made with a sharp, penetrating object (a small knife). The clinician needs to ensure that no part of the object causing the injury is left in the eye.

Differential Diagnosis

■ Differential diagnoses include the following:
  • Conjunctival laceration without scleral injury
  • Intraocular foreign body
  • Clear or hemorrhagic chemosis without obvious scleral injury

Workup

■ As with corneal and conjunctival lacerations, a complete eye examination of both eyes is indicated. If rupture of the globe is suspected, the eye is shielded, no antibiotic ointment or patching is used, and the patient is immediately referred to an ophthalmologist.

■ A diagnosis of scleral rupture or laceration requires a high index of suspicion because these conditions are often obscured by edematous conjunctiva. Minimal manipulation of the globe is prudent in cases in which the diagnosis is uncertain.

■ A CT scan of the globe is indicated if an intraocular foreign body is suspected.

Treatment

■ In cases of partial-thickness lacerations of the sclera (which are rare), the patient is referred to an ophthalmologist for evaluation and possible surgical repair.

■ In cases of suspected or confirmed full-thickness lacerations, intravenous antibiotics are administered and the patient is immediately referred for ophthalmologic evaluation and surgical repair. Topical antibiotics are not used.

■ The patient's tetanus immune status is addressed.

Follow-Up

■ The focus and frequency of follow-up vary depending on the extent of the injury.

CHEMICAL INJURY

Chemical injuries to the eye may be caused by acid, alkali, and other chemically active organic substances such as mace and tear gas. Acid and alkali injuries may cause great visual loss. Organic agents cause severe visual loss less commonly.

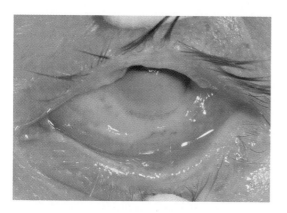

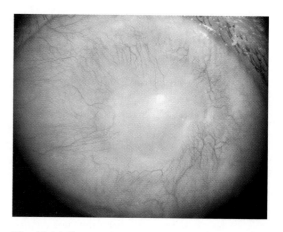

Fig. 15-13 Severe alkali burn with conjunctival and scleral ischemia and marked corneal edema.

Fig. 15-14 Severe alkali burn after 1 year. The cornea is scarred and vascularization is extensive. The prognosis for corneal transplant surgery in these patients is poor.

Symptoms

- Severe pain, redness, blurred vision, and eyelid spasm occur.
- A history of chemical exposure is reported.

Signs

- Signs vary depending on the severity of the injury and the time since the chemical exposure.
- The following apply to mild to moderate injuries:
  - Initial signs include corneal epithelial loss, chemosis and conjunctival hyperemia, subconjunctival hemorrhage, intact episcleral and conjunctival vessels, and mild periocular skin involvement (first-degree burns).
  - Chronic signs include minimal corneal scarring.
- The following apply to severe injuries:
  - Initial signs include severe chemosis; corneal edema and opacification; loss of conjunctival and episcleral vessels, which causes a very white-appearing sclera (Fig. 15-13); severe periocular skin involvement (second- or third-degree burns); and a marked anterior chamber reaction, which may not be visualized.
  - Chronic signs include foreshortened fornices (loss of normal connjunctival cul-de-sac) with symblepharon formation (conjunctival and globe adhesions); severe eyelid abnormalities such as trichiasis (misdirected eyelashes), entropion (lid turned in), and ectropion (lid turned out); severe tear film abnormalities (loss of mucus-producing cells in the conjunctiva); corneal scarring and opacification (Fig. 15-14); and phthisis bulbi (shrunken, nonseeing eye).

Etiology

- The most serious chemical burns to the eye are alkali burns such as lye (NaOH), caustic potash (KOH), and ammonia (NH_4). Fresh lime ($Ca[OH]_2$) and magnesium hydroxide

(Mg[OH]$_2$) are also alkaline but usually cause less severe injury than other alkaline compounds. Household cleaners, fertilizers, and refrigerants contain ammonia. Plaster, cement, mortar, and whitewash contain fresh lime. Sparklers and flares contain magnesium hydroxide. Alkali penetrates rapidly through the cornea and anterior chamber, causing disruption of the cell membrane lipids and secondary cellular necrosis. The degree of alkalinity is correlated with the amount of injury sustained, as is the time from exposure to irrigation.

- Acid burns caused by car batteries (H$_2$SO$_4$), bleach, refrigerant (H$_2$SO$_3$), fruit preservatives, and glass-etching chemicals (HFI) do not penetrate the ocular tissues as readily because of the precipitation of tissue proteins. This acts as a barrier to further tissue penetration.

Workup and Treatment

- As with other ocular injuries, the history guides the evaluation and treatment.
- In cases of severe exposure, initial treatment precedes the ocular evaluation. Copious irrigation with at least 2 L of normal saline solution 0.9% over 1 hour is performed as an initial treatment in the emergency room. Topical anesthetic (e.g., proparacaine) is instilled initially and every 10 to 15 minutes to make this a much less painful procedure. Lid retractors are used if significant orbicularis spasm is present. Various contact lenses that connect to intravenous tubing are available commercially to assist in the irrigation.
- In cases of less severe exposure or questionable history (e.g., the patient reports getting a drop of cleaner in the eye but washing it out at home), less copious irrigation with pH measurement is performed initially.
- The clinician sweeps the conjunctival fornices with a moistened cotton-tipped applicator to remove any retained foreign matter, especially lime, which exists as particulate matter.
- The clinician everts the upper and lower lids to ensure that no retained chemical is present after sweeping the fornices.
- The possibility of a ruptured globe is carefully assessed. Minimal pressure is placed on the globe during lavage when this diagnosis is a possibility or is indicated by the history.
- Irrigation continues until the conjunctival pH normalizes (i.e., 7.3 to 7.6); the pH is checked with the pH section of a urinalysis strip or pH paper. Two to three normal readings should be obtained at 15-minute intervals to ensure stability of the pH.
- Intraocular pressure may fluctuate widely and should be assessed.
- Cycloplegic agents (e.g., homatropine 5%) and mydriatic agents (e.g., phenylephrine 2.5%) are instilled to dilate the pupil. NOTE: In severe injury, some researchers discourage instillation of phenylephrine because of the possibility of further vasoconstricting the conjunctival vessels.
- Antibiotics (e.g., polymyxin B/bacitracin [Polysporin], erythromycin ophthalmic ointment) are instilled and a pressure patch is placed over the eye.
- Immediate referral to an ophthalmologist is needed once the initial lavage is complete. Management of severe burns includes treatment of the intraocular pressure problems, exposure, scarring, and tear film dysfunction; therapy involves corticosteroid administration, ascorbate or citrate supplementation (in cases of alkali burns only), and surgery (e.g., conjunctival grafts, corneal transplants).

Follow-Up

- Patients are usually monitored daily for several days.
- The prognosis mainly depends on the type of injury.
- Even in the most severe alkaline injuries the primary care physician can play a significant role in reducing the chronic sequelae by instructing the patient to irrigate at the place of injury (e.g., home, work) using a sink, shower, or garden hose rather than immediately summoning the patient to the emergency room. As stated, the prognosis is directly affected by the adequacy of the lavage immediately after exposure.

THERMAL INJURY

Symptoms

- Pain, tearing, a foreign body sensation, a red eye, and decreased vision occur.
- A history of exposure to a hot object (e.g., curling iron, tobacco ash, electrical arc, explosion) is reported.

Signs

- Corneal whitening indicates an epithelial or a stromal burn (Fig. 15-15).
- A corneal epithelial defect is evident.
- Conjunctival chemosis and injection occur.
- A minimal anterior chamber reaction is noted.
- Burns of the eyelids and periocular region are evident.

Differential Diagnosis

- Differential diagnoses include the following:
  - Corneal abrasion or infection (especially if no history available)
  - Ultraviolet injury (welder's flash)

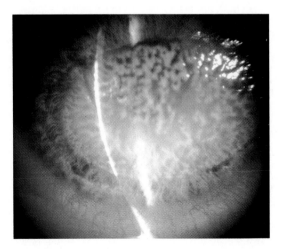

Fig. 15-15 Corneal thermal injury from a curling iron.

Workup

- A complete eye examination of both eyes, intraocular pressure evaluation, and careful notation of depth of burn (if corneal) are needed.
- Fluorescein instillation and a careful description or drawing of the epithelial defect should be performed.
- The diagnosis of ruptured globe should be ruled out or confirmed if this condition is suggested by the history.
- Associated alkaline injury should be ruled out or confirmed if the thermal burn was caused by fireworks or flares (magnesium hydroxide).

Treatment

- In cases of mild injury involving only the superficial cornea, topical antibiotics (e.g., polymyxin B/bacitracin [Polysporin]) are administered and a pressure patch is applied. Symptoms should resolve within 24 to 48 hours. The pressure patch is removed in 24 hours and the cornea is reexamined.
- Cycloplegic agents (e.g., homatropine 5%) are administered before patching.
- In cases of deep burns of the cornea, patients are immediately referred to an ophthalmologist.
- Periocular burns are treated with ophthalmic antibiotic preparations (e.g., polymyxin B/bacitracin [Polysporin], erythromycin ophthalmic ointment). Skin preparations may enter the eye and cause epithelial toxicity.

Follow-Up

- An ophthalmologist or oculoplastic surgeon is consulted if severe periocular injury accompanies the ocular injury. Cicatrization (scarring) of the eyelids from severe burns may lead to exposure and corneal scarring.

HYPHEMA

Hyphema, or blood in the anterior chamber of the eye, is an important indicator of the severity of trauma an eye has sustained. A microhyphema is a condition in which red blood cells are suspended in the aqueous fluid, not yet layered in the dependent portion of the anterior chamber. Hyphemas require ophthalmologic management and follow-up because they can have severe complications. The role of the primary care provider is to confirm the presence of vision if possible and to perform an initial examination with minimal manipulation of the globe, since concomitant ocular injury may be present.

Symptoms

- A history of blunt trauma is usually reported, although the condition may be spontaneous.
- Pain, blurred vision, and a red eye occur.
- Somnolence is noted, especially in children.

Signs

- Red blood cells in the anterior chamber, either suspended (microhyphema) or layered along the dependent portion of the anterior chamber, are noted (Fig. 15-16).

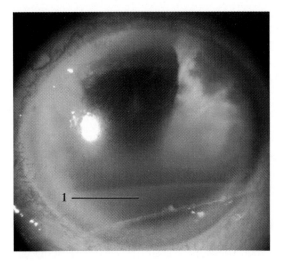

Fig. 15-16 Hyphemas layer with time, much like a hematocrit in a test tube. Here, a 30% hyphema *(1)* is noted.

- The red blood cells are not always found at the 6 o'clock position, because the patient may come for treatment after laying with the head in any position.
- Conjunctival injection, a sluggish or peaked pupil (resulting from a clot), possibly iris tears, and sometimes active bleeding from an iris vessel occur.

Etiology and Differential Diagnosis
- Trauma to the iris or ciliary body can cause a hyphema.
- The hyphema may originate from the iris or a scleral wound after ocular surgery.
- A spontaneous occurrence is possible with intraocular neoplasms (seen in juvenile xanthogranuloma, malignant melanoma, retinoblastoma, and leukemia) and clotting disorders. Spontaneous hyphemas may also result from rubeosis iridis, or new blood vessels growing on the iris. This is seen in ocular ischemic states (e.g., vascular occlusions, proliferative diabetic retinopathy).
- If the hyphema is "spontaneous" in a child, child abuse should be suspected.

Workup
- A history of the exact time and nature of the injury is needed. A ruptured globe must always be ruled out or confirmed.
- Both eyes and periorbital regions are examined. If the patient history suggests a projectile injury, the periorbital skin is assessed for entry wounds.
- The intraocular pressure is measured. Undue manipulation of the globe should be avoided to prevent rebleeding.
- The percentage of the anterior chamber that is filled with clot (e.g., 10%, 20%, 50%) is measured, much like the hematocrit of red blood cells.

- All African-American patients are screened for sickle cell disorders and, after admission, undergo hemoglobin electrophoresis testing. Patients with sickle trait (AS) may be unable to clear the red blood cells from the anterior chamber, resulting in a markedly elevated intraocular pressure 1 to 2 days after injury. This finding is crucial in management because the intraocular pressure must be maintained at a much lower reading in these patients.

Treatment

- Ophthalmologic consultation is mandatory. Accurate evaluation and management of the intraocular pressure is crucial in the care of these patients.
- All patients with severe hyphemas and those in whom patient compliance with follow-up is questionable are admitted.
- The involved eye is kept shielded with no patch, and bed rest is instituted.
- A cycloplegic agent (e.g., atropine sulfate 1%) is administered 2 times a day unless the clot is well established (more than 24 to 48 hours old). An antiemetic (e.g., prochlorperazine [Compazine] 10 mg intramuscularly) and mild analgesia (e.g., acetaminophen [Tylenol]) are used. Aspirin-containing compounds are not used.

Follow-Up

- Daily follow-up for 4 to 5 days is needed and should be performed by an ophthalmologist, who will monitor for intraocular pressure rise, corneal blood staining, and rebleeding. Because a hyphema is a manifestation of significant intraocular injury, regardless of whether the offending agent was sharp or blunt, evaluation for concomitant injury by the ophthalmologist is also crucial.
- The prognosis is generally good for patients with microhyphemas and hyphemas without concomitant injury. Patients with total ("eight-ball") hyphemas, rebleeding, and sickle cell disease have a more guarded prognosis. Long-term complications include glaucoma, corneal blood staining, and retinal injury.

TRAUMATIC IRITIS

Symptoms

- A history of ocular trauma (usually blunt) that occurred up to 2 to 3 days before the symptoms appeared is reported.
- Pain, marked photophobia, a red eye, tearing, and blurred vision occur.

Signs

- Anterior chamber cell (white blood cells in the anterior chamber) and flare (proteinaceous exudate into the anterior chamber) are observed with the use of a thin, bright beam directed obliquely through the anterior chamber.
- Consensual pain (pain from ciliary body spasm in the involved eye) occurs with direct illumination in the uninvolved eye.
- Ciliary flush and conjunctival injection are noted. The pupil may display sluggish movement.

Etiology

- Blunt trauma resulting in intraocular inflammation is a causative agent.

Workup

- A complete eye examination is needed, including a dilated fundus examination and intra-ocular pressure measurement if the history suggests a possible severe ocular injury.

Treatment

- Cycloplegic agents (e.g., homatropine 5% 3 times a day) are administered.
- Corticosteroid drops may be used after consultation with an ophthalmologist. Before they are prescribed, ocular infection must be ruled out and arrangements for adequate follow-up must be in place.

Follow-Up

- The patient is reevaluated 2 days to 1 week after the initial visit depending on the severity of the patient's symptoms and visual acuity. Distance acuity should not be markedly diminished after initial treatment; however, near vision will be poor because of the cycloplegic agent.
- Follow-up with an ophthalmologist is important to rule out any injury to the drainage angle of the eye (angle recession).
- As a rule, the prognosis is excellent. Symptoms should resolve in 7 to 10 days.

TRAUMATIC RETROBULBAR HEMORRHAGE

Symptoms

- A history of significant sharp or blunt trauma to the globe/periorbital region is reported.
- Pain, decreased vision, and a markedly swollen, red eye occur.

Signs

- Proptosis of the involved globe occurs.
- A markedly elevated intraocular pressure and a tense orbit (significant resistance on retropulsion of the globe) are found.
- Diffuse and massive subconjunctival hemorrhage and chemosis are evident. The posterior border of the subconjunctival blood cannot be visualized.
- Eyelid and periorbital ecchymosis occur.
- Extraocular movements may be limited.

Etiology

- Traumatic injury to the arteries within the confines of the orbit cause an abrupt rise in intraorbital pressure and anterior displacement of the globe. The blood can dissect between tissue planes and be visible under the conjunctiva and Tenon's capsule. The elevated pressure is transmitted to the globe itself once the anterior displacement of the eye is limited by the surrounding periocular soft tissues.
- Complications result when the elevated intraocular pressure is not lowered.

Differential Diagnosis

- Differential diagnoses include the following:
  - Orbital cellulitis, which often can be ruled out by the patient history
  - Orbital fracture
  - Carotid-cavernous fistula, which is possible after severe head trauma

Workup

- A complete eye examination with accurate assessment of the intraocular pressure is indicated. The contralateral eye must always be examined in cases of trauma.
- If a ruptured globe is a possible diagnosis, immediate referral to an ophthalmologist is indicated.
- The pupils and extraocular motility are evaluated carefully. The presence or development of a relative afferent pupillary defect may indicate optic nerve injury caused by compression or a traumatic optic neuropathy.
- CT scanning of the orbit is indicated unless the signs suggest a markedly elevated pressure, an impending vascular occlusion, or a nerve dysfunction. CT of the orbit is mandatory but should be delayed until the ophthalmologist has treated the elevated intraocular pressure.
- Intracranial penetration should be suspected in cases in which retrobular hemorrhage resulted from a penetrating injury.

Treatment

- For suspected retrobulbar hemorrhage, patients should be immediately referred to an ophthalmologist.
- Control of intraocular pressure is the first condition to be addressed. Carbonic anhydrase inhibitors (e.g., intravenous acetazolamide [Diamox] 500 mg) and topical β-blockers (e.g., timolol [Timoptic] 0.5%) help control the pressure in patients with limited hemorrhages or hematomas. For patients with active bleeding and worsening retrobular hemorrhages with elevated intraocular pressures (e.g., over 40 mm Hg), an ophthalmologist needs to perform a lateral canthotomy or cantholysis of the lateral canthal tendon. This maneuver decreases the pressure on the globe by increasing the potential volume of the orbit.
- For persistently elevated intraocular pressure despite treatment and cantholysis, emergency orbital decompression may be required. An anterior chamber tap may also decrease the intraocular pressure in an emergency, but this should be performed by the consulting ophthalmologist.

Follow-Up

- Daily follow-up is indicated, with careful monitoring of the intraocular pressure. If a cantholysis was performed, the lateral canthal tendon often needs surgical repair.

GLUE INJURY

Symptoms

- A history of ocular exposure to Super Glue (cyanoacrylate) is reported.
- Immediate closure of the eyelids (usually partial) occurs once exposed to the substance.
- A red eye, a foreign body sensation, pain, and tearing occur.

Signs

- Dried, hardened glue is found at the margin of the approximated eyelids or on the eye (Fig. 15-17).
- The epithelial defect displays diffuse fluorescein staining (toxic epitheliopathy).
- Conjunctival injection is evident.

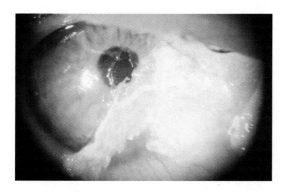

Fig. 15-17 Epoxy glue injury to the cornea. Fortunately, the glue is usually stuck only to the epithelium and does not cause severe scarring.

Workup

■ The patient's visual acuity should be determined and fluorescein staining is performed if possible.

Treatment

■ Prying the lids open causes pain and further superficial injury to the lid margin and should not be attempted. Application of chemicals or solvents to try to break the bond is contraindicated because these substances can cause significant corneal toxic epitheliopathy.

■ Warm compresses are applied, and the glued lids are gently massaged.

■ Warmed topical antibiotic ointments (e.g., erythromycin, polymyxin B/bacitracin [Polysporin] ophthalmic ointments) are placed in the eye several times a day and also rubbed on the lid margin. This treats any epithelial defects and mechanically facilitates lid separation. Artificial tears (e.g., Bion Tears, Celluvisc, Refresh, Tears Naturale) are used as needed for comfort.

■ The patient is reassured that the lids should become "unstuck" within several days of conservative treatment. If not, surgical separation of the lids may be performed.

Follow-Up

■ The focus of follow-up is the same as that for an epithelial defect. The patient is seen in 24 to 48 hours.

INTRAOCULAR FOREIGN BODY

For any patient with a history of metal-on-metal, grinding or hammering, lawn mower, or edger projectile injuries; industrial machinery foreign bodies; explosions or gunshot injury; and any other injury in which high-speed penetration of the globe with foreign material is possible, primary care physicians must be particularly alert. With small intraocular foreign bodies the signs and symptoms may be minimal. Failure to consider the possibility of an intraocular foreign body and making the incorrect diagnosis during the initial examination often results in the patient losing a significant amount of vision and is a common cause of litigation. The presence of an intraocular foreign body must be in the differential diagnosis of primary care providers as they evaluate eye trauma.

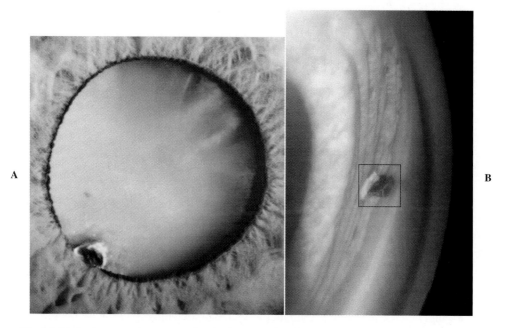

Fig. 15-18 A, A traumatic cataract developed from an iron foreign body that had penetrated the anterior lens capsule. **B,** Gonioscopic view of an iron foreign body that penetrated the globe during a metal-on-metal hammering injury.

Symptoms
- Vision is decreased or may be normal in some patients.
- A history suggestive of penetration of the globe with foreign material is reported.
- Eye pain, photophobia, and a red eye occur. In some patients the eye may be relatively quiet.

Signs
- Conjunctival signs include chemosis, hemorrhage, and laceration. In some patients the conjunctiva is normal.
- Scleral injury manifests as hemorrhage, laceration, and perforation. The sclera can appear normal.
- A periocular entry site is present.
- Foreign material is seen in the anterior segment of the eye; gonioscopic evaluation may be needed to accomplish this (Fig. 15-18).

Etiology
- Types of foreign bodies include metallic (e.g., iron, steel, nickel), nonmetallic (e.g., calcium, vegetable matter), and inert compounds (e.g., glass, plaster, lead, carbon, coal, rubber). "BBs" are composed of various metals, including lead, iron, and brass; they are commonly found as intraocular foreign bodies after an injury.

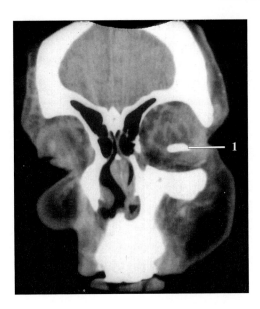

Fig. 15-19 Intraocular foreign body. An intraocular metallic foreign body *(1)*. In this case the globe was hypotonous and disorganized as shown on CT imaging.

Workup

- Both eyes are examined carefully. A ruptured globe is suspected in cases in which uveal prolapse and a very soft eye are evident; a perforation site is noted; a conjunctival, corneal, or scleral laceration is seen; marked conjunctival chemosis and hemorrhage and pupillary or iris abnormalities are evident; and lens opacity or a projectile track is found on slit lamp examination. In these patients the examination is discontinued, the eye is shielded, and the patient is immediately referred to an ophthalmologist.

- A dilated fundus examination with indirect ophthalmoscopy and careful slit lamp examination are mandatory and should be performed by an ophthalmologist. Most anterior segment foreign bodies are visible on slit lamp examination or gonioscopy.

- Plain film imaging may help with the diagnosis, but in general, CT scanning is a much more effective tool to evaluate the globe (and adnexa) for foreign materials (Fig. 15-19). Magnetic resonance imaging (MRI) should not be performed because a small chance of further injury to the globe exists related to the movement of magnetic objects during MRI scanning.

Treatment

- The ophthalmologist should coordinate the patient's care. Surgical intervention is needed in most cases (especially with iron, steel, and copper foreign bodies). The patient is given nothing by mouth, tetanus status is addressed, the eye is shielded, and intravenous antibiotics (gentamicin and cefazolin or gentamicin and clindamycin for vegetable matter) are administered.

- Administration of cycloplegic agents (e.g., homatropine 5%) enhances patient comfort and decreases the chance of posterior adhesions of the iris to the lens (posterior synechiae).

EYELID TRAUMA AND LACERATION

The role of the primary care physician in the evaluation of eyelid trauma is to answer several questions: Is the globe injured? Has the orbit been violated? Is the lid margin (or the body of the eyelid) affected? Has the canalicular system (earliest segment of the lacrimal drainage system) been compromised? Is eyelid closure adequate? If any of these conditions exist or are suspected, the patient should be referred to an ophthalmologist immediately.

Symptoms

- A history of sharp trauma to the eyelid or, in cases of avulsion of the lid, abrasive injury to the eyelid is reported.
- Eye and periorbital pain, a foreign body sensation, and tearing occur.

Signs

- Laceration through the lid margin occurs (Fig. 15-20).
- Conjunctival injection is evident.
- Orbital fat prolapse occurs if the orbital septum has been violated.
- Involvement of the eyelid medial to the superior and inferior puncta suggests canalicular laceration. (For lacrimal system anatomy, see Figs. 12-16 and 13-4.)

Workup

- A complete eye examination of both eyes is indicated. A ruptured globe is ruled out first; an object sharp enough to lacerate the eyelid can easily lacerate the globe as well.

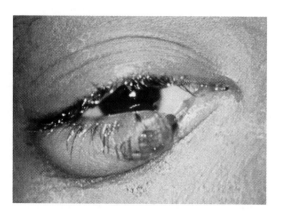

Fig. 15-20 Eyelid margin laceration.

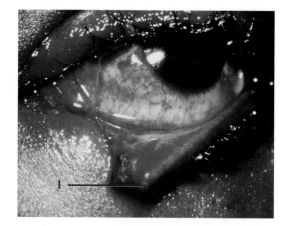

Fig. 15-21 The lower punctum is evident at the extreme cut end of the medial aspect of the lower eyelid *(1)*. Repair should be performed in the operating room with reconstruction of the canalicular system. Careless repair of these injuries could leave the patient with chronic tearing (epiphora).

- For injuries to the medial aspect of the eyelids, evaluation of the canalicular system, lacrimal sac, and medial canthal tendon is needed (Fig. 15-21).
- For patients with injuries to the lateral eyelid, possible involvement of the lateral canthal tendons and lacrimal gland is addressed. This is best performed by an ophthalmologist.
- CT scanning is indicated in any patient in whom injury to the globe is possible or the orbital septum has been violated and the possibility exists for an orbital foreign body.
- The amount of ptosis (drooping of the eyelid) and excursion of the eyelid are evaluated to determine whether any levator muscle injury occurred.

Treatment

- Patients with lid lacerations through the margin of the eyelid should be referred to an ophthalmologist for microscopic repair. Improper repair of the margin may result in corneal exposure, lagophthalmos (incomplete closure of the eyelids), corneal irritation from uneven edges of the margin or improperly tied sutures, and poor cosmesis.
- Lid margin lacerations through the canalicular system (upper and/or lower eyelid) are repaired in the operating room under microscopic conditions. The canalicular system is repaired and cannulated. Improper repair of the canalicular system can result in chronic tearing in addition to complications associated with improper margin repair.
- An avulsive injury of the eyelids necessitates complex operative closure and reconstructive surgery.

Follow-Up

- The time of follow-up is determined by the ophthalmic surgeon but is usually within 7 to 10 days of repair. If a severe eyelid or facial laceration is present, hospitalization with intravenous antibiotics is sometimes needed.
- The prognosis is very good if repairs have been performed properly. Even with proper repair, patients may need additional surgical procedures to correct scarring (cicatricial) changes and to improve cosmesis.

ORBITAL BLOW-OUT FRACTURE

Symptoms

- A history of significant blunt injury to the eye is reported.
- Pain occurs with eye movements.
- Double vision (binocular) is noted.
- Swelling of eyelids occurs after sneezing or blowing nose, which indicates that communication between the orbit and sinus is present.

Signs

- Enophthalmos (posteriorly displaced globe) occurs and is best appreciated by a relative narrowing of the palpebral fissures in the involved eye compared with that of the contralateral side.
- Point tenderness or an irregularity in the orbital rim is noted.
- A numbness or tingling of the upper lip and cheek ipsilateral to the injury indicates an injury to the infraorbital nerve.

■ Subcutaneous emphysema and proptosis are seen if a one-way valve exists between the sinuses (maxillary or ethmoid) and the orbit, trapping air in the orbit. The air dissects anteriorly between the tissue planes.

■ Extraocular movements, especially upgaze, are restricted.

Etiology

■ Orbital blow-out fractures occur in two forms: Direct fractures involve the orbital rim, with extension posteriorly involving the floor of the orbit. Indirect fractures result from compression of the soft tissues of the orbit (e.g., globe, extraocular muscles, fat), generating forces transmitted against the orbital walls. This results in fractures of the walls of the orbit (often the floor) without a fracture of the orbital rim.

Workup

■ A ruptured globe is ruled out, and the contralateral eye is examined. Extraocular motility is often unreliable in the early postinjury period because periorbital edema can restrict motility and affect the position of the globe.

■ The eyelids are examined for crepitus, which may be a sign that intraorbital air is present. These patients need to be monitored for progressive proptosis and visual changes; if tension in the orbit rises because of the increasing orbital air, a compressive or an ischemic optic neuropathy or occlusions of the central retinal vessels may result.

■ The ipsilateral cheek is checked for sensation; infraorbital nerve injury is commonly seen in inferior blow-out fractures.

■ If entrapment of the inferior rectus and inferior oblique muscles is suspected, plain film imaging and/or CT scanning of the orbits are performed to assist in the diagnosis (Fig. 15-22). In severe injuries, CT scanning also aids in the evaluation and management of the anatomic and structural integrity of the globe.

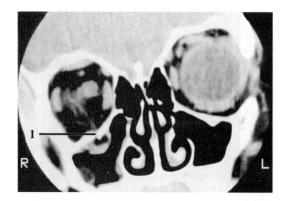

Fig. 15-22 Entrapment of orbital soft tissue in an inferior blow-out fracture. A coronal CT scan shows orbital soft tissue protruding into the superior portion of the maxillary sinus *(1)*.

Treatment

- Referral is indicated for ophthalmologic examination in any case of an orbital blow-out fracture. Any possible injury to the globe is ruled out. The fracture is evidence of extreme shifts in intraocular pressure and force waves through the intraocular tissues. Retinal detachment, vitreous detachment, vitreous hemorrhage, lens subluxation, and damage to the anterior chamber structures are possible consequences of the injury.
- Nasal decongestants (e.g., Afrin) are administered 2 times a day on the involved side.
- Antibiotic coverage (e.g., oral amoxicillin/clavulanate [Augmentin] 500 mg 4 times a day) is instituted for 10 to 14 days to prevent microbial contamination of the orbit from the sinuses.
- Cold compresses or ice packs are applied to the periorbital region to help diminish edema.
- Nose blowing and sneezing are minimized.
- In most patients, surgical repair of the orbit floor is indicated for persistent entrapment, gross enophthalmos, diplopia with motility limitation, and extremely large fractures causing inferior displacement of the globe.

Follow-Up

- Follow-up should begin in conjunction with an oculoplastic surgeon approximately 1 week after the initial injury. At this point the acute edema should be decreased, so the position of the globe can be more accurately assessed. The patient is instructed to watch for any change in the condition's course, specifically periorbital erythema, an increase in pain, and fever, which can be signs of impending orbital cellulitis.

TRAUMATIC OPTIC NEUROPATHY

Symptoms

- A history of traumatic injury to the globe or orbit, causing direct injury of the optic nerve, or to the forehead or temporal region, causing indirect injury of the optic nerve, is reported. Optic nerve injury manifests as a reduction in visual acuity not explained by refractive error or injury to the cornea, lens, or retina.
- Visual acuity is decreased.

Signs

- Color vision and red saturation are decreased and may be accompanied by a visual field defect.
- The optic disc appears normal. If an atrophic disc is seen on examination, a chronic process is ongoing or the nerve sustained injury at least 6 weeks previously.
- Signs of nerve injury such as disc hemorrhage and edema may be seen.
- A new relative afferent pupillary defect in a traumatized eye suggests the diagnosis (i.e., no retinal pathologic conditions or chiasmal damage).

Etiology

- Injury to the optic nerve from a sharp injury or compression by fragments of bone, foreign body, blood, or edema can lead to traumatic optic neuropathy.
- A shearing injury from blunt trauma has also been implicated.

Differential Diagnosis

■ Differential diagnoses include the following:
  • Widespread retinal injury—detachment and subretinal hemorrhage
  • Optic chiasm injury

Workup

■ A ruptured globe is ruled out in the involved eye and the fellow eye is examined. A careful pupillary examination demonstrates a relative afferent defect if an optic neuropathy is present.
■ Color vision, red saturation, and confrontation visual field testing are performed.
■ CT scanning of the head and orbits should pay special attention to the optic chiasm and optic canal to rule out chiasm and compressive injuries if the history is suggestive of these conditions.

Treatment

■ Once the diagnosis is suspected, the patient is immediately referred to an ophthalmologist for complete assessment and management. If a traumatic optic neuropathy is diagnosed, the patient is hospitalized and given intravenous high-dose corticosteroids (e.g., Solu-Medrol 30 mg/kg load, then 15 mg/kg every 6 hours for 72 hours). This is the same dosage of corticosteroids currently recommended for spinal cord trauma.
■ An H_2 blocker (e.g., oral ranitidine [Zantac] 150 mg every day) is administered in conjunction with the corticosteroids for prophylaxis against corticosteroid-induced gastrointestinal bleeding.
■ The patient is reexamined after 2 to 3 days of the corticosteroid regimen. If the visual acuity, color vision, red saturation, and relative afferent defect are improved, the patient begins an oral prednisone taper. If the signs are the same or worse, surgical decompression of the orbit may be indicated.
■ If signs return during the oral prednisone taper, intravenous corticosteroid administration is reinstituted.
■ Serum electrolyte and glucose levels are carefully monitored.

Follow-Up

■ The prognosis depends on the mechanism of injury and degree of damage sustained by the optic nerve. With a clinically evident relative afferent pupillary defect, the optic nerve must have sustained a fairly severe injury; therefore ultimate visual functioning may be poor.

PUPIL ASYMMETRY

See Chapter 11.

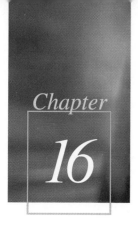

Chapter 16

Guide to Ophthalmic Medications

Michael D. Bennett and Geoffrey Broocker

THIS chapter describes commonly used and prescribed ophthalmic medications. The most common trade names, concentrations, and indications are included, but this is not an official therapeutic document. If discrepancies arise, the reader should obtain official and more complete information from the pharmaceutical manufacturer.

For ease of reference this chapter has been divided into several sections. The first part is an index of medications (Table 16-1). It includes the trade name, generic name, and table containing additional information. The second part discusses diagnostic medications, including stains, anesthetics, and mydriatic and cycloplegic agents (Table 16-2). The third part of this chapter details therapeutic agents. Lubricants (Table 16-3), antibiotics (Table 16-4 and 16-5), antivirals (Table 16-6), antifungals (Table 16-7), antiinflammatory medications (Table 16-8 to 16-11), antiglaucoma medications (Tables 16-12 to 16-18), and agents for relief of seasonal allergic conjunctivitis (Table 16-19) are discussed.

INDEX OF OPHTHALMIC MEDICATIONS

The following guides the reader to additional information about ophthalmic agents.

Table 16-1

Ophthalmic medications

TRADE NAME	GENERIC NAME	ADDITIONAL INFORMATION
Acular	Ketorolac	Tables 16-10, 16-11, 16-19
Adsorbotear	Hydroxyethyl cellulose, povidone	Table 16-3
Akarpine	Pilocarpine hydrochloride	Table 16-14
AK-Chlor	Chloramphenicol	Tables 16-4, 16-5
AK-Cide	Sulfacetamide/prednisolone	Table 16-9
AK-Dex	Dexamethasone sodium phosphate	Tables 16-8, 16-11
AK-Mycin	Erythromycin	Tables 16-4, 16-5
AK-Poly-Bac	Polymyxin B/bacitracin	Tables 16-4, 16-5
AK-Pred	Prednisolone sodium phosphate	Tables 16-8, 16-11
AK-Spore	Polymyxin B/neomycin/gramicidin	Tables 16-4, 16-5
AK-Sulf	Sulfacetamide sodium	Tables 16-4, 16-5
AK-Tracin	Bacitracin zinc	Tables 16-4, 16-5
Alomide	Lodoxamide	Table 16-19
Alphagan	Brimonidine tartrate	Table 16-13
Amphotericin B	Amphotericin B	Table 16-7
Ancobon	Flucytosine	Table 16-7
AquaSite	Polycarbophil, PEG-400, dextran 70	Table 16-3
AquaSite (multidose)	Polycarbophil, PEG-400, dextran 70	Table 16-3
Betagan	Levobunolol hydrochloride	Table 16-12
Betoptic	Betaxolol hydrochloride	Table 16-12
Betoptic S	Betaxolol hydrochloride	Table 16-12
Bion Tears	Hydroxypropyl methylcellulose, dextran 70	Table 16-3
Bleph-10	Sulfacetamide sodium	Tables 16-4, 16-5
Blephamide	Sulfacetamide/prednisolone	Table 16-9
Celluvisc	Carboxymethyl cellulose	Table 16-3
Cetamide	Sulfacetamide sodium	Tables 16-4, 16-5
Chibroxin	Norfloxacin	Tables 16-4, 16-5
Chloramphenicol (generic)	Chloramphenicol	Tables 16-4, 16-5
Chloromycetin	Chloramphenicol	Tables 16-4, 16-5
Chloroptic	Chloramphenicol	Tables 16-4, 16-5
Ciloxan	Ciprofloxacin hydrochloride	Tables 16-4, 16-5
Comfort Tears	Hydroxyethyl cellulose	Table 16-3
Crolom	Cromolyn sodium	Table 16-19
Cytovene	Ganciclovir sodium	Table 16-6
Decadron	Dexamethasone sodium phosphate	Tables 16-8, 16-11
Defy	Tobramycin sulfate	Tables 16-4, 16-5
Dexacidin	Neomycin/polymyxin B/dexamethasone	Table 16-9
Diamox	Acetazolamide	Table 16-16

Table 16-1

Ophthalmic medications—cont'd

TRADE NAME	GENERIC NAME	ADDITIONAL INFORMATION
Econopred	Prednisolone acetate	Tables 16-8, 16-11
Econopred Plus	Prednisolone acetate	Tables 16-8, 16-11
Epifrin	Epinephrine hydrochloride	Table 16-15
Epinal	Epinephrine borate	Table 16-15
Epitrate	Epinephrine bitartrate	Table 16-15
Eppy/n	Epinephrine borate	Table 16-15
Famvir	Famciclovir	Table 16-6
Flarex	Fluorometholone acetate	Tables 16-8, 16-11
Fluor-OP	Fluorometholone	Tables 16-8, 16-11
FML	Fluorometholone	Tables 16-8, 16-11
FML Forte	Fluorometholone	Tables 16-8, 16-11
FML S.O.P.	Fluorometholone	Tables 16-8, 16-11
Foscavir	Foscarnet sodium	Table 16-6
Gantrisin	Sulfisoxazole diolamine	Tables 16-4, 16-5
Garamycin	Gentamicin sulfate	Tables 16-4, 16-5
Genoptic	Gentamicin sulfate	Tables 16-4, 16-5
Gentacidin	Gentamicin sulfate	Tables 16-4, 16-5
Gentak	Gentamicin sulfate	Tables 16-4, 16-5
Gentamicin (generic)	Gentamicin sulfate	Tables 16-4, 16-5
Glaucon	Epinephrine hydrochloride	Table 16-15
Glauctabs	Methazolamide	Table 16-16
Herplex	Idoxuridine	Table 16-6
HMS	Medrysone	Tables 16-8, 16-11
Humorsol	Demecarium bromide	Table 16-4
HypoTears	Polyvinyl alcohol, PEG-400, dextrose	Table 16-3
HypoTears PF	Polyvinyl alcohol, PEG-400, dextrose	Table 16-3
Ilotycin	Erythromycin	Tables 16-4, 16-5
Inflamase	Prednisolone sodium phosphate	Tables 16-8, 16-11
Inflamase Forte	Prednisolone sodium phosphate	Tables 16-8, 16-11
Iopidine	Apraclonidine	Table 16-13
Ismotic	Isosorbide	Table 16-18
Isopto Carbachol	Carbachol	Table 16-14
Isopto Carpine	Pilocarpine hydrochloride	Table 16-14
Isopto Cetamide	Sulfacetamide sodium	Table 16-4, 16-5
Isopto Eserine	Physostigmine	Table 16-4
Isopto Plain	Hydroxypropyl methylcellulose	Table 16-3
Isopto Tears	Hydroxypropyl methylcellulose	Table 16-3
Lacrisert	Hydroxypropyl cellulose	Table 16-3
Livostin	Levocabastine hydrochloride	Table 16-19

Continued

Table 16-1

Ophthalmic medications—cont'd

TRADE NAME	GENERIC NAME	ADDITIONAL INFORMATION
Maxidex	Dexamethasone sodium phosphate	Tables 16-8, 16-11
Maxitrol	Neomycin/polymyxin B/dexamethasone	Table 16-9
Monistat	Miconazole nitrate	Table 16-7
Murine	Polyvinyl alcohol, povidone	Table 16-3
MZM	Methazolamide	Table 16-16
Naphcon-A	Naphazoline/pheniramine	Table 16-19
Natacyn	Natamycin	Table 16-7
Neodecadron	Neomycin/dexamethasone	Table 16-9
Neosporin	Polymyxin B/neomycin/bacitracin	Tables 16-4, 16-5
Neosporin	Polymyxin B/neomycin/gramicidin	Tables 16-4, 16-5
Neotal	Polymyxin B/neomycin/bacitracin	Tables 16-4, 16-5
Neptazane	Methazolamide	Table 16-16
Ocu-Chlor	Chloramphenicol	Tables 16-4, 16-5
Ocufen	Flurbiprofen sodium	Tables 16-10, 16-11
Ocuflox	Ofloxacin	Tables 16-4, 16-5
Ocupress	Carteolol hydrochloride	Table 16-12
Ocusert-Pilo	Pilocarpine hydrochloride	Table 16-14
Opcon-A	Naphazoline/pheniramine	Table 16-19
Ophthacet	Sulfacetamide sodium	Tables 16-4, 16-5
Optipranolol	Metipranolol	Table 16-12
Osmitrol	Mannitol	Table 16-18
Osmoglyn	Glycerin	Table 16-18
Patanol	Olopatadine hydrochloride	Table 16-19
Phospholine iodide	Echothiophate iodide	Table 16-14
Pilagan	Pilocarpine nitrate	Table 16-14
Pilocar	Pilocarpine hydrochloride	Table 16-14
Pilopine HS Gel	Pilocarpine hydrochloride	Table 16-14
Piloptic	Pilocarpine hydrochloride	Table 16-14
Pilostat	Pilocarpine hydrochloride	Table 16-14
Polysporin	Polymyxin B/bacitracin	Tables 16-4, 16-5
Polytrim	Polymyxin B/trimethoprim	Tables 16-4, 16-5
Pred-Forte	Prednisolone acetate	Tables 16-8, 16-11
Pred-G	Prednisolone/gentamicin	Table 16-9
Pred Mild	Prednisolone acetate	Tables 16-8, 16-11

Table 16-1
Ophthalmic medications—cont'd

TRADE NAME	GENERIC NAME	ADDITIONAL INFORMATION
Profenal	Suprofen	Tables 16-10, 16-11
Propine	Dipivefrin hydrochloride	Table 16-14
Refresh	Polyvinyl alcohol, povidone	Table 16-3
Refresh Plus	Carboxymethyl cellulose	Table 16-3
Sodium Sulamyd	Sulfacetamide sodium	Tables 16-4, 16-5
Statrol	Polymyxin B/neomycin	Tables 16-4, 16-5
Storzine	Pilocarpine hydrochloride	Table 16-14
Sulf-10	Sulfacetamide sodium	Tables 16-4, 16-5
Sulfacetamide (generic)	Sulfacetamide sodium	Tables 16-4, 16-5
TearGard	Hydroxyethyl cellulose, polyvinyl alcohol	Table 16-3
Tearisol	Hydroxypropyl methylcellulose	Table 16-3
Tears Naturale II	Hydroxypropyl methylcellulose, dextran 70	Table 16-3
Tears Naturale Free	Hydroxypropyl methylcellulose, dextran 70	Table 16-3
Tears Plus	Polyvinyl alcohol, povidone	Table 16-3
Tears Renewed	Hydroxypropyl methylcellulose, dextran 70	Table 16-3
Terramycin	Polymyxin B/oxytetracycline	Tables 16-4, 16-5
Timoptic	Timolol maleate	Table 16-12
Tobradex	Tobramycin/dexamethasone	Table 16-9
Tobrex	Tobramycin	Table 16-4
Trusopt	Dorzolamide hydrochloride	Table 16-16
Ultra Tears	Hydroxypropyl methylcellulose	Table 16-3
Vasocidin	Sulfacetamide/prednisolone	Table 16-9
Vasocon-A	Naphazoline/antazoline	Table 16-19
Vexol	Rimexolone	Table 16-8
Vira-A	Vidarabine monohydrate	Table 16-6
Viroptic	Trifluridine	Table 16-6
Voltaren	Diclofenac sodium	Tables 16-10, 16-11
Xalatan	Latanoprost	Table 16-17
Zovirax	Acyclovir sodium	Table 16-6

DIAGNOSTIC MEDICATIONS

Diagnostic medications are agents used to facilitate the ophthalmic examination.

Stains

Topical solutions used to highlight epithelial abnormalities, stains used in eye examinations include fluorescein and rose bengal.

Fluorescein. Helpful in diagnosing corneal abrasions, fluorescein stains epithelial basement membranes in areas where the epithelium has been removed. Fluorescein is supplied in sterile paper strips, which is the preferred modality, and as a 2% solution that contains benoxinate, a topical anesthetic. However, the bottle containing the 2% solution is easily contaminated in a clinical setting.

Rose bengal. Rose bengal dye stains sick, devitalized, epithelial cells and is helpful in the diagnosis of herpetic ulcers that may mimic corneal abrasions. Rose bengal is supplied on sterile paper strips.

Anesthetics

Anesthetics are used with diagnostic stains and are essential for intraocular pressure measurements. Tetracaine hydrochloride (Pontocaine) is available in 0.5% and 1.0% solutions, lasts about 15 minutes, and stings. Proparacaine hydrochloride (Ophthetic, Ophthaine) is available in a 0.5% solution, lasts 10 to 15 minutes, and is less irritating.

NOTE: All anesthetics are toxic to epithelial cells and thus will delay or prevent wound healing. Dispensing these agents to patients is a medical legal risk and is strongly discouraged.

Mydriatics and Cycloplegics

Mydriatic and cycloplegic agents can be used for diagnostic and therapeutic purposes. Mydriatics dilate the pupil, and cycloplegic agents paralyze the ciliary muscle. Dilating the pupil is necessary for adequate examination of the internal ocular structures. Therapeutic benefits are numerous: paralyzing the ciliary muscle reduces pain associated with traumatic iritis, prevents posterior synechiae formation (adhesions between the iris and lens), and stabilizes the blood ocular barrier during bouts of intraocular inflammation. These medications usually have a red top.

The typical regimen of mydriatic and cycloplegic agents is as follows:

- Adults—Phenylephrine 2.5%, Tropicamide 0.5%; 1 drop of each; repeated if needed after 20 to 30 minutes
- Children—Phenylephrine 2.5%, Tropicamide 0.5%; 1 drop of each; repeated if needed after 20 to 30 minutes; Cyclopentolate 1% to 2% added if refraction to be performed
- Term infants—Cyclopentolate 0.5%, Phenylephrine 2.5%; 1 drop in each eye; repeated in 5 minutes
- Preterm infants up to 3 months of age—Cyclomidril, 1 drop in each eye; repeated in 5 minutes

Dilating drops are contraindicated in patients with known angle-closure glaucoma. Dilating drops may be less effective in patients with dark irides or intraocular inflammation. Administration of dilating drops to premature infants or children with cardiac disease or hypertension is high risk. These agents should be used cautiously in these patients.

Table 16-2
Dilating drops

AGENT	APPROXIMATE MAXIMUM EFFECT	APPROXIMATE DURATION
Mydriatic		
Phenylephrine 2.5%	20 minutes	3 hours
Cycloplegic/mydriatic		
Tropicamide 0.5%, 1%	20-30 minutes	3-6 hours
Cyclopentolate, 0.5%, 1%, 2%	20-45 minutes	24 hours
Homatropine 2%, 5%	20-40 minutes	2-3 days
Scopolamine 0.25%	20-45 minutes	4-7 days
Atropine 0.5%, 1%, 2%	30-40 minutes	1-2 weeks

THERAPEUTIC MEDICATIONS

Ocular Lubricants

The tear film is a highly complex layer responsible for vision (the primary ocular refractive surface) and ocular comfort. A large percentage of patients have tear film abnormalities and experience symptoms related to "dry eyes." Patients with ocular surface abnormalities usually respond well to artificial lubricants, although the symptomatic relief may be only temporary.

Table 16-3

Artificial tear preparations

GENERIC NAME	TRADE NAME	PRESERVATIVE*
Carboxymethyl cellulose	Refresh Plus	None
	Celluvisc	None
Hydroxyethyl cellulose	Comfort Tears	Benzalkonium chloride, EDTA
Hydroxyethyl cellulose, polyvinyl alcohol	TearGard	Sorbic acid, EDTA
Hydroxyethyl cellulose, povidone	Adsorbotear	Thimerosal, EDTA
Hydroxypropyl cellulose	Lacrisert	None
Hydroxypropyl methylcellulose	Isopto Plain	Benzalkonium chloride
	Isopto Tears	Benzalkonium chloride
	Tearisol	Benzalkonium chloride, EDTA
	Ultra Tears	Benzalkonium chloride
Hydroxypropyl methylcellulose, dextran 70	Bion Tears	None
	Tear Naturale II	Polyquad
	Tears Naturale Fee	None
	Tears Renewed	Benzalkonium chloride, EDTA
Polycarbophil, PEG-400, dextran 70	AquaSite	EDTA
	AquaSite (multidose)	EDTA, sorbic acid
Polyvinyl alcohol, PEG-400, dextrose	HypoTears	Benzalkonium chloride, EDTA
	HypoTears PF	EDTA
Polyvinyl alcohol, povidone	Murine	Benzalkonium chloride, EDTA
	Refresh	None
	Tears Plus	Chlorobutanol

*Preparations containing preservatives should be used no more than 6 to 8 times a day.

Antibiotics

The most common ocular pathogens are usually staphylococci, streptococci and hemophilus. Empiric treatment is generally successful at eradicating most surface infections; however, resistant organisms are becoming more common. Appropriate cultures and susceptibilities should be addressed before the initiation of therapy when clinically indicated.

In general, topical antibiotics are given 4 to 6 times a day for simple infections and during the postoperative period. However, severe infections may require the use of multiple fortified antibiotics every hour around the clock.

Fortified antibiotics. Used by ophthalmologists for serious anterior segment and corneal infections when higher concentrations of drug are needed to fight unusually virulent pathogens, fortified antibiotics are easily prepared by most pharmacies. The most common examples are fortified Tobramycin or Gentamycin, fortified Vancomycin, and fortified Cefazolin.

Table 16-4
Antibiotics

GENERIC NAME	TRADE NAME	BACTERIAL COVERAGE
Bacitracin zinc	AK-Tracin	Most gram-positive organisms, diphtheroids, hemophilus, and actinomyces
Chloramphenicol	AK-Chlor Chloramphenicol (generic) Chloromycetin Chloroptic Ocu-Chlor	Many gram-positive and gram-negative organisms, especially hemophilus, *Moraxella* species, *Staphylococcus aureus,* β-hemolytic streptococci, and diphtheroids
Ciprofloxacin hydrochloride	Ciloxan	Broad spectrum, particularly targeting staphylococci, streptococci, and *Pseudomonas aeruginosa*
Erythromycin	AK-Mycin Erythromycin (generic) Ilotycin	Most gram-positive organisms, diphtheroids, hemophilus, actinomyces, and *Neisseria* species
Gentamicin sulfate	Garamycin Genoptic Gentacidin Gentak Gentamicin (generic)	Broad spectrum, particularly targeting staphylococci (when drug used in high concentrations), and *Pseudomonas aeruginosa*
Norfloxacin	Chibroxin	Broad spectrum, particularly targeting staphylococci, streptococci, and *Pseudomonas aeruginosa*
Ofloxacin	Ocuflox	Broad spectrum, particularly targeting staphylococci, streptococci, and *Pseudomonas aeruginosa*
Polymyxin B/bacitracin	AK-Poly-Bac Polysporin	Some gram-negative organisms and most gram-postive organisms, diphtheroids, hemophilus, and actinomyces

Continued

Table 16-4
Antibiotics—cont'd

GENERIC NAME	TRADE NAME	BACTERIAL COVERAGE
Polymyxin B/neomycin/ bacitracin	AK-Spore Neosporin Neotal Polymyxin B (generic)	Gram-negative organisms and broad spectrum for gram-positive organisms, particularly targeting staphylococci, pseudomonads, diphtheroids, hemophilus, and actinomyces
Polymyxin B/oxytetracycline	Terramycin	Most staphylococci, streptococci, gonococci, *Chlamydia* species and few gram-negative organisms
Polymyxin B/trimethoprim	Polytrim	Most staphylococci, streptococci, and hemophilus
Sulfacetamide sodium	AK-Sulf Bleph-10 Cetamide Isopto Cetamide Ophthacet Sodium Sulamyd Sulf-10 Sulfacetamide (generic)	Wide range of gram-positive and gram- negative organisms; some staphylococci, pneumococci, hemophilus, *Moraxella* species, and *Chlamydia* species
Sulfisoxazole diolamine	Gantrisin	Wide range of gram-positive and gram- negative organisms; some staphylococci, pneumococci, hemophilus, *Moraxella* species, and *Chlamydia* species
Tobramycin sulfate	Defy Tobrex Tobramycin (generic)	Broad spectrum, including staphylococci, streptococci, and hemophilus

Table 16-5

Antibiotic concentrations

GENERIC NAME	TRADE NAME	CONCENTRATION OF SOLUTION	CONCENTRATION OF OINTMENT
Bacitracin zinc	AK-Tracin	NA	50 units/g
Chloramphenicol	AK-Chlor	0.5%	1.0%
	Chloramphenical (generic)	0.5%	1.0%
	Chloromycetin	0.5%	1.0%
	Chloroptic	0.5%	1.0%
	Ocu-Chlor	0.5%	1.0%
Ciprofloxacin hydrochloride	Ciloxan	0.3%	NA
Erythromycin	AK-Mycin	NA	0.5%
	Erythromycin (generic)	NA	0.5%
	Ilotycin	NA	0.5%
Gentamicin sulfate	Garamycin	0.3%	0.3%
	Genoptic	0.3%	0.3%
	Gentacidin	0.3%	0.3%
	Gentak	0.3%	0.3%
	Gentamicin (generic)	0.3%	0.3%
Ofloxacin	Ocuflox	0.3%	NA
Polymyxin B/bacitracin	AK-Poly-Bac	NA	10,000 units, 500 units/g
	Polysporin	NA	10,000 units, 500 units/g
Polymyxin B/neomycin	Statrol	16,250 units, 3.5 mg/ml	10,000 units, 3.5 mg/g
Polymyxin B/neomycin/ bacitracin	Neotal	NA	5000 units, 5 mg, 400 units/g
	Neosporin	NA	NA
	Polymyxin B (generic)	NA	NA
Polymyxin B/neomycin/ gramicidin	AK-Spore	10,000 units	NA
	Neosporin	in 1.75 mg or	NA
	Polymyxin B (generic)	0.025 mg/ml	NA
Polymyxin B/oxytetracycline	Terramycin	NA	10,000 units, 5 mg/g
Polymyxin B/trimethoprim	Polytrim	10,000 units, 1 mg/ml	NA
Sulfacetamide sodium	AK-Sulf	10.0%	10.0%
	Bleph-10	10.0%	10.0%
	Cetamide	NA	10.0%
	Isopto Cetamide	15.0%	NA
	Ophthacet	10.0%	NA
	Sodium Sulamyd	10%, 30%	10.0%
	Sulf-10	10.0%	NA
	Sulfacetamide (generic)	10%, 15%, 30%	10.0%
Sulfisoxazole diolamine	Gantrisin	4.0%	4.0%
Tobramycin sulfate	Defy	0.3%	0.3%
	Tobrex	0.3%	NA
	Tobramycin (generic)	0.3%	0.3%

NA, Not applicable.

Antivirals

Advancements in the chemotherapeutic agents used to fight viral diseases have progressed rather slowly compared with other areas of medicine. This is partly because viruses are obligate intracellular pathogens that use the host's metabolic processes for their survival and replication. Thus antiviral agents need to target the pathogen while leaving uninfected host cells essentially unaffected from their toxic side effects. To date, the most effective antiviral agents target viral enzymes and proteins that are essential for viral assembly.

Table 16-6
Antiviral agents

GENERIC NAME	TRADE NAME	CONCENTRATION	INDICATION
Idoxuridine	Herplex	0.1% Solution	Herpes simplex virus
	Stoxil	0.5% Ointment	Herpes simplex virus
Trifluridine	Viroptic	1.0% Solution	Herpes simplex virus
Vidarabine monohydrate	Vira-A	3.0% Ointment	Herpes simplex virus
Acyclovir sodium	Zovirax	Systemic preparation only	Herpes simplex virus, herpes zoster virus
Foscarnet sodium	Foscavir	Systemic preparation only	Immunocompromised patients with cytolomegalovirus
Famciclovir	Famvir	Systemic preparation only	Herpes zoster virus
Gancyclovir sodium	Cytovene	Systemic preparation only	Immunocompromised patients with cytolomegalovirus

Antifungal agents

Deciding on the appropriate ophthalmic antifungal usually depends on several variables, including the site of primary infection, route of administration, organism involved, and drug sensitivities.

Table 16-7
Antifungal agents

GENERIC NAME	TRADE NAME	TOPICAL CONCENTRATION	SPECTRUM
Amphotericin B	Amphotericin B	0.1-0.5% Solution	Blastomycetes, *Candida* species, *Coccidioides* species, *Histoplasma* species
Flucytosine	Ancobon	1.0% Solution	*Candida* species
Natamycin*	Natacin	5% Suspension	*Candida* species, aspergilli, *Cephalosporium* species, *Fusarium* species, *Penicillium* species
Miconazole nitrate	Monistat	1% Solution	*Candida* species, *Cryptococcus* species, aspergilli

*The drug of choice for most mycotic corneal infections and the only ocular formulation commercially available. The others need to be prepared by the pharmacy.

Antiinflammatory agents

Antiinflammatory agents are used most frequently to suppress immunologic mechanisms of all types, both externally and within the eye. Suppression of severe external inflammation is necessary to prevent corneal scarring and permanent tear film abnormalities. Within the eye, these agents help prevent synechiae (scarring), some forms of glaucoma, and postoperative inflammation. Topical administration allows excellent penetration into the anterior chamber. Some agents penetrate easier than others depending on the chemical composition. Topical corticosteroids should be used with caution because they can cause cataracts and glaucoma and potentiate herpes simplex viral replication.

Table 16-8

Antiinflammatory agents

GENERIC NAME	TRADE NAME	FORMULATION	TOPICAL CONCENTRATION
Dexamethasone	Maxidex	Suspension*	0.1%
Dexamethasone sodium phosphate	AK-Dex	Ointment	0.05%
	Decadron	Ointment	0.05%
	Maxidex	Ointment	0.05%
	Dexamethasone (generic)	Ointment	0.05%
Dexamethasone sodium phosphate	AK-Dex	Solution	0.1%
	Decadron	Solution	0.1%
	Dexamethasone (generic)	Solution	0.1%
Fluorometholone	Fluor-OP	Suspension*	0.1%
	FML	Suspension	0.1%
	FML Forte	Suspension	0.25%
	FML S.O.P.	Ointment	0.1%
Fluorometholone acetate	Flarex	Suspension*	0.1%
Medrysone	HMS	Suspension*	1.0%
Prednisolone acetate	Econopred	Suspension*	0.125%
	Econopred Plus	Suspension	1.0%
	Pred-Forte	Suspension	1.0%
	Pred Mild	Suspension	0.125%
Prednisolone sodium phosphate	AK-Pred	Solution	0.125%, 1.0%
	Inflamase	Solution	0.125%
	Inflamase Forte	Solution	1.0%
	Prednisolone (generic)	Solution	0.125%, 1.0%
Rimexolone	Vexol	Solution	1.0%

*Suspensions need to be shaken before instillation.

Antiinflammatory and antibiotic combinations. Generally, antiinflammatory medications are indicated for steroid-responsive inflammatory ocular conditions for which a corticosteroid is indicated and bacterial infection or risk of bacterial ocular infection exists. These medications are contraindicated in any condition in which an epithelial defect exists, including patients with epithelial herpes simplex keratitis and those who have recently undergone uncomplicated removal of a corneal foreign body.

Table 16-9

Antiinflammatory and antibiotic combinations

GENERIC NAME	TRADE NAME	FORMULATION AND AMOUNT	TYPICAL DOSAGE
Sulfacetamide sodium/ prednisolone acetate	AK-Cide Blephamide Vasocidin	Suspension (5 ml) Ointment (3.5 g)	1 drop 4 times a day At bedtime to 4 times a day
Neomycin/polymyxin B/ dexamethasone	Dexacidin Maxitrol	Suspension (5 ml) Ointment (3.5 g)	1 drop 4 times a day At bedtime to 4 times a day
Neomycin/ dexamethasone	NeoDecadron	Suspension (5 ml) Ointment (3.5 g)	1 drop 4 times a day At bedtime to 4 times a day
Prednisolone acetate/ gentamicin sulfate	Pred-G	Suspension (5 ml) Ointment (3.5 g)	1 drop 4 times a day At bedtime to 4 times a day
Tobramycin/ dexamethasone	Tobradex	Suspension (5 ml) Ointment (3.5 g)	1 drop 4 times a day At bedtime to 4 times a day

Nonsteroidal antiinflammatory agents. Nonsteroidal antiinflammatory agents (NSAIDs) are also used to suppress immunologic mechanisms, both externally and within the eye. They differ from corticosteroids in their effectiveness; however, they do not cause cataracts or glaucoma or potentiate herpes simplex viral replication.

Table 16-10

Nonsteroidal antiinflammatory agents

GENERIC NAME	TRADE NAME	FORMULATION	TOPICAL CONCENTRATION
Diclofenac	Voltaren	Solution	0.1%
Flurbiprofen	Ocufen	Solution	0.03%
Ketorolac	Acular	Solution	0.5%
Suprofen	Profenal	Solution	1.0%

Table 16-11

Comparison of selected antiinflammatory agents

GENERIC NAME	TRADE NAME	COMMENT
NSAIDs	Ocufen Voltaren Acular	Interference with prostaglandin-induced operative miosis, other inflammations (e.g., iritis, cystoid macular edema), and allergy-related irritation; no causation of cataracts or glaucoma; no potentiation of herpes simplex infection
Medrysone	HMS	Weak steroid, very few side effects
Fluorometholone	FML	More potent than medrysone, excellent for external inflammation, fewer side effects than prednisolone and dexamethasone
Prednisolone acetate	Pred-Forte	Potent steroid, highly effective for anterior segment inflammation, higher risk of side effects (IOP elevation, infection, HSV activation)
Dexamethasone sodium phosphate	Decadron	Highly potent and effective, very high risk of side effects
Rimexolone	Vexol	Newer agent, very potent steroid, as potent as prednisolone acetate with very few ocular side effects (similar to those seen with FML)

IOP, Intraocular pressure; *HSV,* herpes simplex virus.

Antiglaucoma medications

Antiglaucoma medications are used to reduce optic nerve damage and visual loss associated with elevated introcular pressure. The seven classes of these medications, which differ in their mechanisms of action, are as follows:

1. β-blocking agents (Table 16-12)
2. Adrenergic agonists (Table 16-13)
3. Cholinergic agonists (Table 16-14)
4. Sympathomimetics (Table 16-15)
5. Carbonic anhydrase inhibitors (Table 16-16)
6. Prostaglandins (Table 16-17)
7. Hyperosmotic agents (Table 16-18)

β-**Blockers.** Historically, the most common first-line treatment for open-angle glaucoma and ocular hypertension, β-blockers work by reducing aqueous humor secretion by the ciliary body. Because of some systemic absorption, they are contraindicated in some patients with heart and respiratory conditions. However, some newer selective β-blockers appear to have less severe side effects. Ocular side effects include stinging and burning.

Table 16-12

Antiglaucoma medications: β-blockers

GENERIC NAME	TRADE NAME	TYPICAL DOSAGE	COMMENTS
Betaxolol hydrochloride	Betoptic-S (0.25%) Betoptic (0.5%)	1 drop 2 times a day 1 drop 2 times a day	β_2 selective, use in patients with cardiac and respiratory conditions
Carteolol hydrochloride	Ocupress (1.0%)	1 drop 2 times a day	Nonselective β-blocker
Levobunolol hydrochloride	Betagan (0.25%, 0.5%) Generic (0.25%, 0.5%)	1 drop 2 times a day 1 drop 2 times a day	Nonselective β-blocker
Metipranolol	Optipranolol (0.3%)	1 drop 2 times a day	Nonselective β-blocker
Timolol maleate	Timoptic (0.25%, 0.5%)	1 drop 2 times a day	Nonselective β-blocker
Timolol maleate	Timoptic XE	Once a day (0.25%, 0.5%)	Nonselective β-blocker; solution becoming a gel once in contact with the eye, increasing period of drug delivery
Timolol hemihydrate	Betimol (0.25%, 0.5%)	1 drop 2 times a day	Nonselective β-blocker

α Agonists. α Agonists reduce intraocular pressure by increasing uveoscleral and conventional outflow. This class may prove to be effective at reducing intraocular pressure without the cardiac side effects of β-blockers. Currently, two drugs are on the market. The most common side effect is an allergic reaction developing with long-term use.

Table 16-13
Antiglaucoma medications: α agonists

GENERIC NAME	TRADE NAME	TYPICAL DOSAGE	COMMENTS
Apraclonidine	Iopidine (0.5%, 1%)	1 drop 3 times a day	Short-term adjuvant for patients on maximal medical therapy, approximately 1 month to be effective
Alphagan	Brimonide tartrate (0.2%)	1 drop 3 times a day	Newer agent with seemingly better toleration than its predecessor, less tachyphylaxis noted

Cholinergics. Parasympathomimetic agents are divided into direct-acting (cholinergic) and indirect-acting (anticholinesterase) agents. Used primarily for glaucoma and control of accommodative esotropia, they reduce intraocular pressure by causing contraction on the ciliary muscle. This contraction pulls on the trabecular meshwork and facilitates aqueous outflow. Acute poisoning with these agents can produce the cholinergic crisis syndrome, which includes sweating, gastrointestinal disturbances, bradycardia, and paralysis of the respiratory muscles.

Table 16-14
Antiglaucoma medications: cholinergic agents

GENERIC NAME	TRADE NAME	TYPICAL DOSAGE	CONCENTRATION
Cholinergic agents			
Carbachol	Isopto Carbachol	1 drop 3 times a day	1.5%, 3%
Pilocarpine hydrochloride	Akarpine	1 drop 4 times a day	1%, 2%, 4%
	Isopto Carpine	1 drop 4 times a day	0.5%, 1%-6%, 8%, 10%
	Ocusert-Pilo	1 per week	20-40 mg/hr/week
	Pilocar	1 drop 4 times a day	0.5%, 1%-4%, 6%
	Pilopine HS Gel	½ inch every hour	4%
	Piloptic	1 drop 4 times a day	0.5%, 1%-4%, 6%
	Pilostat	1 drop 4 times a day	1%, 2%, 4%
	Storzine	1 drop 4 times a day	1%, 2%, 4%
	Generic	1 drop 4 times a day	0.5%, 1%-4%, 6%
Pilocarpine nitrate	Pilagan	1 drop 4 times a day	1%, 2%, 4%
Anticholinesterase agents			
Physostigmine	Isopto Eserine	1 drop 4 times a day	0.25%, 0.5%
	Generic (ointment)	½ inch every hour	0.25%
Demecarium	Humorsol	1 drop 2 times a day to 1 drop a week	0.25%, 0.5%
Echothiophate iodide	Phospholine iodide	1 drop 2 times a day	0.125%, 0.25%

Sympathomimetics. Sympathomimetics have been of limited usefulness in the general population due to the numerous side effects associated with their use. However, a certain subset of the population tolerates these medications. These agents reduce intraocular pressure by increasing aqueous outflow.

Table 16-15
Antiglaucoma medications: sympathomimetics

GENERIC NAME	TRADE NAME	TYPICAL DOSAGE	CONCENTRATION
Epinephrine bitartrate	Epitrate	1 drop every day	2%
	Eppy/n	or 2 times a day	1%, 2%
Epinephrine hydrochloride	Epifrin	1 drop every day	0.5%, 1%, 2%
	Glaucon	or 2 times a day	1%, 2%
Dipivefrin hydrochloride	Propine	1 drop 2 times a day	0.10%

Carbonic anhydrase inhibitors. Carbonic anhydrase inhibitors (CAIs) reduce aqueous formation by direct inhibition of carbonic anhydrase within the ciliary body. Oral CAIs are highly effective but can also result in serious side effets such as paresthesias, anorexia, gastrointestinal disturbances, headaches, altered taste and smell, and sodium and potassium depletion. Currently, one topical CAI appears to be much better tolerated, with a lower side-effect profile.

Table 16-16
Antiglaucoma medications: carbonic anhydrase inhibitors

GENERIC NAME	TRADE NAME	TYPICAL DOSAGE	COMMENTS
Dorzolamide hydrochloride	Trusopt (2%)	1 drop 3 times a day	Only topical CAI
Acetazolamide	Diamox Generic	250 mg tablet 4 times a day (oral) or 500 mg sequel 2 times a day (oral)	Numerous systemic side effects
Methazolamide	Neptazane Glauctabs MZM Generic	50 mg tablets 2 times a day (oral)	Not as effective as Diamox but appears to be better tolerated by some patients

Prostaglandins. This new class of agents is used to treat open-angle glaucoma and ocular hypertension. The mechanism of action is to increase uveoscleral outflow, thus reducing intraocular pressure. Currently, only one drug is on the market. The most common side effect is an increase in iris pigmentation.

Table 16-17
Antiglaucoma medications: prostaglandins

GENERIC NAME	TRADE NAME	TYPICAL DOSAGE	COMMENTS
Latanoprost	Xalatan (0.005%)	1 drop a day (evening)	New agent, increase in uveoscleral outflow to lower intraocular pressure, side effect of increased iris pigmentation in some patients

Hyperosmotic agents. Given systemically, hyperosmotic agents increase the osmolality of the blood. This creates an osmotic gradient between the blood and vitreous cavity and effectively pulls fluid from the vitreous and aqueous humors into the bloodstream. These medications are used to lower the intraocular pressure in an attack of angle-closure glaucoma and to produce a soft eye during surgery.

Table 16-18
Antiglaucoma medications: hyperosmotic agents

GENERIC NAME	TRADE NAME	TYPICAL DOSAGE	CONCENTRATION/COMMENTS
Glycerin	Osmoglyn (50%)	1-1.5 g/kg	Oral agent
Isosorbide	Ismotic (45%)	1.5 g/kg	Oral agent; 30 min to onset, 5-6 hr duration
Mannitol	Osmitrol (5%-20%)	0.5-2 g/kg	IV drug, adult dose ranging from 20-200 g/24 hr

Seasonal allergic conjunctivitis

Ocular allergy encompasses a broad spectrum of diseases characterized by a marked type I hypersensitivity response. Exposure to environmental allergens such as animal dander, pollens, and dust can cause symptoms in sensitized individuals. An allergic response is typically characterized by conjunctival injection, chemosis (swelling of the conjunctiva), tearing, eyelid swelling, burning, and ocular and periocular itching. Treatment of allergic ocular disease ideally entails removing the offending agent or modifying the patient's environment and treating the patient topically to provide symptomatic relief.

Table 16-19

Agents for relief of allergy symptoms

GENERIC NAME	TRADE NAME	TYPICAL DOSAGE	MECHANISM OF ACTION
Cromolyn	Crolom	1 drop 4 times a day	Mast-cell inhibitor
Ketorolac	Acular	1 drop 4 times a day	NSAID
Levocabastin	Livostin	1 drop 4 times a day	H_1 antagonist
Lodoxamide	Alomide	1 drop 4 times a day	Mast-cell inhibitor
Naphazoline/ antazoline	Vasocon-A	1 drop 4 times a day	Antihistamine/ decongestant
Naphazoline/ pheniramine	Naphcon-A Opcon-A	1 drop 4 times a day	Antihistamine/ decongestant
Olopatadine hydrochloride	Patanol	1 drop 2 times a day	Antihistamine and mast-cell stabilizer

Index